COLOR ATLAS OF
HUMAN ANATOMY

THIRD EDITION

R.M.H. McMinn

MD, PhD, FRCS (Eng.)
Emeritus Professor of Anatomy,
Royal College of Surgeons of England
and University of London

R.T. Hutchings

Freelance Photographer
Formerly Chief Medical Laboratory
Scientific Officer, Royal College
of Surgeons of England

J. Pegington

MB, BCh, FRCS (Eng.)
Emeritus Professor of Anatomy
University College London

P.H. Abrahams

MB, BS, FRCS (Ed), FRCR
Clinical Anatomist, University of Cambridge
Family Practitioner, Brent
Fellow of Girton College, Cambridge
Mosby–Wolfe

M Mosby-Wolfe

London Baltimore Bogotá Boston Buenos Aires Caracas Carlsbad, CA Chicago Madrid Mexico City Milan Naples, FL New York Philadelphia St. Louis Sydney Tokyo Toronto Wiesbaden

Mosby–Year Book Inc.
11830 Westline Drive
St Louis, MO 63146

Copyright © 1993 Mosby–Year Book Europe Limited
All rights reserved.
Published in 1993 with rights in the USA, Canada and Puerto Rico by Mosby–Year
Book, Inc.
Reprinted 1994 &1995 by Mosby–Wolfe, an imprint of Times Mirror International
Publishers Limited, Lynton House, 7–12 Tavistock Square, London WC1E 9LB, UK
Printed in Hong Kong by Mandarin Offset Ltd.

10   9   8   7   6   5   4

ISBN 0–8151–5851–3 (Hard cover)
ISBN 0–8151–5858–0 (Paperback)

English edition first published in 1977 by Wolfe Publishing
Second edition published 1988

Library of Congress Cataloging-in-Publication Data

McMinn, R.M.H. (Robert Matthew Hay)
        A colour atlas of human anatomy/Robert M.H. McMinn, Ralph T.
Hutchings, Peter H. Abrahams.—3rd ed.
                p. cm.
        Includes index.
        ISBN 0–8151–5858–0 (pbk.).—ISBN 0–8151–5851–3 (hardcover)
        I. Human anatomy—Atlases. I. Pegington, John. II. Abrahams,
    Peter H. III. Title
        [DNLM: 1. Anatomy—atlases. QS 17 M4785ca]
    QM25.M23 1993
    611'.022'2—dc20
    DNLM/DLC
    for Library of Congress   92-48935
                                                            CIP

Contents

Preface

For this Third Edition of 'A Colour Atlas of Human Anatomy', the original authors are pleased to welcome as their editorial colleagues John Pegington and Peter Abrahams, who bring with them many years of experience in Clinical Anatomy teaching at both undergraduate and postgraduate levels.

The general order of presentation has been preserved, but there are numerous changes and additions, designed to clarify and explain a subject which is not the easiest to understand for newcomers.

Orientation is a major problem, particularly in some complex areas. Line drawings have therefore been added where necessary to reinforce understanding.

Also, there are now included more than 80 new examples of modern imaging techniques, which allow side-by-side comparison with anatomical specimens. This correlation of anatomy with investigative procedures routinely being used on patients bridges the gap between preclinical and clinical studies.

Further notes, particularly of a clinical nature, have been added and, in the sections on bones, colour distinctions have been made to emphasize the differences between joint capsules and epiphysial lines.

We hope that these additions will render the Atlas even more helpful to Anatomy students in the future than it has been in the past.

R M H McMinn
R T Hutchings
J Pegington
P H Abrahams

Introduction

The body is made up of the head, trunk and limbs. The trunk consists of the neck, thorax (chest) and abdomen (belly). The lower part of the abdomen is the pelvis, but this word is also used to refer just to the bones of the pelvis. The lowest part of the pelvis (and lowest part of the trunk) is the perineum. The central axis of the trunk is the vertebral column (spine), and the upper part of it (cervical part) supports the head.

The main parts of the upper limb are the arm, forearm and hand. Note that in strict anatomical terms the word 'arm' means the upper arm, the part between the shoulder and elbow, although the word is commonly used to mean the whole of the upper limb.

The main parts of the lower limb are the thigh, leg and foot. Note that in strict anatomical terms the word 'leg' means the lower leg, the part between the knee and foot, although the word is commonly used to mean the whole of the lower limb.

For the description of the positions of structures in human anatomy, the body is assumed to be standing upright with the feet together and the head and eyes looking to the front, with the arms straight by the side and the palms of the hands facing forwards. This is the 'anatomical position' (see the illustrations below), and structures are always described relative to one another using this as the 'standard' position, even when the body is, for example, lying on the back in bed or on a dissecting room table.

The 'median sagittal plane' is an imaginary vertical, longitudinal line through the middle of the body from front to back, dividing the body into right and left halves. The adjective 'medial' means nearer the median plane, and 'lateral' means farther from it. Thus, in the anatomical position, the little finger is on the medial side of the hand and the thumb is on the lateral side; the great toe is on the medial side of the foot and the little toe on the lateral side.

In the forearm where there are two bones, the radius on the lateral (thumb) side and the ulna on the medial side, the adjectives 'radial' and 'ulnar' can be used instead of lateral and medial. Similarly in the lower leg where there are two bones, the fibula on the lateral side and the tibia on the medial side, 'fibular' and 'tibial' are alternative adjectives.

'Anterior' and 'posterior' mean nearer the front or nearer the back of the body respectively. Thus on the face the nose is anterior to the ears, and the ears are posterior to the nose. Sometimes 'ventral' is used instead of anterior, and 'dorsal' instead of posterior (terms from comparative anatomy which are appropriate for four-footed animals).

The hand and foot have special terms applied to them. The anterior or ventral surface of the hand is usually called the palm or palmar surface, and the posterior or dorsal surface is the dorsum. But in the foot the upper surface is the dorsal surface or dorsum, and the undersurface or sole is the plantar surface.

'Superior' and 'inferior' mean nearer the upper or lower end of the body respectively; the nose is superior to the mouth and inferior to the forehead (even if the body is upside down; the upright 'anatomical position' is always the reference position).

'Superficial' means near the skin surface, and 'deep' means farther away from the surface.

'Proximal' and 'distal' mean nearer to and farther from the root of the structure: in the upper limb, the forearm is distal to the elbow and proximal to the hand.

The words 'sagittal' and 'coronal' describe certain planes of section, most often used in the head and brain. The 'sagittal plane' is any front-to-back plane that is parallel to the median plane, and the 'coronal plane' (sometimes called the frontal plane) is a vertical plane at right angles to the median plane.

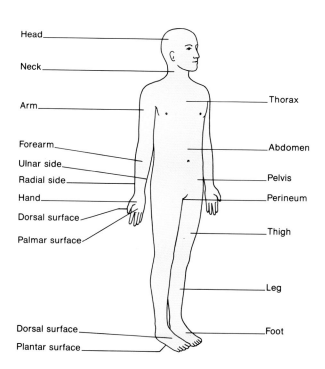

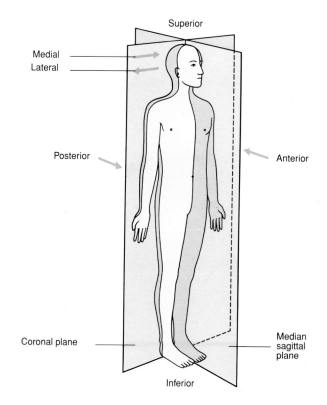

The book is arranged in the general order 'head to toe'—head and neck (including the brain), followed by the vertebral column and spinal cord, thorax, upper limb, abdomen and pelvis, and lower limb. In each section the bones are considered first, followed by dissections and other illustrations.

Structures are labelled by overlying numbers which are identified in the key lists. The numbers on the pictures are generally arranged in a clockwise order starting at the top of the picture, although it has not always seemed appropriate to stick rigidly to this pattern. Sometimes in crowded areas or for small structures, leader lines are necessary; an arrowhead at the end of a leader indicates that the item is just out of view beyond the tip of the arrow. Self-testing can be carried out by covering up the key.

For bones, the parts of each are first named, and then the pictures are repeated indicating the sites of attachments of muscles and ligaments. Although the details of individual skull bones are included, for most students knowledge of the skull as a whole is much more important.

Dissections and other items are introduced by a short commentary which draws attention to the most significant features, so helping to sort out 'the wood from the trees'. The commentary is supplemented by notes which again emphasize the more important features or help to explain difficult topics, but they are not intended to give a comprehensive description of everything seen. The book is designed to supplement existing texts, not to substitute for them.

The Appendix at the back of the book contains reference lists of vessels, nerves, muscles and skull foramina, with illustrations of the whole skeleton and of the principal vessels and nerves. The diagram of the arteries, for example, shows at a glance which are the main vessels of the upper limb, and in the reference lists their branches are named.

Acknowledgements

For the preparation of new dissections for this edition we are most grateful to Bari Logan, Prosector to the University of Cambridge. For new artwork we are much indebted to Rosemary Watts, with additional material from Philip Ball. We also thank our models for surface anatomy, and Dr Umraz Khan and Dr Ravinder Ranger for all their valuable help in proofing the Atlas.

In addition to imaging material from Dr Oscar Craig, Dr Paul Grech, Dr Kim Fox and Dr Richard Underwood, new material has generously been provided by Dr Niall Moore, Professor Jamie Weir, Dr Philip Owen, Dr Phil Gishen and Dr Anna-Maria Belli, and endoscopic views of the knee and hip joints by Mr David J. Dandy and Mr Richard R. Villar, respectively. For the endoscopic views of the nose and larynx we are grateful to Mr J.D. Shaw and Mr J.M. Lancer, and for the ophthalmoscopic view we thank Miss Erna Kritzinger.

We renew our thanks to all those who over many years contributed specimens to the Anatomy Museum of the Royal College of Surgeons of England, and especially to the late Dr D.H. Tompsett who also prepared the corrosion casts (full details of the methods used can be found in his book *Anatomical Techniques*, 2nd edition, 1970, Livingstone), and to the late Sir Edward Muir, who, as President of the College, allowed us to reproduce the illustrations of museum specimens; to Dr J.L. Cordingley, Professor T.W. Glenister, and Professor F.R. Johnson for the loan of osteological material; and to Mr V.H. Oswal for the coloured dissections of the ear.

We also wish to thank the staff of Mosby–Year Book Europe Limited who have been so enthusiastically involved in this book, especially Rachael Miller and Patrick Daly.

To the memory of Peter Wolfe

Sabrina Carswell (619)263-2725

Skull, from the front

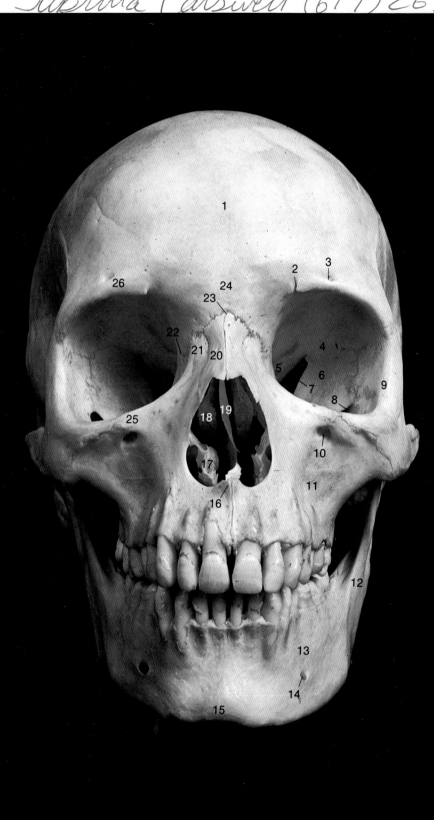

1 Frontal bone
2 Frontal notch
3 Supra-orbital foramen
4 Orbit (orbital cavity)
5 Lesser ⎫
6 Greater ⎭ wing of sphenoid bone
7 Superior ⎫
8 Inferior ⎭ orbital fissure
9 Zygomatic bone
10 Infra-orbital foramen
11 Maxilla
12 Ramus ⎫
13 Body ⎭ of mandible
14 Mental foramen
15 Mental protuberance
16 Anterior nasal spine
17 Inferior ⎫
18 Middle ⎭ nasal concha
19 Nasal septum
20 Nasal bone
21 Frontal process of maxilla
22 Lacrimal bone
23 Nasion
24 Glabella
25 Infra-orbital margin
26 Supra-orbital margin

● The term 'skull' includes the mandible, and 'cranium' refers to the skull without the mandible, but these definitions are not always strictly observed.
● The calvaria is the vault of the skull (cranial vault or skull-cap) and is the upper part of the cranium that encloses the brain.
● The front part of the skull forms the facial skeleton.
● The supra-orbital, infra-orbital and mental foramina (3, 10 and 14) lie in approximately the same vertical plane.
● Details of individual skull bones are given on pages 26 to 35, of the bones of the orbit and nose on page 20, and of the teeth on page 21.

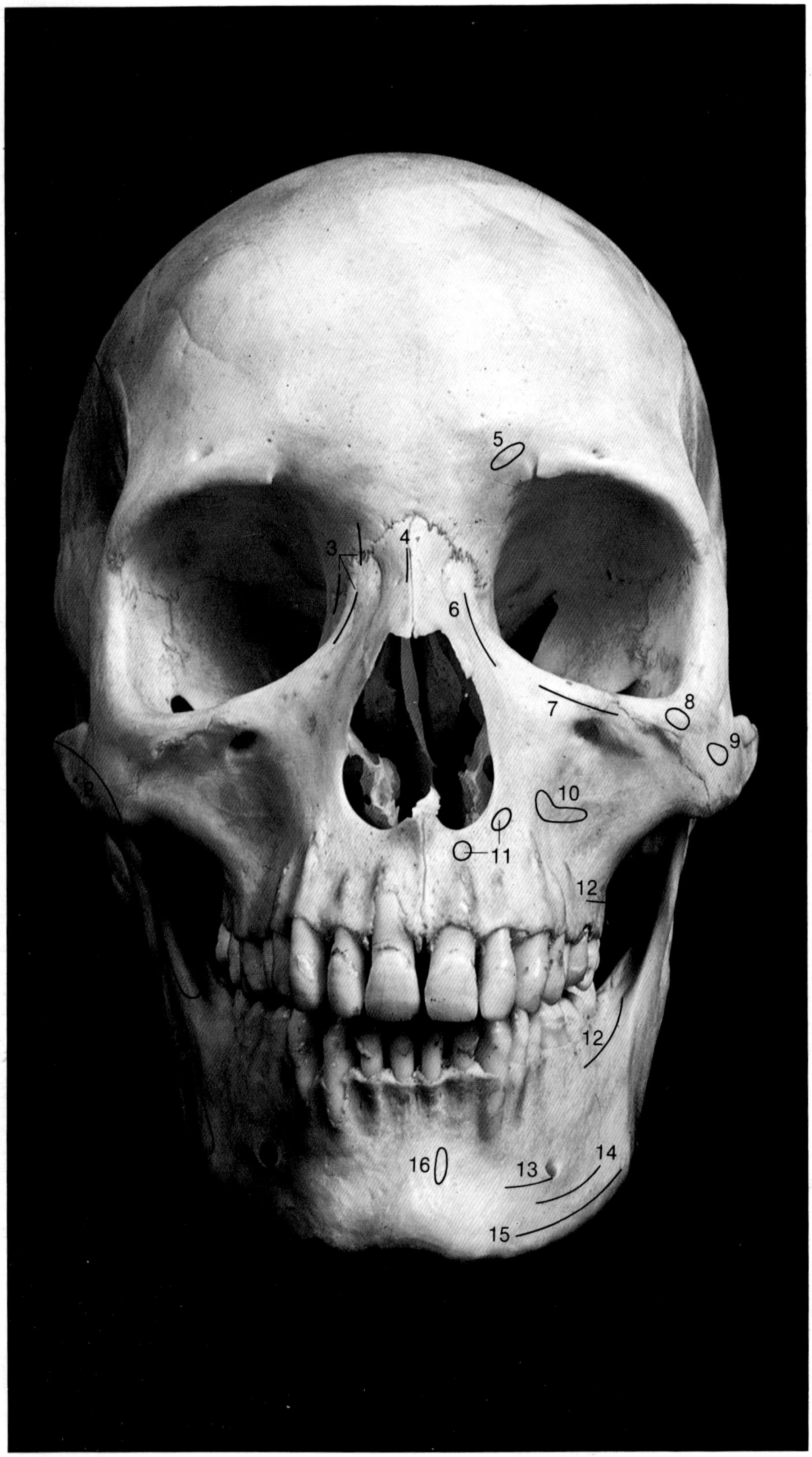

A Skull, from the front. Muscle attachments

1	Temporalis
2	Masseter
3	Orbicularis oculi
4	Procerus
5	Corrugator supercilii
6	Levator labii superioris alaeque nasi
7	Levator labii superioris
8	Zygomaticus minor
9	Zygomaticus major
10	Levator anguli oris
11	Nasalis
12	Buccinator
13	Depressor labii inferioris
14	Depressor anguli oris
15	Platysma
16	Mentalis

• The attachment of levator labii superioris (7) is above the infra-orbital foramen and that of levator anguli oris (10) is below it.
• The attachment of depressor labii inferioris (13) is in front of the mental foramen and that of depressor anguli oris (14) is below it.

B Skull radiograph. Occipitofrontal projection

1 Frontal bone
2 Supra-orbital margin
3 Lesser wing of sphenoid bone
4 Superior orbital fissure
5 Zygomatic bone
6 Infra-orbital margin
7 Nasal septum
8 Anterior nasal spine
9 Ramus } of mandible
10 Body

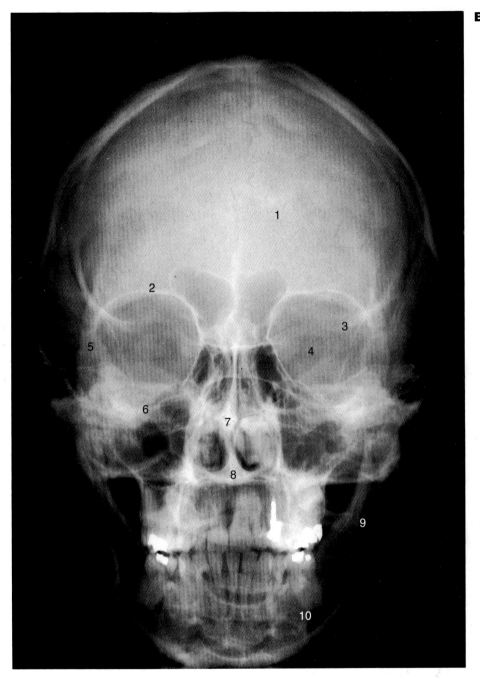

A

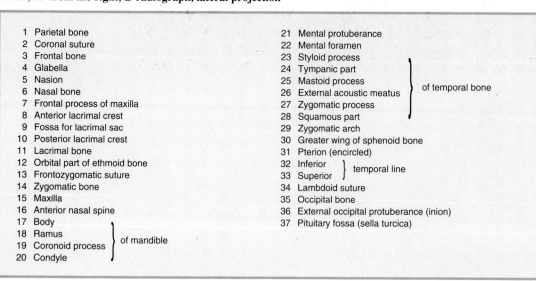

Skull, A from the right, B radiograph, lateral projection

1	Parietal bone	21	Mental protuberance	
2	Coronal suture	22	Mental foramen	
3	Frontal bone	23	Styloid process	
4	Glabella	24	Tympanic part	
5	Nasion	25	Mastoid process	
6	Nasal bone	26	External acoustic meatus	of temporal bone
7	Frontal process of maxilla	27	Zygomatic process	
8	Anterior lacrimal crest	28	Squamous part	
9	Fossa for lacrimal sac	29	Zygomatic arch	
10	Posterior lacrimal crest	30	Greater wing of sphenoid bone	
11	Lacrimal bone	31	Pterion (encircled)	
12	Orbital part of ethmoid bone	32	Inferior	temporal line
13	Frontozygomatic suture	33	Superior	
14	Zygomatic bone	34	Lambdoid suture	
15	Maxilla	35	Occipital bone	
16	Anterior nasal spine	36	External occipital protuberance (inion)	
17	Body	37	Pituitary fossa (sella turcica)	
18	Ramus	of mandible		
19	Coronoid process			
20	Condyle			

• Pterion (31) is not a single point but an *area* where the frontal (3), parietal (1), squamous part of the temporal (28) and greater wing of the sphenoid bone (30) adjoin one another. It is an important landmark for the anterior branch of the middle meningeal artery which underlies this area on the inside of the skull (page 25, 45).

B

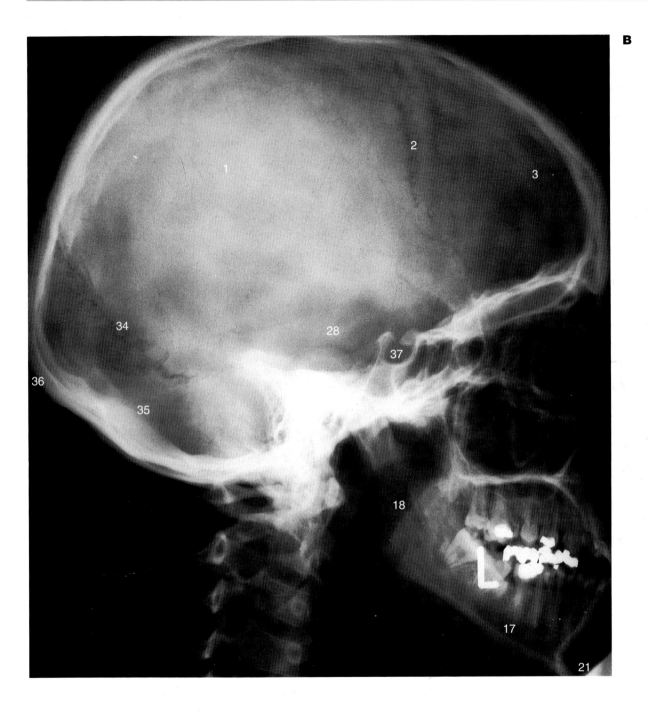

A

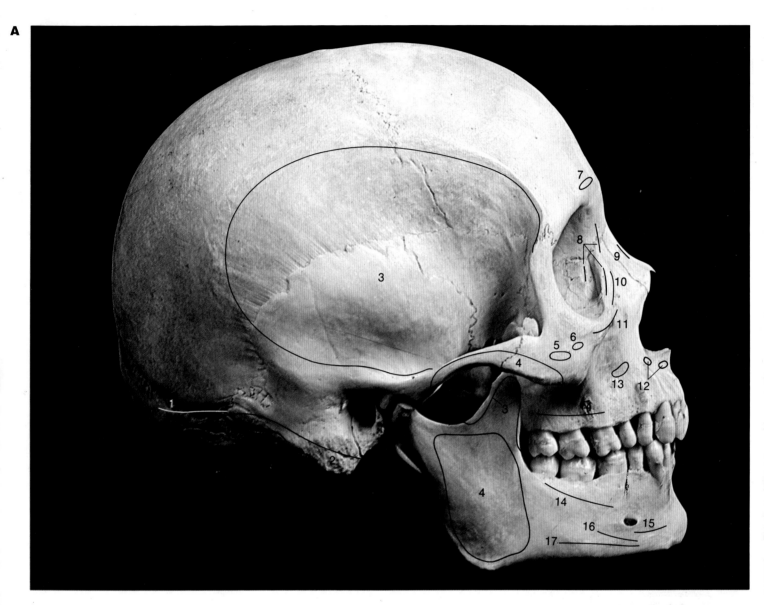

A Skull, from the right. Muscle attachments

1	Occipital part of occipitofrontalis
2	Sternocleidomastoid
3	Temporalis
4	Masseter
5	Zygomaticus major
6	Zygomaticus minor
7	Corrugator supercilii
8	Orbicularis oculi
9	Procerus
10	Levator labii superioris alaeque nasi
11	Levator labii superioris
12	Nasalis
13	Levator anguli oris
14	Buccinator
15	Depressor labii inferioris
16	Depressor anguli oris
17	Platysma

• The bony attachments of the buccinator muscle (14) are to the upper and lower jaws (maxilla and mandible) opposite the three molar teeth. (The teeth are identified on page 21, C.)

• The upper attachment of temporalis (upper 3) occupies the temporal fossa (the narrow space above the zygomatic arch at the side of the skull). The lower attachment of temporalis (lower 3) extends from the lowest part of the mandibular notch of the mandible, over the coronoid process and down the front of the ramus almost as far as the last molar tooth.

• Masseter (4) extends from the zygomatic arch to the lateral side of the ramus of the mandible.

B Skull, from behind

1 Parietal bone
2 Sagittal suture
3 Parietal foramen
4 Lambda
5 Lambdoid suture
6 Sutural bone
7 Occipital bone
8 External occipital protuberance (inion)
9 Highest ⎫
10 Superior ⎬ nuchal line
11 Inferior ⎭

● This cranium shows several sutural bones (6) in the lambdoid suture (5) and one of them (lower left) is unusually large.

C Skull. Right infratemporal region, obliquely from below

1 Mastoid process
2 External acoustic meatus
3 Mandibular fossa
4 Articular tubercle
5 Zygomatic arch
6 Infratemporal crest
7 Infratemporal surface of greater wing of sphenoid bone
8 Pterygomaxillary fissure and pterygopalatine fossa
9 Inferior orbital fissure
10 Infratemporal (posterior) surface of maxilla
11 Third molar tooth
12 Tuberosity of maxilla
13 Pyramidal process ⎫ of palatine
14 Horizontal plate ⎬ bone
15 Lateral ⎫
16 Medial ⎬ pterygoid plate
17 Pterygoid hamulus
18 Vomer
19 Spine of sphenoid bone
20 Styloid process and sheath
21 Occipital condyle
22 Occipital groove
23 Mastoid notch

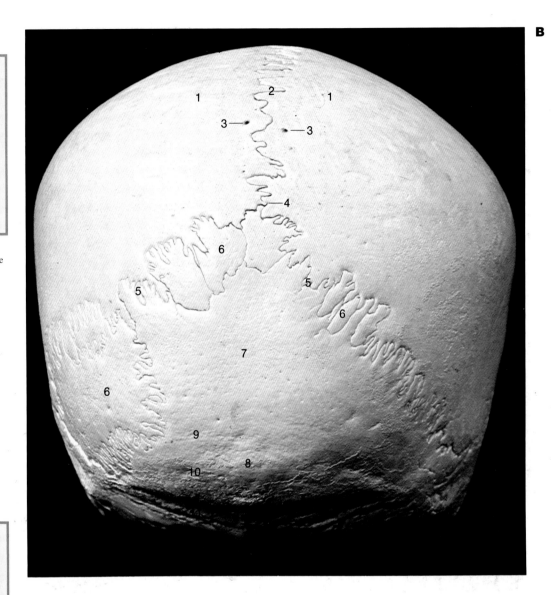

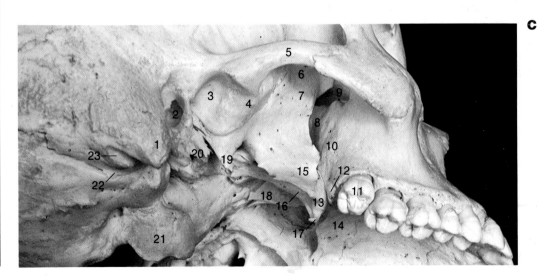

A

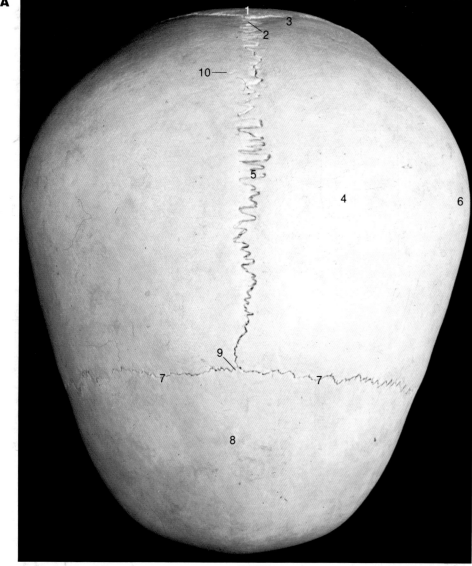

FRONT

A Skull, from above

1	Occipital bone
2	Lambda
3	Lambdoid suture
4	Parietal bone
5	Sagittal suture
6	Parietal eminence
7	Coronal suture
8	Frontal bone
9	Bregma
10	Parietal foramen

• In this skull the parietal eminences are prominent (A6).

• The point where the sagittal suture (A5) meets the coronal suture (A7) is the bregma (A9). At birth the unossified parts of the frontal and parietal bones in this region form the membranous anterior fontanelle (page 22, D5).

• The point where the sagittal suture (A5) meets the lambdoid suture (A3) is the lambda (A2). At birth the unossified parts of the parietal and occipital bones in this region form the membranous posterior fontanelle (page 22, C19).

• The label 8 in the centre of the frontal bone indicates the line of the frontal suture in the fetal skull (page 22, A6). The suture may persist in the adult skull and is sometimes known as the metopic suture.

B

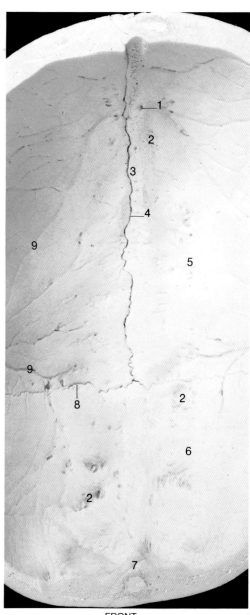

FRONT

B Skull. Internal surface of the cranial vault, central part

1	Parietal foramen
2	Depressions for arachnoid granulations
3	Groove for superior sagittal sinus
4	Sagittal suture
5	Parietal bone
6	Frontal bone
7	Frontal crest
8	Coronal suture
9	Grooves for middle meningeal vessels

• The arachnoid granulations (page 69, A5), through which cerebrospinal fluid drains into the superior sagittal sinus, cause the irregular depressions (B2) on the parts of the frontal and parietal bones (B6 and 5) that overlie the sinus.

C Skull. External surface of the base

1 Incisive fossa
2 Palatine process of maxilla
3 Horizontal plate of palatine bone
4 Greater palatine foramen
5 Lesser palatine foramina
6 Tuberosity of maxilla
7 Pterygoid hamulus
8 Medial pterygoid plate
9 Pyramidal process of palatine bone
10 Lateral pterygoid plate
11 Inferior orbital fissure
12 Infratemporal crest of greater wing of
sphenoid bone
13 Zygomatic arch
14 Squamous part of temporal bone
15 Articular tubercle
16 Mandibular fossa
17 Petrosquamous fissure
18 Edge of tegmen tympani
19 Petrotympanic fissure
20 Squamotympanic fissure
21 Tympanic part of temporal bone
22 External acoustic meatus
23 Styloid process
24 Stylomastoid foramen
25 Mastoid process
26 Mastoid notch
27 Occipital groove
28 Mastoid foramen
29 Superior nuchal line
30 External occipital protuberance
31 External occipital crest
32 Inferior nuchal line
33 Foramen magnum
34 Condylar canal
35 Occipital condyle
36 Hypoglossal canal
37 Jugular foramen
38 Carotid canal
39 Apex of petrous part of temporal bone
40 Spine of sphenoid bone
41 Foramen spinosum
42 Foramen ovale
43 Foramen lacerum
44 Pharyngeal tubercle
45 Scaphoid fossa
46 Palatinovaginal canal
47 Vomerovaginal canal
48 Posterior border of vomer
49 Posterior nasal aperture (choana)
50 Posterior nasal spine
51 Palatine grooves and spines
52 Transverse palatine suture
53 Median palatine suture

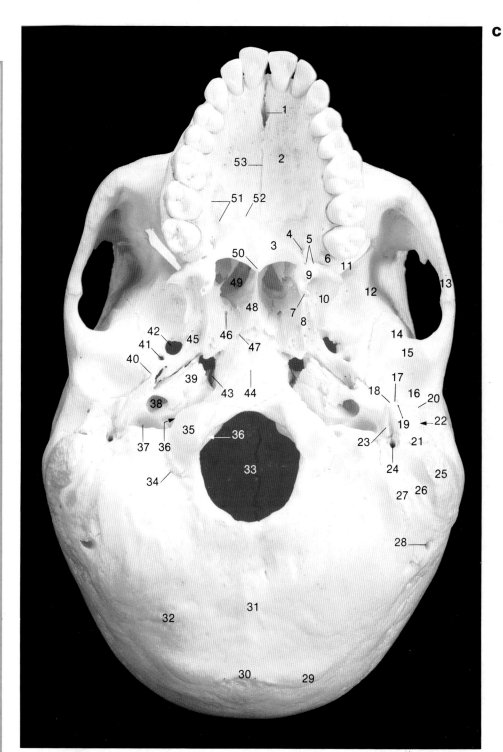

- The palatine process of the maxilla (2) and the horizontal plate of the palatine bone (3) form the hard palate (roof of the mouth and floor of the nose).
- The spaces on either side of the vomer (48) leading forwards into the nasal cavity are the posterior nasal apertures or choanae (49).
- The gap medial to the zygomatic arch (13) indicates the lower part of the temporal fossa, where it merges with the upper lateral part of the infratemporal fossa.
- The carotid canal (38), recognized by its round shape in the inferior surface of the petrous part of the temporal bone, does not pass straight upwards to open into the inside of the skull but takes a right-angled turn forwards and medially within the petrous temporal to open into the back of the foramen lacerum (43).
- For the contents of skull foramina see page 339.

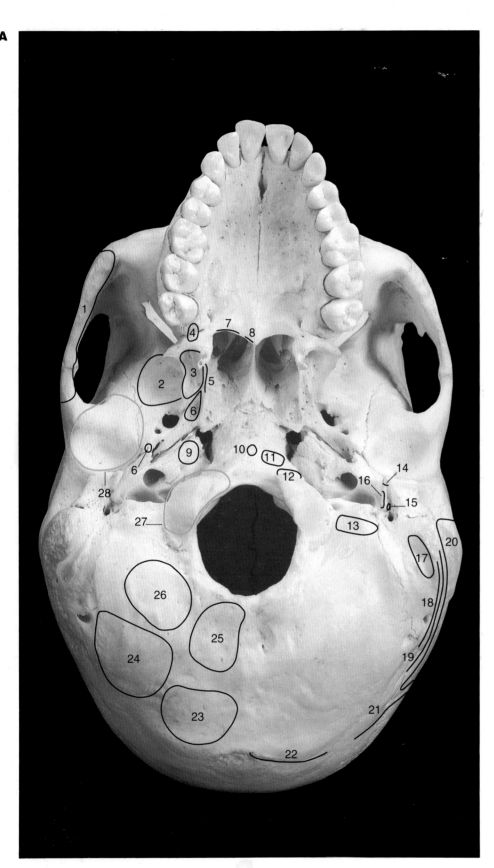

A Skull. External surface of the base. Muscle attachments

Green line = capsule attachments of atlanto-occipital and temporomandibular joints

1	Masseter
2	Upper head of lateral pterygoid
3	Deep head of medial pterygoid
4	Superficial head of medial pterygoid
5	Superior constrictor
6	Tensor veli palatini
7	Palatopharyngeus
8	Musculus uvulae
9	Levator veli palatini
10	Pharyngeal raphe
11	Longus capitis
12	Rectus capitis anterior
13	Rectus capitis lateralis
14	Styloglossus
15	Stylohyoid
16	Stylopharyngeus
17	Posterior belly of digastric
18	Longissimus capitis
19	Splenius capitis
20	Sternocleidomastoid
21	Occipital part of occipitofrontalis
22	Trapezius
23	Semispinalis capitis
24	Superior oblique
25	Rectus capitis posterior minor
26	Rectus capitis posterior major
27	Capsule attachment of atlanto-occipital joint
28	Capsule attachment of temporo-mandibular joint

• The medial pterygoid plate has no pterygoid muscles attached to it. It passes straight backwards, giving origin at its lower end to part of the superior constrictor of the pharynx (5).
• The lateral pterygoid plate has both pterygoid muscles attached to it: medial and lateral muscles from the medial and lateral surfaces respectively (3 and 2). The plate becomes twisted slightly laterally because of the constant pull of these muscles which pass backwards and laterally to their attachments to the mandible (page 27).

B Skull. Internal surface of the base (cranial fossae)

1 Diploë
2 Frontal sinus
3 Frontal crest
4 Foramen caecum
5 Crista galli
6 Cribriform plate of ethmoid bone
7 Groove for anterior ethmoidal nerve and vessels
8 Orbital part of frontal bone
9 Lesser wing of sphenoid bone
10 Jugum of sphenoid bone
11 Prechiasmatic groove
12 Tuberculum sellae
13 Pituitary fossa (sella turcica)
14 Dorsum sellae
15 Optic canal
16 Anterior clinoid process
17 Foramen rotundum
18 Venous foramen
19 Foramen ovale
20 Foramen spinosum
21 Greater wing of sphenoid bone
22 Grooves for middle meningeal vessels
23 Squamous part of temporal bone
24 Tegmen tympani
25 Petrous part of temporal bone
26 Groove for superior petrosal sinus
27 Arcuate eminence
28 Groove for sigmoid sinus
29 Groove for transverse sinus
30 Groove for superior sagittal sinus
31 Internal occipital protuberance
32 Parietal bone
33 Occipital bone
34 Foramen magnum
35 Hypoglossal canal
36 Jugular foramen
37 Groove for inferior petrosal sinus
38 Internal acoustic meatus
39 Clivus
40 Posterior clinoid process
41 Carotid groove
42 Foramen lacerum
43 Trigeminal impression
44 Hiatus and groove for greater petrosal nerve
45 Hiatus and groove for lesser petrosal nerve
46 Superior orbital fissure

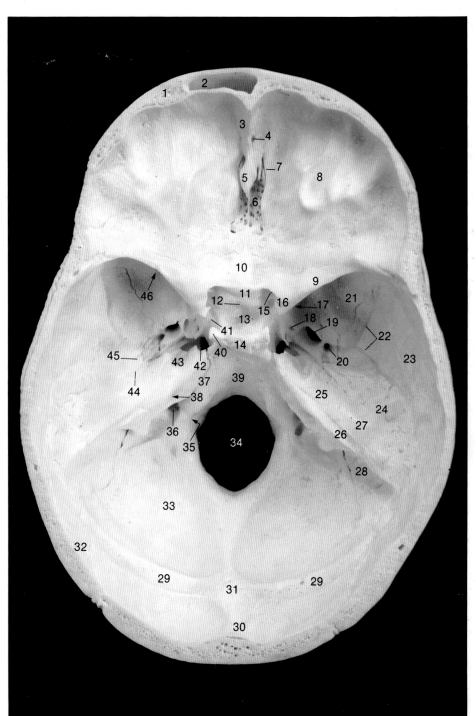

B

- The anterior cranial fossa is limited posteriorly on each side by the free margin of the lesser wing of the sphenoid (9) with its anterior clinoid process (16), and centrally by the anterior margin of the prechiasmatic groove (11).
- The middle cranial fossa is butterfly-shaped and consists of a central or median part and right and left lateral parts. The central part includes the pituitary fossa (13) on the upper surface of the body of the sphenoid, with the prechiasmatic groove (11) in front and the dorsum sellae (14) with its posterior clinoid processes (40) behind. Each lateral part extends from the posterior border of the lesser wing of the sphenoid (9) to the groove for the superior petrosal sinus (26) on the upper edge of the petrous part of the temporal bone.
- The posterior cranial fossa, whose most obvious feature is the foramen magnum (34), is behind the dorsum sellae (14) and the grooves for the superior petrosal sinuses (26) which are on the upper edges of the petrous parts of the temporal bones (25).

A Skull. Bones of the left orbit

The bones forming the roof, lateral wall, floor and medial wall of the orbit are indicated in the list below by being bracketed together

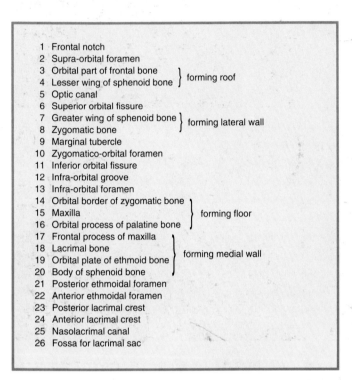

A

1 Frontal notch
2 Supra-orbital foramen
3 Orbital part of frontal bone ⎫
4 Lesser wing of sphenoid bone ⎬ forming roof
5 Optic canal
6 Superior orbital fissure
7 Greater wing of sphenoid bone ⎫ forming lateral wall
8 Zygomatic bone ⎭
9 Marginal tubercle
10 Zygomatico-orbital foramen
11 Inferior orbital fissure
12 Infra-orbital groove
13 Infra-orbital foramen
14 Orbital border of zygomatic bone ⎫
15 Maxilla ⎬ forming floor
16 Orbital process of palatine bone ⎭
17 Frontal process of maxilla ⎫
18 Lacrimal bone ⎪
19 Orbital plate of ethmoid bone ⎬ forming medial wall
20 Body of sphenoid bone ⎭
21 Posterior ethmoidal foramen
22 Anterior ethmoidal foramen
23 Posterior lacrimal crest
24 Anterior lacrimal crest
25 Nasolacrimal canal
26 Fossa for lacrimal sac

• The fossa for the lacrimal sac (A26) is formed partly by the lacrimal groove of the frontal process of the maxilla (A17) and partly by the similar groove on the lacrimal bone (A18).

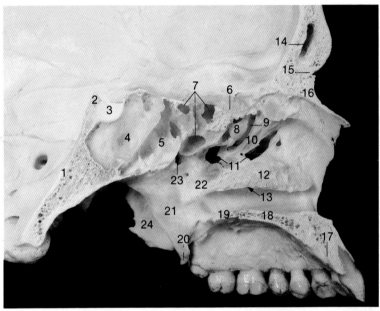

B

B Lateral wall of the left nasal cavity

In this midline sagittal section of the skull, with the nasal septum removed, the superior and middle nasal conchae have been dissected away to reveal the air cells of the ethmoidal sinus, in particular the ethmoidal bulla (8). Compare this bony background with A on page 52

1 Clivus
2 Dorsum sellae
3 Pituitary fossa (sella turcica)
4 Right sphenoidal sinus
5 Left sphenoidal sinus
6 Cribriform plate of ethmoid bone
7 Air cells of ethmoidal sinus
8 Ethmoidal bulla
9 Semilunar hiatus
10 Uncinate process of ethmoid bone
11 Opening of maxillary sinus
12 Inferior nasal concha
13 Inferior meatus
14 Frontal sinus
15 Nasal spine of frontal bone
16 Nasal bone
17 Incisive canal
18 Palatine process of maxilla
19 Horizontal plate of palatine bone
20 Pterygoid hamulus
21 Medial pterygoid plate
22 Perpendicular plate of palatine bone
23 Sphenopalatine foramen
24 Lateral pterygoid plate

• The roof of the nasal cavity consists mainly of the cribriform plate of the ethmoid bone (B6) with the body of the sphenoid containing the sphenoidal sinuses (B4 and 5) behind, and the nasal bone (B16) and the nasal spine of the frontal bone (B15) at the front.
• The floor of the cavity consists of the palatine process of the maxilla (B18) and the horizontal plate of the palatine bone (B19).
• The medial wall is the nasal septum (page 25) which is formed mainly by two bones—the perpendicular plate of the ethmoid and the vomer—and the septal cartilage.
• The lateral wall is the most interesting and complicated, consisting of the medial surface of the maxilla with its large opening (B11), overlapped from above by parts of the ethmoid (B7, 8 and 10) and lacrimal bones, from behind by the perpendicular plate of the palatine (B22), and below by the inferior concha (B12).
• When covered by mucous membrane, the ethmoidal bulla (B8) and the uncinate process of the ethmoid (B10) form the upper and lower boundaries respectively of the semilunar hiatus (page 52, A7).

C

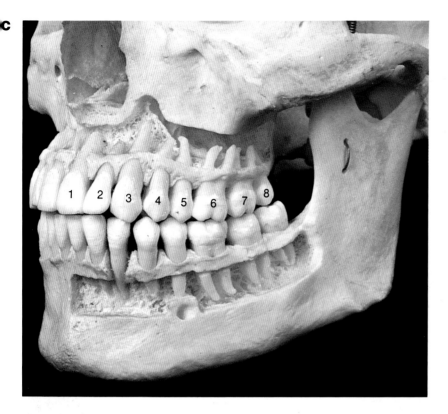

D

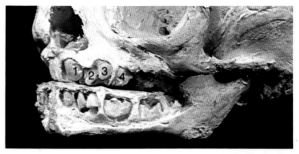

E

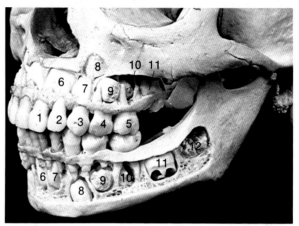

C Skull.
**Permanent teeth,
from the left and
in front**
The alveolar bone has
been partially removed
to show the roots of
the teeth, which are
numbered and named
on the left side

1	First (central)	} incisor
2	Second (lateral)	
3	Canine	
4	First	} premolar
5	Second	
6	First	} molar
7	Second	
8	Third	

● The corresponding teeth of the upper and lower jaws have similar
names. In clinical dentistry the teeth are often identified by the numbers 1
to 8 (as listed here) rather than by name.
● The third molar is sometimes called the wisdom tooth.

**Skull. Upper and lower jaws
from the left and in front, D
in the newborn with
unerupted deciduous teeth,
E in a four-year-old child
with erupted deciduous teeth
and unerupted permanent
teeth**

● The deciduous molars occupy the
positions of the premolars of the
permanent dentition.

1	First (central)	} incisor	
2	Second (lateral)		of deciduous
3	Canine		dentition
4	First	} molar	
5	Second		
6	First (central)	} incisor	
7	Second (lateral)		
8	Canine		
9	First	} premolar	of permanent
10	Second		dentition
11	First	} molar	
12	Second		

F

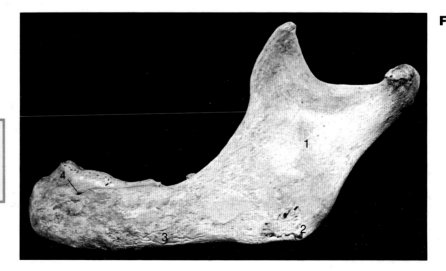

F Skull.
**Edentulous
mandible in old
age, from the left**

1	Ramus
2	Angle
3	Body
4	Mental foramen

● With the loss of teeth the alveolar bone becomes absorbed, so that the mental
foramen (4) and mandibular canal lie near the upper margin of the bone.
● The angle (2) between the ramus (1) and body (3) becomes more obtuse,
resembling the infantile angle (as in D and E, above).

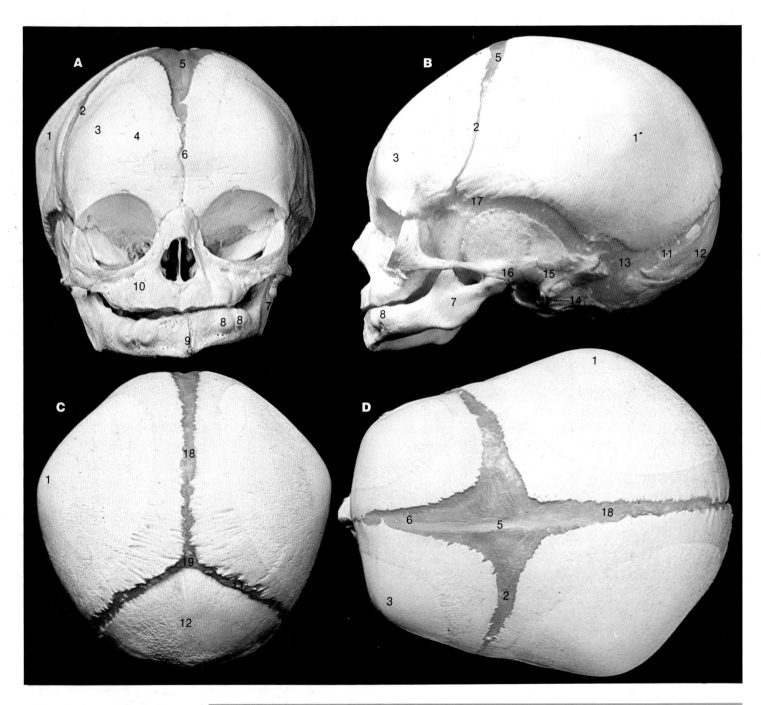

Skull of a full-term fetus, **A** from the front, **B** from the left and slightly below, **C** from behind, **D** from above. Fetal skull radiographs, **E** frontal projection, **F** lateral projection

1 Parietal tuberosity	11 Lambdoid suture
2 Coronal suture	12 Occipital bone
3 Frontal tuberosity	13 Mastoid fontanelle
4 Half of frontal bone	14 Stylomastoid foramen
5 Anterior fontanelle	15 External acoustic meatus
6 Frontal suture	16 Tympanic ring
7 Ramus of mandible	17 Sphenoidal fontanelle
8 Elevations over deciduous teeth in body of mandible	18 Sagittal suture
9 Symphysis menti	19 Posterior fontanelle
10 Maxilla	

E

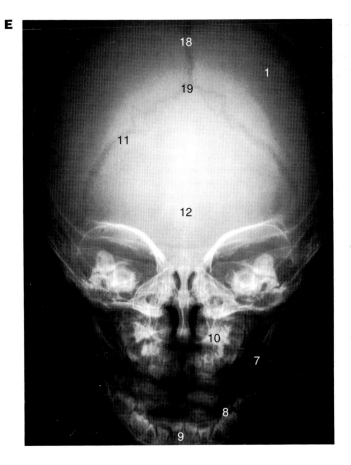

F

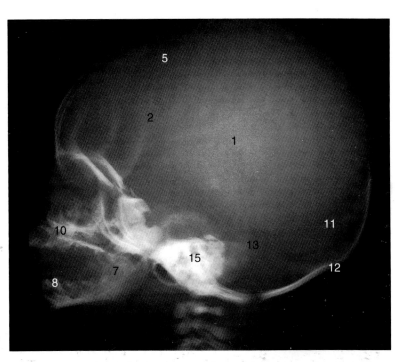

G

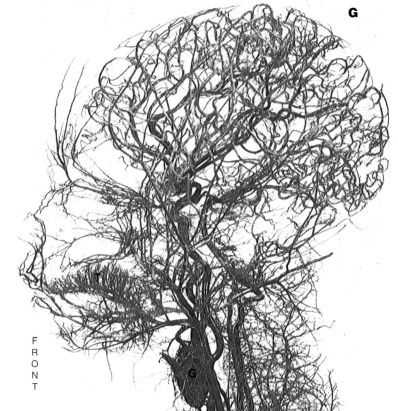

• The face at birth forms a relatively smaller proportion of the cranium than in the adult (about one eighth compared with one half) because of the small size of the nasal cavity and maxillary sinuses and the lack of erupted teeth.

• The posterior fontanelle (C19, E19) closes about two months after birth, the anterior fontanelle (A5, D5, F5) in the second year.

• Due to the lack of the mastoid process (which does not develop until the second year) the stylomastoid foramen (B14) and the emerging facial nerve are relatively near the surface and unprotected.

G Cast of the head and neck arteries of a full-term fetus, from the left

In this cast of fetal arteries, note in the front of the neck the dense arterial pattern indicating the thyroid gland (G), and above and in front of it the fine vessels outlining the tongue (T)

FRONT

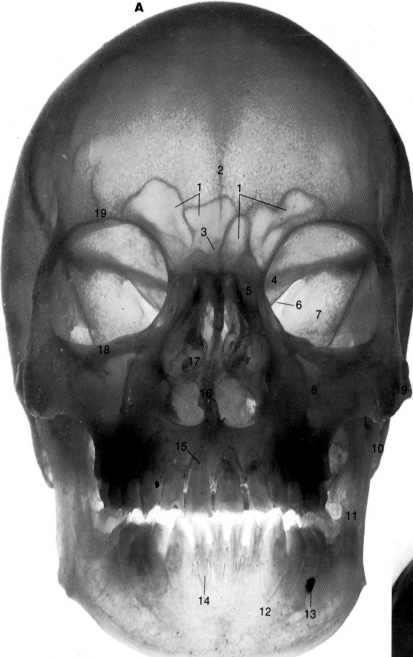

A

Skull, A cleared specimen from the front, illuminated from behind, **B** radiograph of facial bones, occipitofrontal view

1 Frontal sinus
2 Frontal crest
3 Crista galli
4 Lesser wing of sphenoid bone
5 Ethmoidal sinus
6 Superior orbital fissure
7 Greater wing of sphenoid bone
8 Maxillary sinus
9 Zygomatic arch
10 Mastoid process
11 Ramus
12 Body } of mandible
13 Mental foramen
14 Root of lower lateral incisor
15 Root of upper central incisor
16 Nasal septum
17 Inferior nasal concha
18 Infra-orbital margin
19 Supra-orbital margin

• Compare with the skull on page 9.

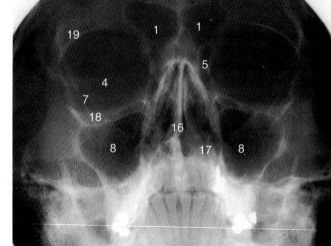

B

Left half of the skull. Sagittal section

The inside of the left half of the skull is seen from the right, with the bony part of the nasal septum (8 and 9) preserved

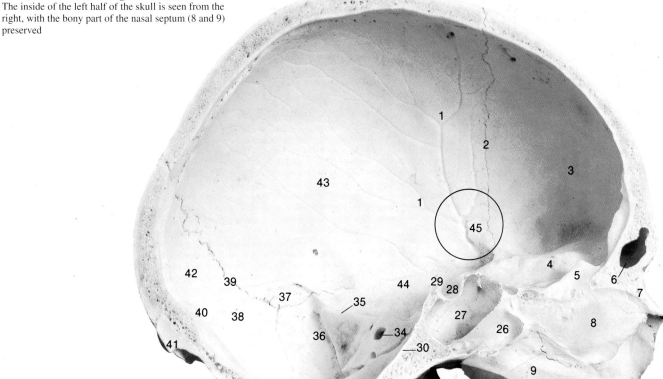

1 Grooves for middle meningeal vessels	25 Posterior nasal aperture (choana)
2 Coronal suture	26 Right sphenoidal sinus
3 Squamous part of frontal bone	27 Left sphenoidal sinus
4 Orbital part of frontal bone	28 Pituitary fossa (sella turcica)
5 Crista galli of ethmoid bone	29 Dorsum sellae
6 Frontal sinus	30 Clivus
7 Nasal bone	31 Margin of foramen magnum
8 Perpendicular plate of ethmoid bone	32 Occipital condyle
9 Vomer	33 Hypoglossal canal
10 Incisive canal	34 Internal acoustic meatus in petrous part of temporal bone
11 Palatine process of maxilla	35 Groove for superior petrosal sinus
12 Horizontal plate of palatine bone	36 Groove for sigmoid sinus
13 Alveolar process of maxilla	37 Mastoid (posterior inferior) angle of parietal bone
14 Mental protuberance	38 Groove for transverse sinus
15 Body of mandible	39 Lambdoid suture
16 Mylohyoid line	40 Internal occipital protuberance
17 Groove for mylohyoid nerve	41 External occipital protuberance
18 Angle of mandible	42 Occipital bone
19 Mandibular foramen	43 Parietal bone
20 Lingula	44 Squamous part of temporal bone
21 Ramus of mandible	45 Pterion (encircled)
22 Lateral pterygoid plate	
23 Pterygoid hamulus of medial pterygoid plate	
24 Medial pterygoid plate	

- The bony part of the nasal septum consists of the vomer (9) and the perpendicular plate of the ethmoid bone (8). The anterior part of the septum consists of the septal cartilage (page 51, C6).
- The palatine process of the maxilla (11) and the horizontal plate of the palatine bone (12) form the hard palate. Its lower surface is the roof of the mouth; its upper surface is the floor of the nasal cavity.
- In this skull the sphenoidal sinuses (26 and 27) are large, and the right one (26) has extended to the left of the midline. The pituitary fossa (28) projects down into the left sinus (27).
- The internal acoustic meatus (34) is in approximately the same vertical plane as the hypoglossal canal (33).
- The grooves for the middle meningeal vessels (1) pass upwards and backwards. The circle (45) marks the region of the pterion, and corresponds to the position shown on the outside of the skull on page 12, A31.
- The groove for the transverse sinus (38) on the occipital bone (42) extends on to the mastoid angle (37) of the parietal bone (43), and then curls downwards on the temporal bone as the groove for the sigmoid sinus (36) to reach the jugular foramen (page 19, B36).
- The external occipital protuberance (41) is not on the most posterior part of the back of the skull but some distance below and in front of it.

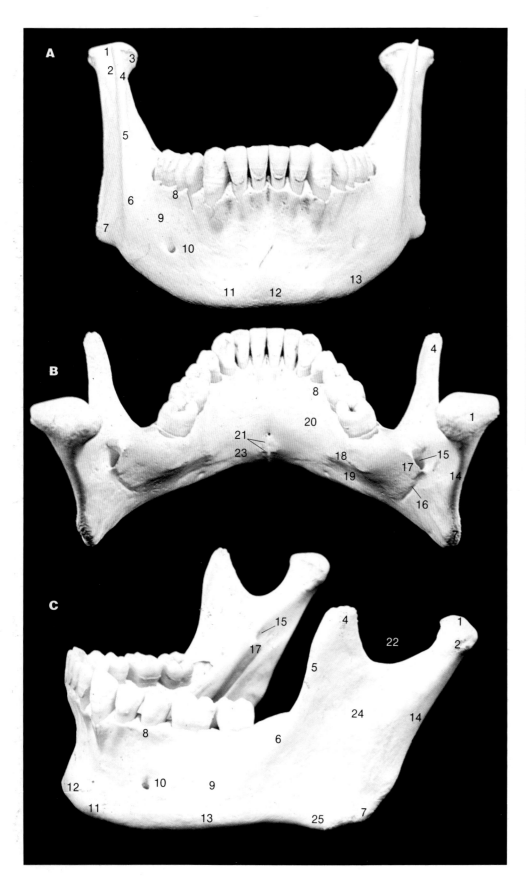

Mandible, A from the front, B from behind and above, C from the left and front

1 Head
2 Neck
3 Pterygoid fovea
4 Coronoid process
5 Anterior border of ramus
6 Oblique line
7 Angle
8 Alveolar part
9 Body
10 Mental foramen
11 Mental tubercle
12 Mental protuberance
13 Base
14 Posterior border of ramus
15 Mandibular foramen
16 Mylohyoid groove
17 Lingula
18 Mylohyoid line
19 Submandibular fossa
20 Sublingual fossa
21 Superior and inferior mental
   spines
22 Mandibular notch
23 Digastric fossa
24 Ramus
25 Inferior border of ramus

● The head (1) and the neck (2, including the pterygoid fovea, 3) constitute the condyle.
● The alveolar part (8) contains the sockets for the roots of the teeth.
● The base (13) is the inferior border of the body (9), and becomes continuous with the inferior border (25) of the ramus (24).
● In this mandible (also shown with muscle attachments on the next page) the third molar teeth are unerupted.

Mandible, A from the front, B from behind and above, C from the left and front. Muscle attachments

Green line = capsule attachment of temporomandibular joint; blue line = limit of attachment of the oral mucous membrane, pale green line = ligament attachment

1	Temporalis
2	Masseter
3	Lateral pterygoid
4	Buccinator
5	Depressor labii inferioris
6	Depressor anguli oris
7	Platysma
8	Mentalis
9	Medial pterygoid
10	Pterygomandibular raphe and superior constrictor
11	Mylohyoid
12	Anterior belly of digastric
13	Geniohyoid
14	Genioglossus
15	Sphenomandibular ligament
16	Stylomandibular ligament

• The lateral pterygoid (A3) is attached to the pterygoid fovea on the neck of the mandible (and also to the capsule of the temporomandibular joint and the articular disc—see page 40, A7 and B23).
• The medial pterygoid (B9, C9) is attached to the medial surface of the angle of the mandible, below the groove for the mylohyoid nerve.
• Masseter (C2) is attached to the lateral surface of the ramus.
• Temporalis (C1) is attached over the coronoid process, extending back as far as the deepest part of the mandibular notch and downwards over the front of the ramus almost as far as the last molar tooth. Note that in this mandible the last molar has not erupted.
• Buccinator (C4) is attached opposite the three molar teeth, at the back reaching the pterygomandibular raphe (C10).
• Genioglossus (B14) is attached to the upper mental spine and geniohyoid (B13) to the lower.
• Mylohyoid (11) is attached to the mylohyoid line.

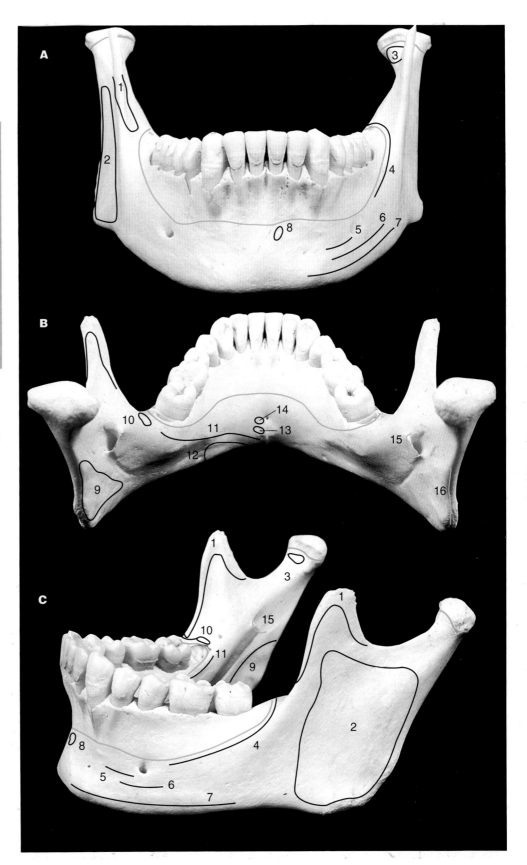

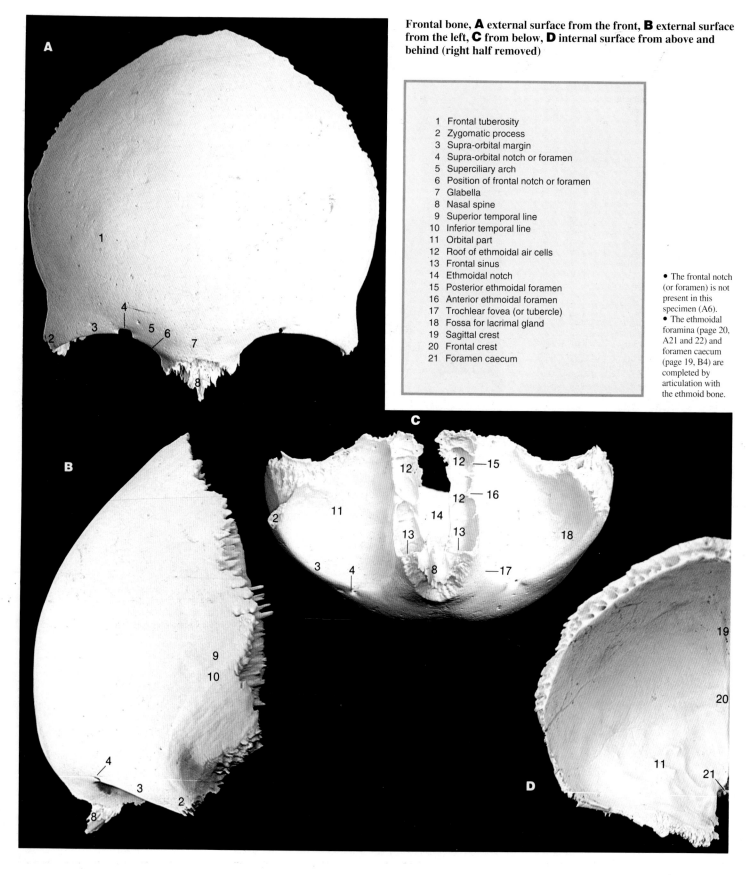

Frontal bone, A external surface from the front, **B** external surface from the left, **C** from below, **D** internal surface from above and behind (right half removed)

1 Frontal tuberosity
2 Zygomatic process
3 Supra-orbital margin
4 Supra-orbital notch or foramen
5 Superciliary arch
6 Position of frontal notch or foramen
7 Glabella
8 Nasal spine
9 Superior temporal line
10 Inferior temporal line
11 Orbital part
12 Roof of ethmoidal air cells
13 Frontal sinus
14 Ethmoidal notch
15 Posterior ethmoidal foramen
16 Anterior ethmoidal foramen
17 Trochlear fovea (or tubercle)
18 Fossa for lacrimal gland
19 Sagittal crest
20 Frontal crest
21 Foramen caecum

● The frontal notch (or foramen) is not present in this specimen (A6).
● The ethmoidal foramina (page 20, A21 and 22) and foramen caecum (page 19, B4) are completed by articulation with the ethmoid bone.

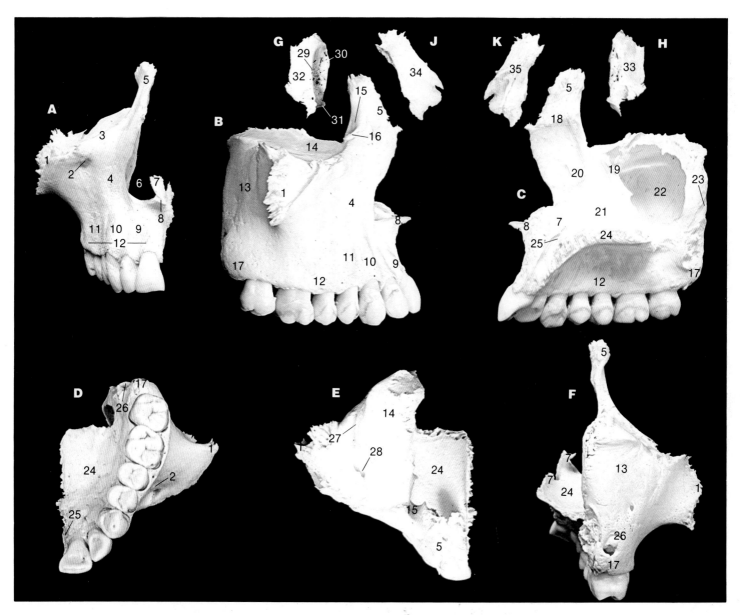

Right maxilla, **A** from the front, **B** from the lateral side, **C** from the medial side, **D** from below, **E** from above, **F** from behind

Right lacrimal bone, **G** from the lateral side, **H** from the medial side

Right nasal bone, **J** from the lateral side, **K** from the medial side

1 Zygomatic process	15 Lacrimal groove
2 Infra-orbital foramen	16 Anterior lacrimal crest
3 Infra-orbital margin	17 Tuberosity
4 Anterior surface	18 Ethmoidal crest
5 Frontal process	19 Middle meatus
6 Nasal notch	20 Conchal crest
7 Nasal crest	21 Inferior meatus
8 Anterior nasal spine	22 Maxillary hiatus and sinus
9 Incisive fossa	23 Greater palatine canal
10 Canine eminence	24 Palatine process
11 Canine fossa	25 Incisive canal
12 Alveolar process	26 Unerupted third molar tooth
13 Infratemporal surface	27 Infra-orbital groove
14 Orbital surface	28 Infra-orbital canal

29 Posterior lacrimal crest	32 Orbital surface
30 Lacrimal groove	33 Nasal surface
31 Lacrimal hamulus	

34 Lateral surface and vascular foramen
35 Internal surface and groove for anterior ethmoidal nerve

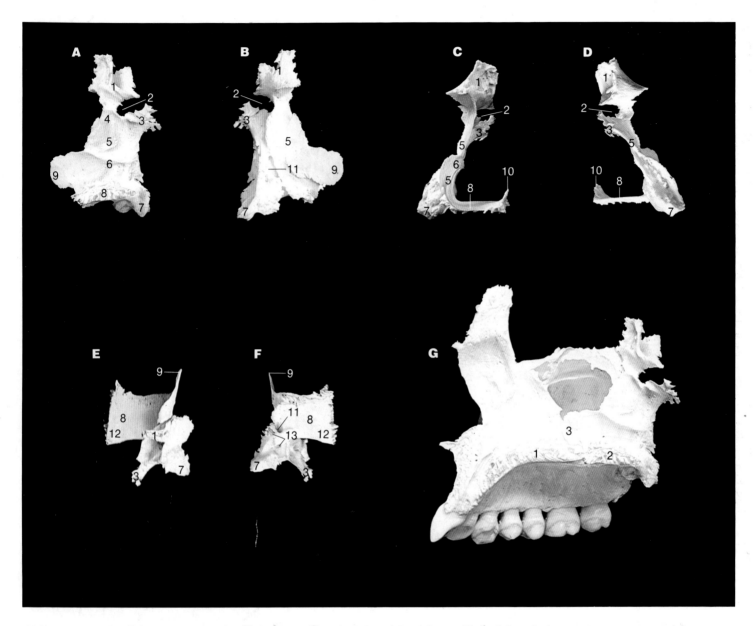

Right palatine bone, **A** from the medial side, **B** from the lateral side, **C** from the front, **D** from behind, **E** from above, **F** from below

G Articulation of the right maxilla and the palatine bone, from the medial side

1 Orbital process
2 Sphenopalatine notch
3 Sphenoidal process
4 Ethmoidal crest
5 Perpendicular plate
6 Conchal crest
7 Pyramidal process
· 8 Horizontal plate
9 Maxillary process
10 Nasal crest
11 Greater palatine groove
12 Posterior nasal spine
13 Lesser palatine canals

1 Palatine process of maxilla
2 Horizontal plate ⎱
3 Maxillary process ⎰ of palatine

● Compare G with C on page 29.

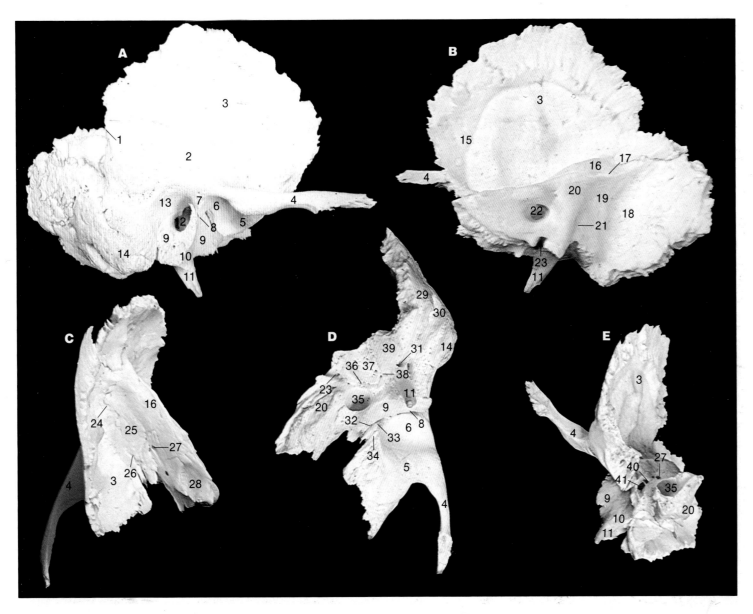

Right temporal bone, A external aspect, **B** internal aspect, **C** from above, **D** from below, **E** from the front

1	Parietal notch	16	Arcuate eminence
2	Groove for middle temporal artery	17	Groove for superior petrosal sinus
3	Squamous part	18	Groove for sigmoid sinus
4	Zygomatic process	19	Subarcuate fossa
5	Articular tubercle	20	Petrous part
6	Mandibular fossa	21	Aqueduct of vestibule
7	Postglenoid tubercle	22	Internal acoustic meatus
8	Squamotympanic fissure	23	Cochlear canaliculus
9	Tympanic part	24	Petrosquamous fissure (from above)
10	Sheath of styloid process	25	Tegmen tympani
11	Styloid process	26	Hiatus and groove for lesser petrosal nerve
12	External acoustic meatus	27	Hiatus and groove for greater petrosal nerve
13	Suprameatal triangle	28	Trigeminal impression on apex of petrous part
14	Mastoid process	29	Occipital groove
15	Grooves for branches of middle meningeal vessels	30	Mastoid notch

31	Stylomastoid foramen
32	Petrotympanic fissure
33	Edge of tegmen tympani
34	Petrosquamous fissure (from below)
35	Carotid canal
36	Canaliculus for tympanic branch of glossopharyngeal nerve
37	Jugular fossa
38	Mastoid canaliculus for auricular branch of vagus nerve
39	Jugular surface
40	Canal for tensor tympani
41	Auditory tube

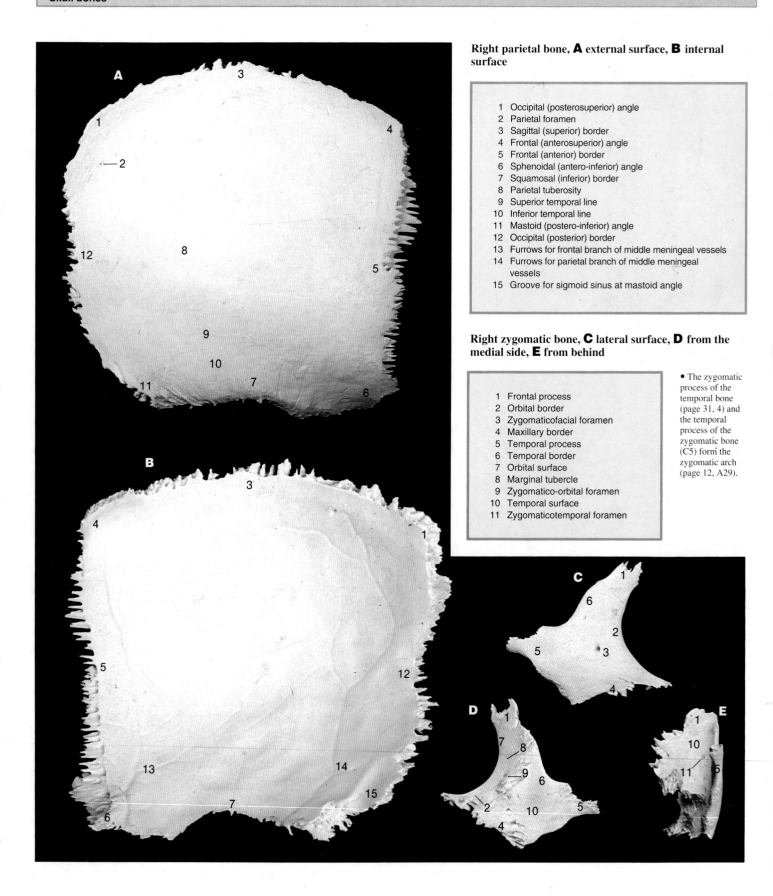

Right parietal bone, A external surface, B internal surface

1 Occipital (posterosuperior) angle
2 Parietal foramen
3 Sagittal (superior) border
4 Frontal (anterosuperior) angle
5 Frontal (anterior) border
6 Sphenoidal (antero-inferior) angle
7 Squamosal (inferior) border
8 Parietal tuberosity
9 Superior temporal line
10 Inferior temporal line
11 Mastoid (postero-inferior) angle
12 Occipital (posterior) border
13 Furrows for frontal branch of middle meningeal vessels
14 Furrows for parietal branch of middle meningeal vessels
15 Groove for sigmoid sinus at mastoid angle

Right zygomatic bone, C lateral surface, D from the medial side, E from behind

1 Frontal process
2 Orbital border
3 Zygomaticofacial foramen
4 Maxillary border
5 Temporal process
6 Temporal border
7 Orbital surface
8 Marginal tubercle
9 Zygomatico-orbital foramen
10 Temporal surface
11 Zygomaticotemporal foramen

• The zygomatic process of the temporal bone (page 31, 4) and the temporal process of the zygomatic bone (C5) forni the zygomatic arch (page 12, A29).

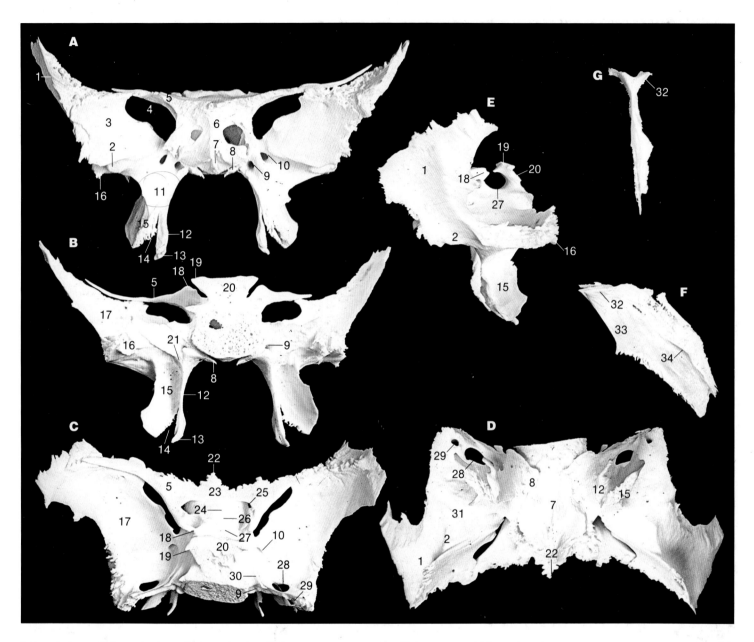

Sphenoid bone, **A** from the front, **B** from behind, **C** from above and behind, **D** from below, **E** from the left.
Vomer, **F** from the right, **G** from behind

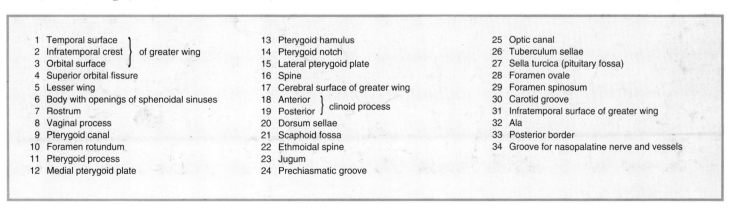

1	Temporal surface	} of greater wing	13	Pterygoid hamulus	25	Optic canal
2	Infratemporal crest		14	Pterygoid notch	26	Tuberculum sellae
3	Orbital surface		15	Lateral pterygoid plate	27	Sella turcica (pituitary fossa)
4	Superior orbital fissure		16	Spine	28	Foramen ovale
5	Lesser wing		17	Cerebral surface of greater wing	29	Foramen spinosum
6	Body with openings of sphenoidal sinuses		18	Anterior	} clinoid process	30	Carotid groove
7	Rostrum		19	Posterior		31	Infratemporal surface of greater wing
8	Vaginal process		20	Dorsum sellae		32	Ala
9	Pterygoid canal		21	Scaphoid fossa		33	Posterior border
10	Foramen rotundum		22	Ethmoidal spine		34	Groove for nasopalatine nerve and vessels
11	Pterygoid process		23	Jugum			
12	Medial pterygoid plate		24	Prechiasmatic groove			

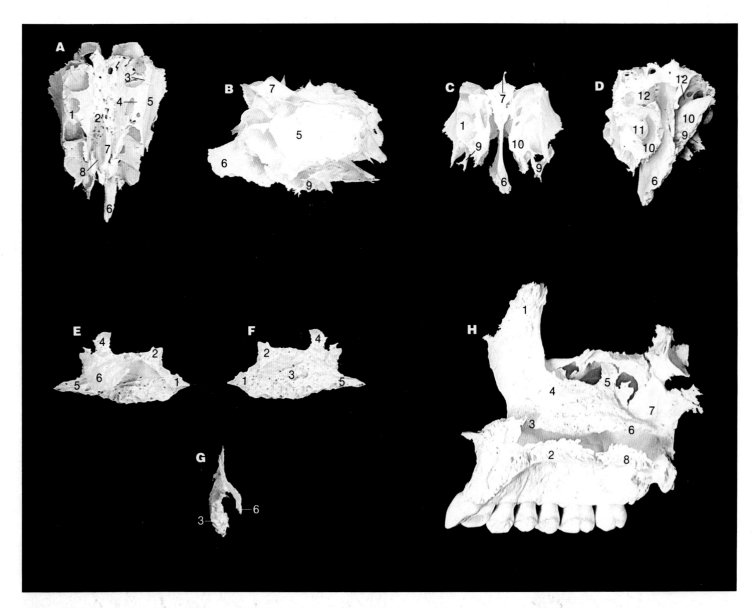

Ethmoid bone, **A** from above, **B** from the left, **C** from the front, **D** from the left, below and behind

Right inferior nasal concha, **E** from the lateral side, **F** from the medial side, **G** from behind

H Articulation of right maxilla, palatine bone and inferior nasal concha, from the medial side

1	Ethmoidal labyrinth (containing ethmoidal air cells)
2	Cribriform plate
3	Posterior ⎫
4	Anterior ⎬ ethmoidal groove
5	Orbital plate
6	Perpendicular plate
7	Crista galli
8	Ala of crista galli
9	Uncinate process
10	Middle nasal concha
11	Ethmoidal bulla
12	Superior nasal concha

1	Anterior end
2	Lacrimal process
3	Medial surface
4	Ethmoidal process
5	Posterior end
6	Maxillary process

1	Frontal process ⎫
2	Palatine process ⎬ of maxilla
3	Anterior end ⎫
4	Lacrimal process ⎪ of inferior nasal
5	Ethmoidal process ⎬ concha
6	Posterior end ⎪
7	Perpendicular ⎫ plate of palatine
8	Horiz... ⎬

• Compare with G on page 30 and C on page 29.

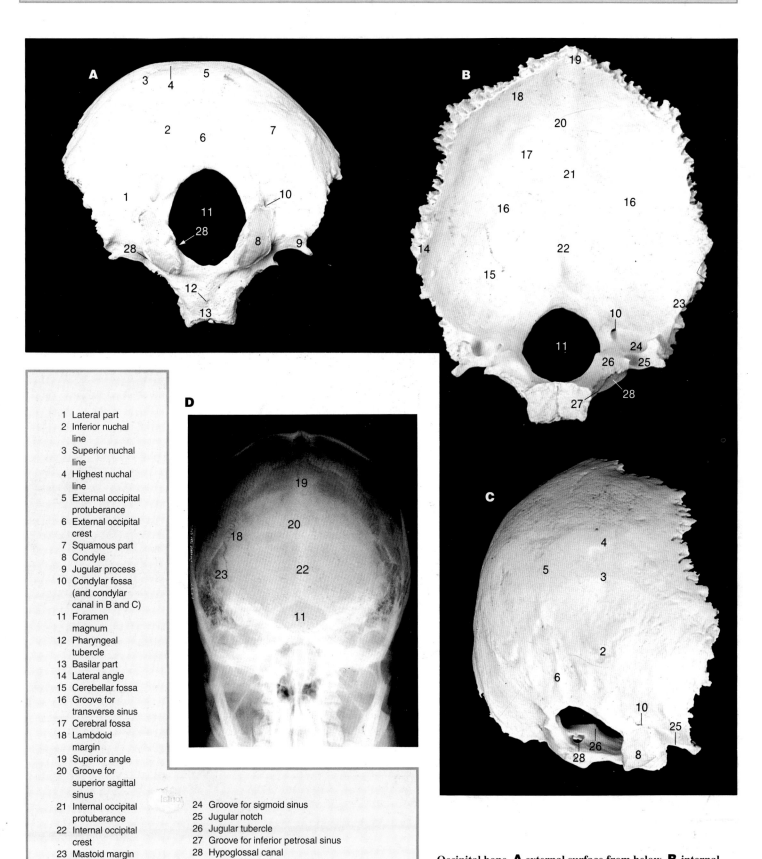

1 Lateral part
2 Inferior nuchal line
3 Superior nuchal line
4 Highest nuchal line
5 External occipital protuberance
6 External occipital crest
7 Squamous part
8 Condyle
9 Jugular process
10 Condylar fossa (and condylar canal in B and C)
11 Foramen magnum
12 Pharyngeal tubercle
13 Basilar part
14 Lateral angle
15 Cerebellar fossa
16 Groove for transverse sinus
17 Cerebral fossa
18 Lambdoid margin
19 Superior angle
20 Groove for superior sagittal sinus
21 Internal occipital protuberance
22 Internal occipital crest
23 Mastoid margin
24 Groove for sigmoid sinus
25 Jugular notch
26 Jugular tubercle
27 Groove for inferior petrosal sinus
28 Hypoglossal canal

Occipital bone, **A** external surface from below, **B** internal surface, **C** external surface from the right and below. **D** radiograph of the skull, fronto-occipital projection (Townes')

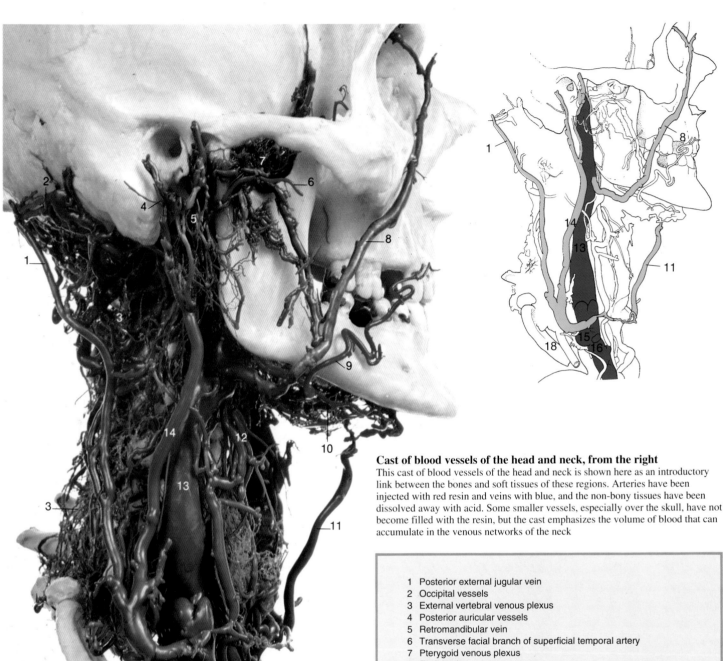

Cast of blood vessels of the head and neck, from the right

This cast of blood vessels of the head and neck is shown here as an introductory link between the bones and soft tissues of these regions. Arteries have been injected with red resin and veins with blue, and the non-bony tissues have been dissolved away with acid. Some smaller vessels, especially over the skull, have not become filled with the resin, but the cast emphasizes the volume of blood that can accumulate in the venous networks of the neck

• Over the body of the mandible, the (tortuous) facial artery (9) lies in front of the (straight) facial vein (8).

1 Posterior external jugular vein
2 Occipital vessels
3 External vertebral venous plexus
4 Posterior auricular vessels
5 Retromandibular vein
6 Transverse facial branch of superficial temporal artery
7 Pterygoid venous plexus
8 Facial vein
9 Facial artery
10 Submental artery
11 Anterior jugular vein
12 Superior thyroid vessels
13 Internal jugular vein
14 External jugular vein
15 Subclavian vein
16 Brachiocephalic vein
17 Subclavian artery
18 First rib
19 Internal thoracic artery

Face. Surface markings on the front and left side

Compare many of the features noted here with the dissection on page 38. Details of the eye are given on page 62, and of the ear on page 65. For surface markings of the neck see page 45

- The external apertures of the nose (7, the nares) are commonly called the nostrils.
- The inner end of the eyebrow overlies the supra-orbital margin (as at 9 and 10) but the outer end lies above the margin (11).
- The pulsation of the superficial temporal artery (17) is palpable in front of the tragus of the ear (18).
- The parotid duct (19 and 20) lies under the middle third of a line drawn from the tragus of the ear (18) to the midpoint of the philtrum (27).
- The pulsation of the facial artery (23) is palpable where the vessel crosses the lower border of the mandible at the anterior margin of the masseter muscle, about 2.5 cm (1 in) in front of the angle of the mandible (21).
- The infra-orbital foramen (14) is about 0.5 cm below the infra-orbital margin (13).

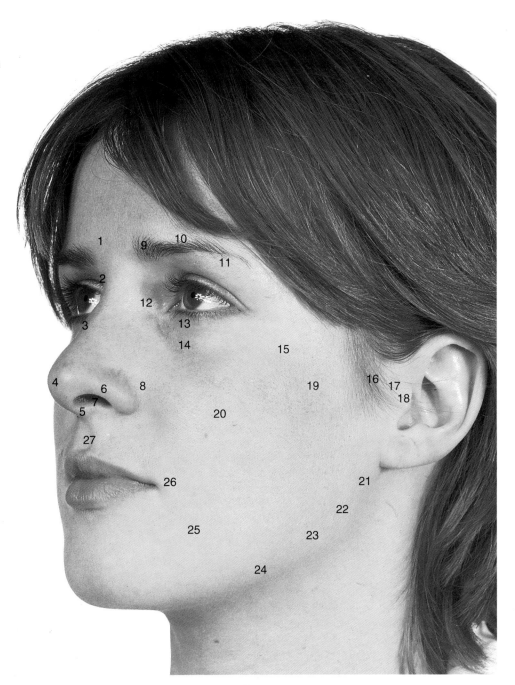

1 Glabella	11 Lateral part of supra-orbital margin	20 Parotid duct turning medially at anterior border of masseter
2 Root	12 Medial palpebral ligament in front of lacrimal sac	21 Angle of mandible
3 Dorsum	13 Infra-orbital margin	22 Lower border of ramus of mandible
4 Apex	14 Infra-orbital foramen, nerve and vessels	23 Anterior border of masseter and facial artery and vein
5 Septum ⎫ of external nose	15 Zygomatic arch	24 Lower border of body of mandible
6 Ala ⎬	16 Head of mandible	25 Mental foramen, nerve and vessels
7 External aperture ⎭	17 Auriculotemporal nerve and superficial temporal vessels	26 Lateral angle of mouth
8 Alar groove	18 Tragus	27 Philtrum
9 Frontal notch and supratrochlear nerve and vessels	19 Parotid duct emerging from gland	
10 Supra-orbital notch (or foramen), nerve and vessels		

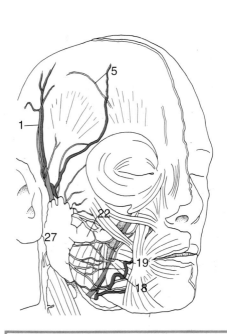

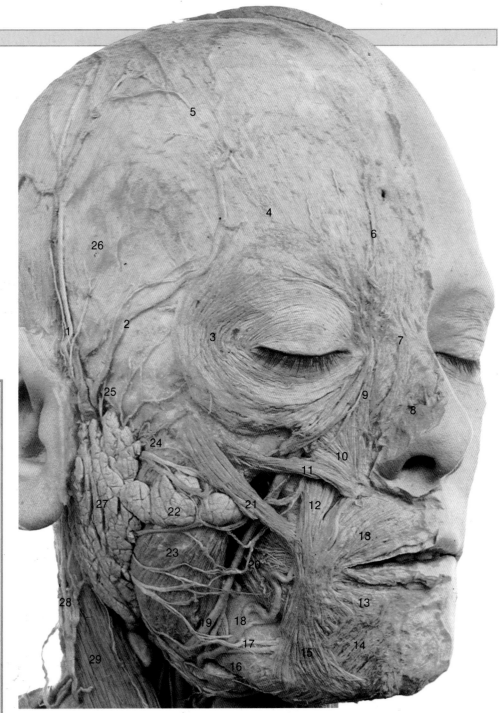

1 Auriculotemporal nerve and superficial temporal vessels
2 Anterior branch of superficial temporal artery
3 Orbicularis oculi
4 Frontalis part of occipitofrontalis
5 Supra-orbital nerve
6 Supratrochlear nerve
7 Procerus
8 Nasalis
9 Levator labii superioris alaeque nasi
10 Levator labii superioris
11 Zygomaticus minor
12 Levator anguli oris
13 Orbicularis oris
14 Depressor labii inferioris
15 Depressor anguli oris
16 Body of mandible
17 Marginal mandibular branch of facial nerve
18 Facial artery
19 Facial vein
20 Buccinator and buccal branches of facial nerve
21 Zygomaticus major
22 Accessory parotid gland overlying parotid duct
23 Masseter
24 Zygomatic ⎱ branches of facial nerve
25 Temporal ⎰
26 Temporalis underlying temporal fascia
27 Parotid gland
28 Great auricular nerve
29 Sternocleidomastoid

Face. Superficial dissection, from the front and the right

The facial muscles are displayed but the platysma, which extends from the mandible into the neck, has been removed with the skin. The largest facial muscles are orbicularis oculi (3), orbicularis oris (13) and buccinator (20). The facial artery and vein (18 and 19) pass from the neck on to the face at the lower anterior angle of the masseter muscle (23), and branches of the facial nerve (25, 24, 20 and 17) fan out from below the anterior margin of the parotid gland (27). This gland has an unusually large accessory part (22) which extends forwards over the masseter and obscures the parotid duct (which can be seen on page 39, A15)

● The facial artery (18) is tortuous and lies anterior to the facial vein (19) which is straight. Both vessels pass deep to the zygomaticus muscles (21 and 11).
● The facial expression group of muscles, which includes those of the mouth, eyelids, nose and scalp (except the occipitalis part of occipitofrontalis) (see Appendix, page 338), is supplied by the facial nerve.
● The muscles of mastication, which include masseter (23), temporalis (26) and the medial and lateral pterygoids, are supplied by the mandibular branch of the trigeminal nerve.

Right lower face and upper neck, A parotid and upper cervical regions, B submandibular region

All fascia has been removed, together with part of platysma in A and the whole of it in B. In A the various branches of the facial nerve (see note) emerge from beneath the anterior border of the parotid gland (11). The parotid duct (15) crosses the masseter muscle (16) before piercing the buccinator (18), and a large accessory parotid gland (14) lies just above the duct. In B the facial vein (17) has formed a plexus as it crosses the lower border of the mandible and overlies the submandibular gland (31). The facial artery (19) has been deep to the gland and appears at its upper border to run on to the face in front of the vein. On the face the facial vessels are superficial to buccinator (18) but deep to other facial muscles such as zygomaticus major (20)

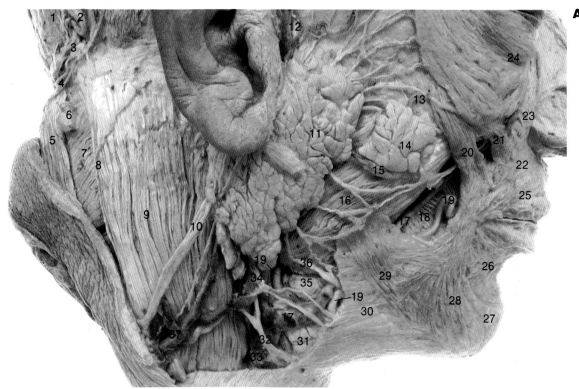

A

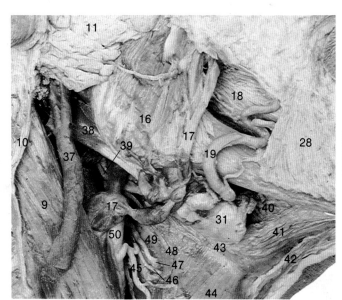

B

FRONT

1 Occipitalis part of occipitofrontalis	25 Orbicularis oris
2 Occipital artery	26 Depressor labii inferioris
3 Greater occipital nerve	27 Mentalis
4 Third occipital nerve	28 Depressor anguli oris
5 Trapezius	29 Risorius (aberrant)
6 An occipital lymph node	30 Platysma
7 Splenius capitis	31 Submandibular gland
8 Lesser occipital nerve	32 Transverse cervical nerve
9 Sternocleidomastoid	33 Internal jugular vein
10 Great auricular nerve	34 Cervical branch of facial nerve
11 Parotid gland and facial nerve branches at anterior border	35 Submandibular lymph nodes
12 Superficial temporal vessels and auriculotemporal nerve	36 Marginal mandibular branch of facial nerve
13 Transverse facial vessels	37 External jugular vein
14 Accessory parotid gland	38 Posterior belly of digastric
15 Parotid duct	39 Hypoglossal nerve
16 Masseter	40 Mylohyoid
17 Facial vein	41 Anterior belly of digastric
18 Buccinator	42 Anterior jugular vein
19 Facial artery	43 Greater horn of hyoid bone
20 Zygomaticus major	44 Superior belly of omohyoid
21 Zygomaticus minor	45 Superior thyroid artery
22 Levator labii superioris	46 Superior laryngeal artery
23 Levator labii superioris alaeque nasi	47 Internal laryngeal nerve
24 Orbicularis oculi	48 Thyrohyoid
	49 Thyrohyoid membrane
	50 External carotid artery

• The risorius muscle (29) has no bony attachment. It normally passes from the parotid fascia to the skin at the angle of the mouth, but is at a lower level in this specimen.
• The five branches of the facial nerve on the face fan out from below the anterior border of the parotid gland (A11). The first three are usually multiple. Several temporal and zygomatic branches are seen between labels A12 and 13. Buccal branches overlie the masseter muscle (A16), and the marginal mandibular and cervical branches are separately labelled (A36 and 34).
• The marginal mandibular branch (A36) of the facial nerve sometimes runs just below the lower border of the mandible for part of its course instead of just above it, and so may overlie the submandibular gland (B31).
• Embedded within the parotid gland are the facial nerve (A11), the retromandibular vein, the external carotid artery and its terminal branches (maxillary and superficial temporal, page 40, B35, 9 and 24), filaments from the auriculotemporal nerve (A12) which convey to the gland secretomotor fibres from the otic ganglion (page 53, E29), and lymph nodes.

39

A

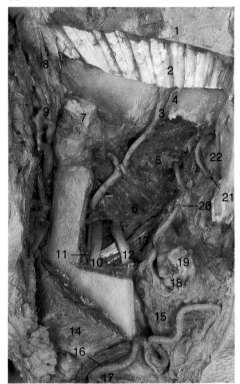

B

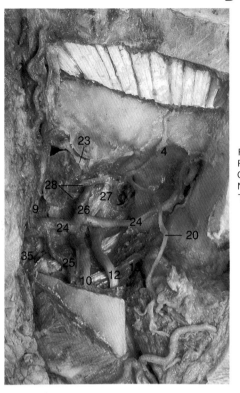

Right infratemporal fossa, A with the pterygoid muscles intact, B after removal of the lateral pterygoid, C after removal of the lateral and medial pterygoids

In A the zygomatic arch and the lower part of the temporalis muscle (2) with the coronoid process and part of the ramus of the mandible have been removed to display the two pterygoid muscles (5 and 6, 13), with the inferior alveolar and lingual nerves (10 and 12) emerging between the lateral and medial pterygoids, and more anteriorly the buccal nerve (20) emerging between the two heads of the lateral pterygoid (5 and 6). In B, removal of the lateral pterygoid reveals the maxillary artery (24) and two of its largest branches—the inferior alveolar (25) passing downwards to the mandibular foramen and the middle meningeal (26) passing upwards between the roots of the auriculotemporal nerve (28) to the foramen spinosum. In C (a different specimen from A and B) both pterygoid muscles and the mandible have been removed to show the lateral pterygoid plate (29), with tensor veli palatini (30) behind it and the chorda tympani (32) joining the lingual nerve (12) superficial to the muscle. The styloid process (36) is also seen with its three attached muscles—stylohyoid (37), styloglossus (40) and stylopharyngeus (41)

C

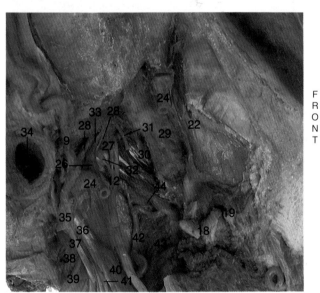

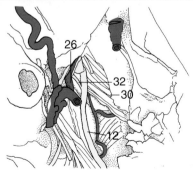

1	Temporal fascia	23	Articular disc
2	Temporalis	24	Maxillary artery
3	Deep temporal artery	25	Inferior alveolar artery
4	Deep temporal nerve	26	Middle meningeal artery
5	Upper head ⎫ of lateral	27	Mandibular nerve
6	Lower head ⎭ pterygoid	28	Roots of auriculotemporal nerve
7	Capsule of temporomandibular joint	29	Lateral pterygoid plate
8	Auriculotemporal nerve	30	Tensor veli palatini
9	Superficial temporal artery	31	Nerve to medial pterygoid
10	Inferior alveolar nerve	32	Chorda tympani
11	Nerve to mylohyoid	33	Accessory meningeal artery
12	Lingual nerve	34	External acoustic meatus
13	Medial pterygoid	35	External carotid artery
14	Masseter	36	Styloid process
15	Buccinator	37	Stylohyoid
16	Facial vein	38	Internal jugular vein
17	Facial artery	39	Accessory nerve
18	Molar glands	40	Styloglossus
19	Parotid duct	41	Stylopharyngeus and glosso-pharyngeal nerve
20	Buccal nerve	42	Ascending pharyngeal artery
21	Posterior superior alveolar artery	43	Superior constrictor of pharynx
22	Infratemporal surface of maxilla	44	Levator veli palatini

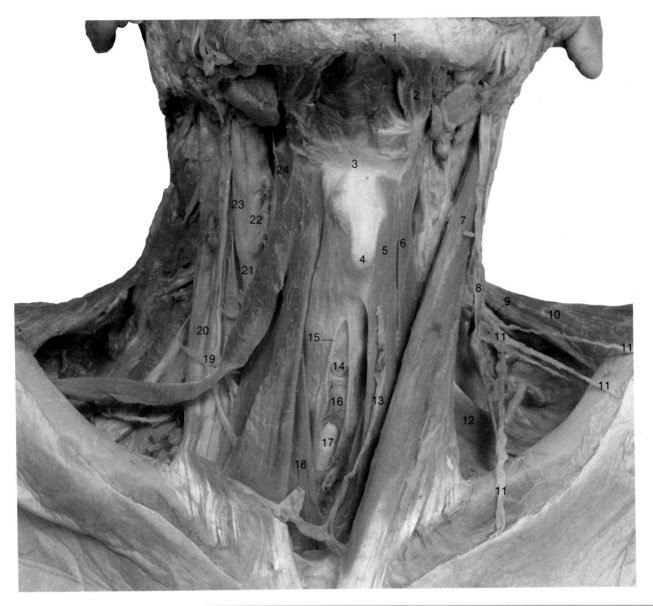

Front of the neck. Superficial dissection
The right sternocleidomastoid, carotid sheath and the investing layer of deep cervical fascia have been removed. The pretracheal fascia (15) is being incised to show the isthmus of the thyroid gland (16)

1	Lower border of mandible	13	Anterior jugular vein
2	Anterior belly of digastric	14	Arch of cricoid cartilage
3	Hyoid bone	15	Pretracheal fascia (cut edge)
4	Laryngeal prominence (Adam's apple)	16	Isthmus of thyroid gland
5	Sternohyoid	17	Trachea
6	Superior belly of omohyoid	18	Sternothyroid
7	Sternocleidomastoid	19	Ansa cervicalis
8	External jugular vein	20	Internal jugular vein
9	Accessory nerve	21	Common carotid artery
10	Trapezius	22	External carotid artery
11	Supraclavicular nerve	23	Internal carotid artery
12	Inferior belly of omohyoid	24	Thyrohyoid

• Midline landmarks in the neck include the body of the hyoid bone (3), the laryngeal prominence (Adam's apple, 4), the arch of the cricoid cartilage (14) and the trachea (17). Many of the features shown here can be seen again when looking at the neck from the side (pages 43 to 47).
• Sternocleidomastoid (7) completely overlaps the internal jugular vein (20) but the bifurcation of the common carotid artery (21) into the internal and external carotids (23 and 22) is just in front of the anterior border of the muscle (between labels 6 and 7, where the connective tissue of the carotid sheath is intact; on the other side the sheath has been removed).
• The site for feeling the carotid pulse (pulsation of the common carotid artery) is in the lower front part of the neck, between the anterior border of sternocleidomastoid and the side of the larynx, as indicated on page 45, B12. In this specimen the bifurcation of the common carotid is lower than usual; it is often level with the hyoid bone (3).
• Sternohyoid (5) and the superior belly of omohyoid (6) lie superficial to sternothyroid (18) and thyrohyoid (24).

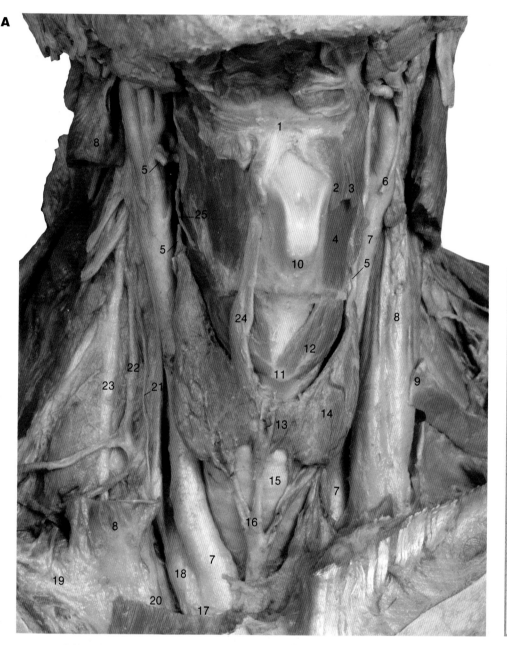

A Front of the neck. Superficial dissection
Most of both sternocleidomastoids, the right internal jugular vein (8) and part of the right clavicle have been removed. The lateral lobes of the thyroid gland (14) overlap the common carotid arteries (7), and a pyramidal lobe is present (24). The inferior thyroid veins (16) run down in front of the trachea (15). On the right side a segment of the superior thyroid artery (5) has been cut out to show the external laryngeal nerve (25) which runs down immediately behind the artery. On the left the artery has an unusually high origin

1	Body of hyoid bone
2	Sternohyoid
3	Superior belly of omohyoid
4	Thyrohyoid
5	Superior thyroid artery
6	Upper root of ansa cervicalis
7	Common carotid artery
8	Internal jugular vein
9	Tendon of omohyoid
10	Laryngeal prominence (Adam's apple)
11	Arch of cricoid cartilage
12	Cricothyroid
13	Isthmus of thyroid gland
14	Lateral lobe of thyroid gland
15	Trachea
16	Inferior thyroid veins
17	Brachiocephalic trunk
18	Subclavian artery
19	Subclavian vein
20	Right brachiocephalic vein
21	Carotid sheath (cut edge)
22	Ascending cervical artery
23	Phrenic nerve behind prevertebral fascia
24	Pyramidal lobe of thyroid gland
25	External laryngeal nerve

• The upper end of the brachiocephalic trunk (17) divides into the right common carotid and right subclavian arteries (7 and 18).
• The phrenic nerve (23) runs down over scalenus anterior under cover of the prevertebral fascia.
• The internal jugular vein (8) and the subclavian vein (19) unite (behind the sternoclavicular joint) to form the brachiocephalic vein (20).
• The tendon of omohyoid (9) is a guide to the underlying internal jugular vein (8).
• The pyramidal lobe of the thyroid gland (24) is more common on the left side than on the right, as here. It represents the remains of the thyroglossal duct from the pharynx, from which the gland develops. The duct may also form cysts or a fibrous cord; if muscle fibres are present in the latter they constitute the levator of the thyroid gland.
• Cricothyroid (12) is the only intrinsic muscle of the larynx to be seen on the outside of the larynx.
• For the back of the thyroid gland see page 54.

B Left side of the neck, from the left and front

In this superficial dissection, platysma and most of the investing layer of the deep cervical fascia have been removed. The accessory nerve (9) emerges from within the substance of sternocleidomastoid (2) to pass beneath the anterior border of trapezius (8). It must be distinguished from cervical nerves to trapezius (10) which emerge from behind sternocleidomastoid

1 Parotid gland
2 Sternocleidomastoid
3 External jugular vein
4 Great auricular nerve
5 Prevertebral fascia overlying levator
   scapulae
6 Lesser occipital nerve
7 Splenius capitis
8 Trapezius
9 Accessory nerve
10 Cervical nerves to trapezius
11 Superficial cervical vein
12 Branches of supraclavicular nerve
13 Clavicle
14 Anterior jugular vein
15 Investing layer of deep cervical fascia
16 Laryngeal prominence (Adam's apple)
17 Transverse cervical nerve
18 Submandibular gland
19 Lower border of mandible

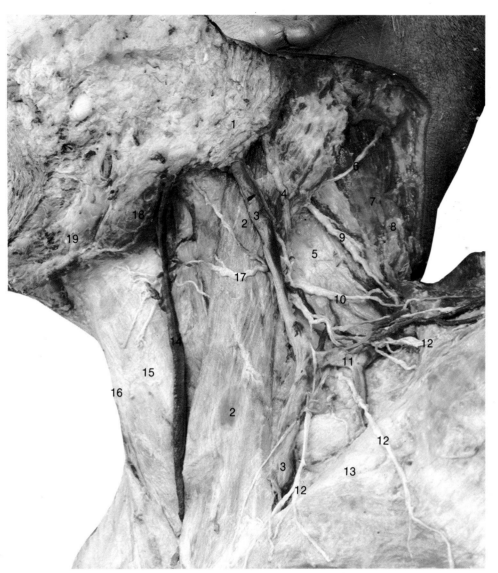

• The nerve commonly known in English as the accessory nerve (or spinal part of the accessory nerve) is in official anatomical nomenclature the ramus externus of the truncus nervi accessorii. The cells of origin are in the anterior horn of the upper five or six cervical segments of the spinal cord, and the fibres supply sternocleidomastoid and trapezius. (The cranial part of the accessory nerve, ramus internus of the truncus nervi accessorii, is derived from the nucleus ambiguus in the medulla oblongata and joins the vagus nerve to supply muscles of the soft palate and larynx.)
• The motor nerve supply of trapezius (8) is usually the accessory nerve (9), with the branches from the cervical plexus to the muscle (10) being afferent only, but in some cases the cervical branches do appear to be motor.
• The motor nerve supply of sternocleidomastoid (2) is the accessory nerve (9). The cervical branches to the muscle (10) are afferent.

A Left side of the neck, from the left and front

Platysma and the deep cervical fascia have been removed. The external jugular vein (14) crosses sternocleidomastoid (15) to pass behind the clavicle near the front corner of the posterior triangle and the brachial plexus (27), and the accessory nerve (18) emerges from the muscle to cross the posterior triangle and enter trapezius (19) about 5 cm above the clavicle. The common carotid artery (41) divides into the external and internal carotids (43 and 42) below the level of the greater horn of the hyoid bone (50), and at about this same level the internal laryngeal nerve (48) and the superior laryngeal artery (47) pierce the thyrohyoid membrane (49). The lower pole of the parotid gland (5) lies behind the angle of the mandible covered by masseter (1), and the submandibular gland (59) is below the mandible and crossed by the marginal mandibular branch of the facial nerve (3)

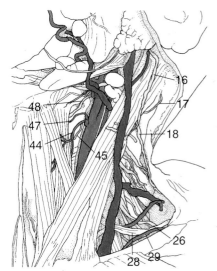

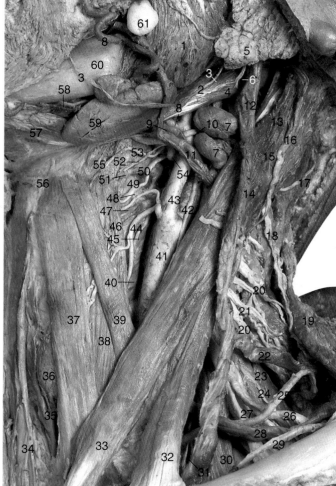

• The external jugular vein (14) is formed by the union of the posterior branch of the retromandibular vein (12) and the posterior auricular vein (13).
• The accessory nerve (18) emerges into the posterior triangle from within the substance of sternocleidomastoid (15); the cervical nerves to trapezius (20) and other cervical plexus branches emerge from behind the muscle.
• The dorsal scapular nerve (24) emerges from scalenus medius (23); the suprascapular nerve (26) is a larger nerve arising from the upper trunk of the brachial plexus (27).
• The suprascapular artery (29) runs across the lowest part of the posterior triangle (often behind the clavicle) at a lower level than the superficial cervical artery (25).
• The internal laryngeal nerve (48) and the superior laryngeal artery (47, a branch of the superior thyroid) pierce the thyrohyoid membrane (49) to enter the larynx.
• Sternohyoid (37) and the superior belly of omohyoid (39) overlie sternothyroid (38) and thyrohyoid (46).
• In 20 per cent of faces, as in this specimen, the marginal mandibular branch of the facial nerve (3) arches downwards off the face for part of its course and overlies the submandibular gland (59).

1 Masseter	23 Scalenus medius	44 Superior thyroid artery
2 Stylohyoid	24 Dorsal scapular nerve	45 External laryngeal nerve
3 Marginal mandibular branch of facial nerve	25 Superficial cervical artery	46 Thyrohyoid
4 Posterior belly of digastric	26 Suprascapular nerve	47 Superior laryngeal artery
5 Parotid gland	27 Upper trunk of brachial plexus	48 Internal laryngeal nerve
6 Cervical branch of facial nerve	28 Inferior belly of omohyoid	49 Thyrohyoid membrane
7 Jugulodigastric lymph nodes	29 Suprascapular artery	50 Greater horn of hyoid bone
8 Facial artery	30 Scalenus anterior	51 Nerve to thyrohyoid
9 Lingual vein	31 Phrenic nerve	52 Hyoglossus
10 Hypoglossal nerve	32 Clavicular head } of sternocleidomastoid	53 Suprahyoid artery
11 Facial vein	33 Sternal head	54 Lingual artery
12 Posterior branch of retromandibular vein	34 Anterior jugular vein	55 Mylohyoid
13 Posterior auricular vein	35 Inferior thyroid vein	56 Body of hyoid bone
14 External jugular vein	36 Thyroid gland	57 Anterior belly of digastric
15 Sternocleidomastoid	37 Sternohyoid	58 Submental artery and vein
16 Great auricular nerve	38 Sternothyroid	59 Submandibular gland
17 Lesser occipital nerve	39 Superior belly of omohyoid	60 Body of mandible
18 Accessory nerve	40 Inferior constrictor of pharynx	61 Buccal fat pad
19 Trapezius	41 Common carotid artery	
20 Cervical nerves to trapezius	42 Internal carotid artery and superior root of ansa cervicalis	
21 Supraclavicular nerve (cut upper edge)		
22 Superficial cervical vein	43 External carotid artery	

B Neck. Surface markings of the front and right side
Compare many of the features noted here with the dissection opposite, and with those on pages 41 to 43

B

1 Mastoid process
2 Tip of transverse process of atlas
3 Sternocleidomastoid
4 External jugular vein
5 Lowest part of parotid gland
6 Angle of mandible
7 Anterior border of masseter and facial artery
8 Submandibular gland
9 Tip of greater horn of hyoid bone
10 Hypoglossal nerve
11 Internal laryngeal nerve
12 Site for palpation of common carotid artery
13 Anterior jugular vein
14 Body of hyoid bone
15 Laryngeal prominence (Adam's apple)
16 Vocal fold
17 Arch of cricoid cartilage
18 Isthmus of thyroid gland
19 Jugular notch and trachea
20 Sternal head } of sterno-
21 Clavicular head } cleidomastoid
22 Sternoclavicular joint and union of internal jugular and subclavian veins to form brachiocephalic vein
23 Clavicle
24 Pectoralis major
25 Infraclavicular fossa and cephalic vein
26 Deltoid
27 Inferior belly of omohyoid
28 Upper trunk of brachial plexus
29 Accessory nerve passing under anterior border of trapezius
30 Accessory nerve emerging from sternocleidomastoid

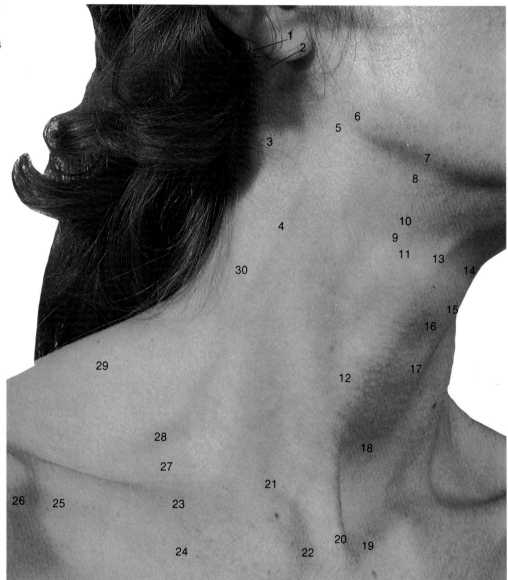

- The accessory nerve (A18) emerges from the posterior border of sternocleidomastoid (B30) at about the junction of the upper and middle thirds of the muscle and crosses the posterior triangle to pass beneath the anterior border of trapezius (A19, B29) at a point 5 cm (2 in) above the clavicle (B23).
- The hypoglossal nerve (A10, B10) curves forwards just above the tip of the greater horn of the hyoid bone (A50, B9), and the internal laryngeal nerve (A48, B11) runs downwards and forwards just below it.
- The pulsation of the common carotid artery (A41, B12) can be felt by backward pressure in the angle between the lower anterior border of sternocleidomastoid and the side of the larynx and trachea.
- The cricoid cartilage (B17) is about 5 cm (2 in) above the

jugular notch of the manubrium of the sternum (B19).
- The lower end of the internal jugular vein lies behind the interval between the sternal (B20) and clavicular (B21) heads of sternocleidomastoid (when viewed from the front), just above the point where it joins the subclavian vein to form the brachiocephalic vein (B22).
- The external jugular vein (A14, B4) passes obliquely downwards and backwards over the upper part of sternocleidomastoid (B3), and then crosses the posterior triangle to enter the subclavian vein below and behind the clavicle (near the label B23).
- The uppermost part of the brachial plexus (A27, B28) can be felt as a cord-like structure in the lower part of the posterior triangle.

A Right side of the neck. Deep dissection

Parts of the mandible, the parotid and submandibular glands, mylohyoid and sternocleidomastoid have been removed. Key features of this dissection are the posterior belly of digastric (64) and the posterior border of hyoglossus (18). For further dissection of this specimen see opposite

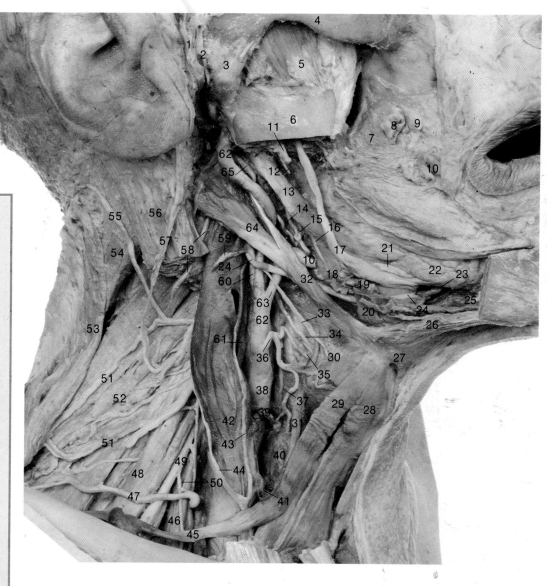

1 Auriculotemporal nerve
2 Superficial temporal artery
3 Capsule of temporomandibular joint
4 Zygomatic arch
5 Temporalis
6 Ramus of mandible
7 Buccinator
8 Molar glands
9 Parotid duct
10 Facial artery
11 Inferior alveolar nerve
12 Nerve to mylohyoid
13 Styloglossus
14 Glossopharyngeal nerve
15 Ascending palatine artery
16 Stylohyoid ligament
17 Lingual nerve
18 Hyoglossus
19 Deep part of submandibular gland
20 Mylohyoid and nerve
21 Submandibular duct
22 Sublingual gland
23 Deep lingual artery
24 Hypoglossal nerve
25 Geniohyoid
26 Anterior belly of digastric and nerve
27 Hyoid bone
28 Sternohyoid
29 Superior belly of omohyoid
30 Thyrohyoid and nerve
31 Sternothyroid
32 Stylohyoid
33 Thyrohyoid membrane
34 Internal laryngeal nerve
35 Superior laryngeal artery
36 Superior thyroid artery
37 External laryngeal nerve
38 Common carotid artery
39 Superior thyroid vein
40 Lateral lobe of thyroid gland
41 Middle thyroid vein
42 Internal jugular vein
43 Upper root ⎫ of ansa
44 Lower root ⎬ cervicalis
45 Inferior belly of omohyoid
46 Scalenus anterior
47 Superficial cervical artery
48 Scalenus medius

49 Ventral ramus of fifth cervical nerve
50 Roots of phrenic nerve
51 Cervical nerves to trapezius
52 Levator scapulae
53 Trapezius
54 Splenius capitis
55 Lesser occipital nerve
56 Sternocleidomastoid
57 Great auricular nerve
58 Accessory nerve
59 Sternocleidomastoid branch of occipital artery
60 Occipital artery
61 Vagus nerve
62 External carotid artery
63 Linguofacial trunk
64 Posterior belly of digastric
65 Posterior auricular artery

- The hypoglossal nerve (24) curls forwards round the sternocleido-mastoid branch (59) of the occipital artery (60) to run forwards into the tongue superficial to the hyoglossus (18) and deep to mylohyoid (20).
- The lingual nerve (17) lies superficial to hyoglossus (18) and at this level is a flattened band rather than a typical round nerve, with the deep part of the submandibular gland (19) below it. The nerve crosses underneath the submandibular duct (21), lying first lateral to the duct and then medial to it.
- Omohyoid (29, 45) is of little functional importance, but the tendon joining the two bellies (adjacent to the label 45) is a useful landmark in dissections and operations—it overlies the lower part of the internal jugular vein (42).
- The deep lingual artery (23) is the name given to the lingual artery distal to the anterior border of hyoglossus (18).
- The thyrohyoid membrane (33) is pierced by the internal laryngeal nerve (34) and the superior laryngeal artery (35).
- Apart from supplying muscles of the tongue, the hypoglossal nerve (24) gives branches to geniohyoid (25) and thyrohyoid (30) and forms the upper root of the ansa cervicalis (43). These three branches consist of the fibres from the first cervical nerve that have joined the hypoglossal nerve higher in the neck; they are not derived from the hypoglossal nucleus.

B

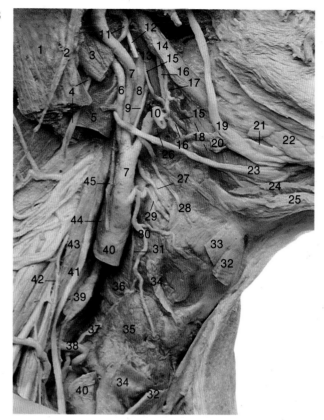
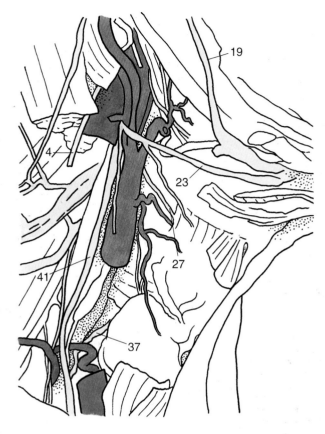

B Right side of the neck. Deep dissection

This dissection is similar to A on page 46 but after the removal of parts of the great vessels, posterior belly of digastric, stylohyoid and infrahyoid muscles. The lingual (26) and facial (10) branches of the external carotid artery (7) arise from a common trunk. The hypoglossal nerve (23) hooks forwards round the occipital artery (6), and the glossopharyngeal nerve (15) curls round stylopharyngeus (13)

1 Sternocleidomastoid	24 Mylohyoid
2 Great auricular nerve	25 Anterior belly of digastric
3 Posterior belly of digastric	26 Lingual artery
4 Accessory nerve	27 Internal laryngeal nerve
5 Internal jugular vein	28 Thyrohyoid and nerve
6 Occipital artery	29 Superior laryngeal artery
7 External carotid artery	30 Superior thyroid artery
8 Internal carotid artery	31 External laryngeal nerve
9 Ascending pharyngeal artery	32 Sternohyoid
10 Facial artery	33 Superior belly of omohyoid
11 Posterior auricular artery	34 Sternothyroid
12 Stylohyoid (cut end displaced medially)	35 Lateral lobe of thyroid gland
13 Stylopharyngeus	36 Inferior constrictor
14 Styloglossus	37 Recurrent laryngeal nerve
15 Glossopharyngeal nerve	38 Inferior thyroid artery
16 Stylohyoid ligament	39 Middle cervical sympathetic ganglion
17 Ascending palatine artery	40 Common carotid artery
18 Hyoglossus	41 Vagus nerve
19 Lingual nerve	42 Phrenic nerve
20 Submandibular ganglion	43 Scalenus anterior
21 Submandibular duct	44 Carotid sinus
22 Sublingual gland	45 Upper root of ansa cervicalis
23 Hypoglossal nerve	

- The glossopharyngeal nerve (15) passes downwards and forwards, curling round the lateral side of stylopharyngeus (13).
- The vagus nerve (41) runs straight downwards between the internal jugular vein (5) laterally and the internal (8) and common carotid (40) arteries medially.
- The accessory nerve (4) passes downwards and backwards behind the posterior belly of digastric (3) and (usually) in front of the internal jugular vein (5) before entering sternocleidomastoid (1).
- The hypoglossal nerve (23) passes forwards by hooking underneath the sternocleidomastoid branch of the occipital artery (6); this unlabelled branch overlies the cut end of the internal jugular vein (5).
- Lying superficial to hyoglossus (18) are, in order from above downwards, the lingual nerve (19) with the attached submandibular ganglion (20), the submandibular duct (21) and the hypoglossal nerve (23).
- Passing deep to the posterior border of hyoglossus (18), in order from above downwards, are the glossopharyngeal nerve (15), the stylohyoid ligament (16) and the lingual artery (26).
- The removal of parts of the sternohyoid (32), omohyoid (33) and sternothyroid (34) displays the lateral lobe of the thyroid gland (35). Note the inferior thyroid artery (38) behind the lower part of the lobe, with the recurrent laryngeal nerve (37) passing deep to this looping vessel to enter the pharynx beneath the inferior constrictor (36). The nerve may lie behind or in front of the artery or pass between branches of it.

A

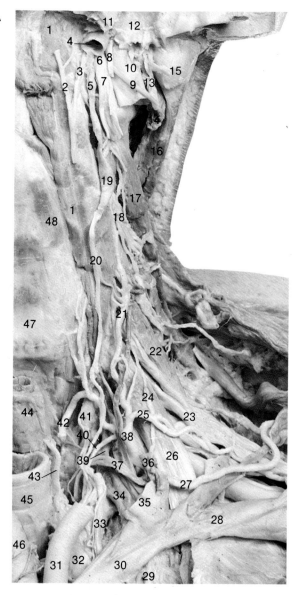

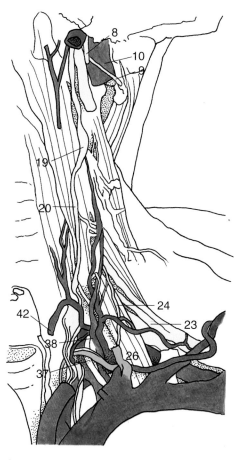

A Left prevertebral region

In this deep dissection of the left side of the neck seen from the front, the main muscles are longus capitis (1) and scalenus anterior (26). In the upper part of the specimen note the cut ends of the internal carotid artery (4) and internal jugular vein (10) with their associated nerves. In the lower part, the thyrocervical trunk (38) arises from the subclavian artery (32) medial to scalenus anterior (26), and the thoracic duct (37) enters the left side of the junction of the internal jugular vein (35) with the subclavian vein (28)

1 Longus capitis	17 Levator scapulae	34 Vertebral vein
2 Ascending pharyngeal artery	18 Ventral ramus of third cervical nerve	35 Internal jugular vein
3 Meningeal branch of ascending pharyngeal artery	19 Superior cervical ganglion	36 Jugular lymphatic trunk
4 Internal carotid artery	20 Sympathetic trunk	37 Thoracic duct
5 Internal carotid nerve	21 Ascending cervical artery and vein	38 Thyrocervical trunk
6 Vagus nerve	22 Scalenus medius	39 Vertebral artery
7 Inferior vagal ganglion	23 Upper trunk of brachial plexus	40 A large oesophageal branch of inferior thyroid artery
8 Glossopharyngeal nerve	24 Phrenic nerve	41 Middle cervical ganglion
9 Accessory nerve	25 Superficial cervical artery	42 Inferior thyroid artery
10 Internal jugular vein	26 Scalenus anterior	43 Recurrent laryngeal nerve
11 Spine of sphenoid bone	27 Suprascapular artery	44 Oesophagus
12 Tympanic part of temporal bone	28 Subclavian vein	45 Trachea
13 Occipital artery	29 Internal thoracic artery	46 Brachiocephalic trunk
14 Posterior belly of digastric	30 Left brachiocephalic vein	47 Anterior longitudinal ligament
15 Mastoid process	31 Left common carotid artery	48 Longus colli
16 Sternocleidomastoid	32 Left subclavian artery	
	33 Vagus nerve	

B Right trigeminal nerve branches, from the left

This dissection of right-sided structures (in a sagittal section of the head) is seen from the left side after removal of part of the base of the skull (mainly the petrous part of the temporal bone), so giving an unusual view of the medial or deep aspect of the ophthalmic (11), maxillary (12) and mandibular (13) branches of the trigeminal nerve (17) which are usually seen and dissected only from their lateral sides. Part of the medial pterygoid (30) has been cut away to show the lingual nerve (31) lying in front of the inferior alveolar nerve (32); compare with the lateral view of these structures on page 40, 10 and 12. In the mouth, where much of the tongue has been removed, the lingual nerve (31) is seen curling under the submandibular duct (44). The cut ends of the hypoglossal nerve (45) and lingual artery (37) are separated by hyoglossus (38)

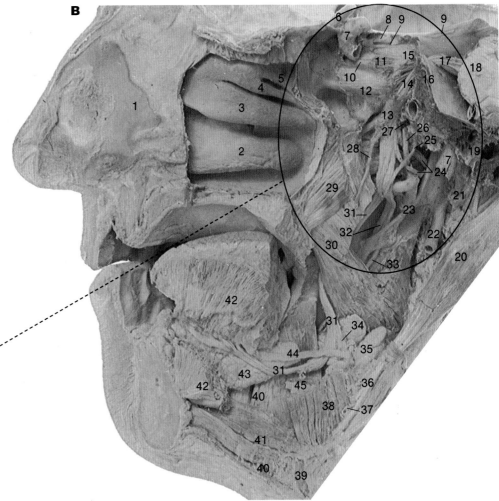

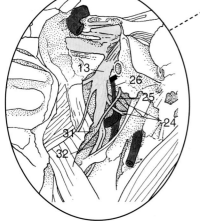

• The occasional supreme (highest) nasal concha (5) is present in this specimen.
• The chorda tympani (25) leaves the skull through the petrotympanic fissure and joins the posterior aspect of the lingual nerve (31) about 2 cm below the skull.
• The right cavernous sinus has been opened up from the medial side, so revealing from this aspect the nerves that lie in the sinus—the ophthalmic (11), maxillary (12), oculomotor (8), trochlear (9) and abducent (10).
• The lower end of the lingual nerve (31, in the mouth) is seen hooking under the submandibular duct (44), lying first lateral to the duct and then medial to it.
• The mandibular nerve (13) is labelled just after it has passed through the foramen ovale and where it divides into its various branches. Note the inferior alveolar nerve (32) entering the mandibular foramen after giving off the nerve to mylohyoid (33), with the lingual nerve (31) anterior to it and being joined by the chorda tympani (25).
• The middle meningeal artery (26) runs upwards between the two roots of the auriculotemporal nerve (24) to reach the foramen spinosum.

1	Nasal septum	24 Roots of auriculotemporal nerve
2	Inferior ⎫	25 Chorda tympani
3	Middle ⎬ nasal concha	26 Middle meningeal artery
4	Superior ⎪	27 Marker in auditory tube
5	Supreme ⎭	28 Nerve to medial pterygoid
6	Optic nerve	29 Tensor veli palatini
7	Internal carotid artery	30 Medial pterygoid
8	Oculomotor nerve	31 Lingual nerve
9	Trochlear nerve	32 Inferior alveolar nerve
10	Abducent nerve	33 Nerve to mylohyoid
11	Ophthalmic ⎫	34 Submandibular ganglion
12	Maxillary ⎬ branches of trigeminal nerve	35 Submandibular gland
13	Mandibular ⎭	36 Stylohyoid ligament
14	Motor root of trigeminal nerve	37 Lingual artery
15	Trigeminal ganglion	38 Hyoglossus
16	Petrous part of temporal bone	39 Body of hyoid bone
17	Trigeminal nerve	40 Mylohyoid
18	Pons	41 Geniohyoid
19	Jugular bulb	42 Genioglossus
20	Posterior belly of digastric	43 Sublingual gland
21	Parotid gland	44 Submandibular duct
22	External carotid artery	45 Hypoglossal nerve
23	Sphenomandibular ligament and maxillary artery	

Sagittal section of the head, A right half, from the left, B MR (magnetic resonance) image

The section has been cut slightly to the left of the midline and shows the right half of the head with the nasal septum intact. The hard palate (31) forms the roof of the mouth and the floor of the nose, and is a little below the level of the foramen magnum (17). The pons (14), medulla oblongata (16) and cerebellum (11) are on approximately the same level as the nose. The inlet of the larynx (23) is below and behind the epiglottis (26), in the front of the laryngeal part of the pharynx (22). Compare many of the features seen in the cut section with the MR image in B

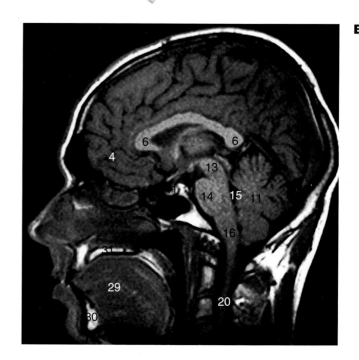

A

B

1	Left frontal sinus	22	Laryngeal part of pharynx
2	Left ethmoidal air cells	23	Inlet of larynx
3	Falx cerebri	24	Thyroid cartilage
4	Medial surface of right	25	Hyoid bone
	cerebral hemisphere	26	Epiglottis
5	Anterior cerebral artery	27	Vallecula
6	Corpus callosum	28	Oral part of pharynx
7	Arachnoid granulations	29	Tongue
8	Superior sagittal sinus	30	Mandible
9	Tentorium cerebelli	31	Hard palate
10	Straight sinus	32	Soft palate
11	Cerebellum	33	Nasopharynx
12	Great cerebral vein	34	Dens of axis
13	Midbrain	35	Anterior arch of atlas
14	Pons	36	Pharyngeal tonsil
15	Fourth ventricle	37	Opening of auditory tube
16	Medulla oblongata	38	Choana (posterior nasal
17	Margin of foramen magnum		aperture)
18	Cerebellomedullary cistern	39	Nasal septum
	(cisterna magna)	40	Sphenoidal sinus
19	Posterior arch of atlas	41	Pituitary gland
20	Spinal cord	42	Optic chiasma
21	Intervertebral disc between		
	axis and third cervical		
	vertebra		

• The falx cerebri (3) separates the two cerebral hemispheres. The tentorium cerebelli (9) separates the posterior parts of the cerebral hemispheres from the cerebellum (11).

Nose, mouth, pharynx and larynx in sagittal section, from the right, C with the nasal septum intact, D with the nasal septum removed

Removal of the nasal septum (C4 to 6) reveals the superior, middle and inferior nasal conchae (D47, 49 and 51) on the lateral wall of the left half of the nasal cavity. The auditory tube (C12) opens into the upper part of the nasal part of the pharynx (C36). The palatoglossal folds (C20) form the boundary between the mouth (beneath the palate, C9 and 10) and the oral part of the pharynx (C35). The palatine tonsils lie between the palatoglossal and palatopharyngeal folds (C20 and 18)

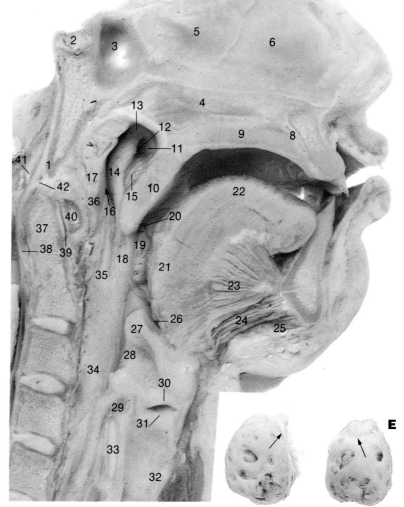

C

D

E

1	Anterior margin of foramen magnum	29	Arytenoid cartilage
2	Pituitary gland	30	Vestibular fold
3	Left sphenoidal sinus	31	Vocal fold
4	Vomer	32	Arch } of cricoid cartilage
5	Perpendicular plate of ethmoid } nasal septum	33	Lamina
6	Septal cartilage	34	Laryngeal } part of pharynx
7	Frontal sinus	35	Oral
8	Incisive canal	36	Nasal
9	Hard palate	37	Dens of axis
10	Soft palate	38	Transverse ligament of atlas
11	Salpingopalatal fold	39	Median atlanto-axial joint
12	Opening of auditory tube	40	Anterior arch of atlas
13	Tubal elevation	41	Tectorial membrane
14	Salpingopharyngeal fold	42	Apical ligament of dens
15	Levator elevation	43	Intercavernous venous sinus
16	Pharyngeal recess	44	Optic nerve
17	Pharyngeal tonsil	45	Right sphenoidal sinus
18	Palatopharyngeal fold	46	Spheno-ethmoidal recess
19	Palatine tonsil	47	Superior nasal concha
20	Palatoglossal fold	48	Superior meatus
21	Pharyngeal } part of dorsum of tongue	49	Middle nasal concha
22	Oral	50	Middle meatus
23	Genioglossus	51	Inferior nasal concha
24	Geniohyoid	52	Inferior meatus
25	Mylohyoid	53	Atrium
26	Vallecula	54	Vestibule
27	Epiglottis		
28	Aryepiglottic fold		

• The palatoglossal folds (20) form the boundary between the mouth and the oral part of the pharynx (35). The (palatine) tonsils (19) which lie between the palatoglossal (20) and palatopharyngeal folds (18) are therefore in the oral part of the pharynx, not in the mouth.
• In C the cricoid cartilage (32, 33) is lying at a higher level than normal (opposite the fourth and fifth cervical vertebrae, instead of the sixth).

• In D the sphenoidal air sinuses (3, 45) are large, and both have extended across the midline.
• The sphenopalatine artery (the termination of the maxillary artery), supplying much of the lateral wall of the nose and nasal septum, enters the nasal cavity through the sphenopalatine foramen (page 20, B23) which lies immediately behind the posterior end of the middle nasal concha.

E Palatine tonsils
The pits on the medial surfaces of these operation specimens from a child aged 14 years are the openings of the tonsillar crypts. The arrows indicate the intratonsillar clefts (the remains of the embryonic second pharyngeal pouch)

• The palatine tonsils (commonly called simply 'the tonsils', C19) are masses of lymphoid tissue that are frequently enlarged in childhood but become much reduced in size in later life. Together with the lymphoid tissue in the posterior part of the tongue (lingual tonsil, at C21) and in the posterior wall of the nasopharynx (pharyngeal tonsil, C17), they form a protective 'ring' of lymphoid tissue at the upper end of the respiratory and alimentary tracts.

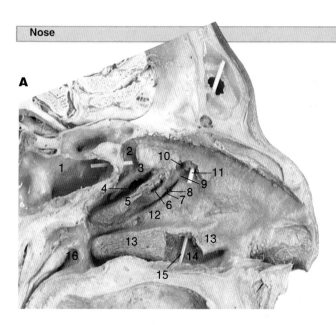

A

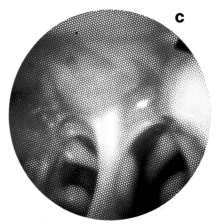

B

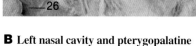

C

A Lateral wall of the left nasal cavity

The middle nasal concha (5) and part of the inferior concha (13) have been removed, and markers have been placed in the openings of the sphenoidal sinus (1), frontal sinus (11) and nasolacrimal duct (15)

1 Left sphenoidal sinus (marker in opening)
2 Spheno-ethmoidal recess
3 Superior nasal concha
4 Superior meatus
5 Cut edge of middle nasal concha
6 Ethmoidal bulla and opening of middle ethmoidal air cells
7 Semilunar hiatus
8 Marker in opening of maxillary sinus
9 Ethmoidal infundibulum
10 Opening of anterior ethmoidal air cells
11 Marker in frontonasal duct (opening of frontal sinus)
12 Middle meatus
13 Inferior nasal concha
14 Inferior meatus
15 Marker in opening of nasolacrimal duct
16 Opening of auditory tube

• The sites of the various openings into the different parts of the nasal cavity (referred to in the five notes below) can be summarized as follows:
Into the spheno-ethmoidal recess: the sphenoidal sinus.
Into the superior meatus: the posterior ethmoidal air cells.
Into the middle meatus: the middle and anterior ethmoidal air cells and the maxillary sinus.
Into the inferior meatus: the nasolacrimal duct.
• The sphenoidal sinus (A1) opens into the spheno-ethmoidal recess (A2).
• The posterior ethmoidal air cells open into the superior meatus (A4), the middle cells on or above the ethmoidal bulla (A6), in the middle meatus (A12), and the anterior cells into the infundibulum (A9) or frontonasal duct (A11), also in the middle meatus (A12).
• The frontal sinus opens into the middle meatus by the frontonasal duct (A11) or via the infundibulum (A9), which is the upward and anterior continuation of the semilunar hiatus (A7).
• The maxillary sinus opens into the semilunar hiatus (A7) of the middle meatus; occasionally there are two openings, one of which may be below the hiatus (as in the specimen on the page opposite, D14).
• The nasolacrimal duct (A15) opens into the inferior meatus (A14).

B Left nasal cavity and pterygopalatine ganglion, from the right

Behind the nasal cavity the perpendicular plate of the palatine bone (page 20, B22) has been removed to open up the greater palatine canal containing the greater palatine nerve and vessels (17). The left sphenoidal sinus has been dissected away to show the nerve of the pterygoid canal (7); the canal is below the floor of the sinus in the body of the sphenoid bone (page 33, A9)

• The olfactory area of the nasal mucosa occupies the mucosa overlying the superior nasal concha (A3), the corresponding part of the septum and the adjacent part of the roof of the nose.
• The nerve of the pterygoid canal (B7) is formed by the union of the greater petrosal nerve (B6, from the facial) and the deep petrosal nerve (B5, from the sympathetic plexus round the internal carotid artery—the internal carotid nerve, B4).

1 Arcuate eminence
2 Internal acoustic meatus and facial nerve
3 Internal carotid artery
4 Internal carotid (sympathetic) nerve
5 Deep petrosal nerve
6 Greater petrosal nerve
7 Nerve of pterygoid canal
8 Trigeminal ganglion
9 Maxillary nerve
10 Abducent nerve
11 Oculomotor nerve
12 Optic nerve
13 Olfactory nerve filaments
14 Frontal sinus and marker
15 Anterior ethmoidal nerve
16 Left nasopalatine nerve
17 Greater palatine nerve and vessels
18 Lesser palatine nerves
19 Inferior nasal concha
20 Marker emerging from frontonasal duct in middle meatus
21 Artificial opening into maxillary sinus and marker
22 Opening of maxillary sinus and marker
23 Pterygopalatine ganglion
24 Opening of auditory tube and marker
25 Inferior ganglion of vagus nerve
26 Vertebral artery
27 Internal jugular vein

C Endoscopic view of the posterior nasal apertures (choanae) of the nose

The nasal septum is seen in the midline, with conchae projecting from the lateral wall into the nasal cavity on each side.

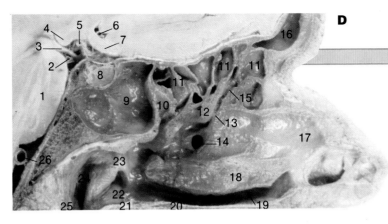

D Lateral wall of the left nasal cavity

In this sagittal section through the nose the superior and middle nasal conchae have been removed and the ethmoidal air cells (11) opened up

1	Pons	15	Ethmoidal infundibulum
2	Superior cerebellar artery	16	Frontal sinus
3	Oculomotor nerve	17	Atrium
4	Mamillary body	18	Inferior nasal concha
5	Posterior cerebral artery	19	Inferior meatus
6	Anterior cerebral artery	20	Hard palate
7	Optic nerve	21	Soft palate
8	Pituitary gland	22	Opening of auditory tube
9	Sphenoidal sinus	23	Tubal elevation
10	Spheno-ethmoidal recess	24	Pharyngeal recess
11	Ethmoidal air cells	25	Pharyngeal tonsil
12	Ethmoidal bulla	26	Basilar artery (tortuous)
13	Semilunar hiatus		
14	Opening of maxillary sinus (unusually low)		

• When enlarged the lymphoid tissue of the pharyngeal tonsil constitutes the adenoids.

• The opening of the auditory tube lies over 1 cm behind the posterior end of the inferior nasal concha.

E Right trigeminal nerve, petrosal nerves and associated ganglia

Viewed from the right, much of the right side of the skull has been removed, leaving the medial sides of the right orbit (13) and maxillary sinus (22). Behind the sinus are seen the three branches of the trigeminal nerve: ophthalmic (7), maxillary (6) and mandibular (5)

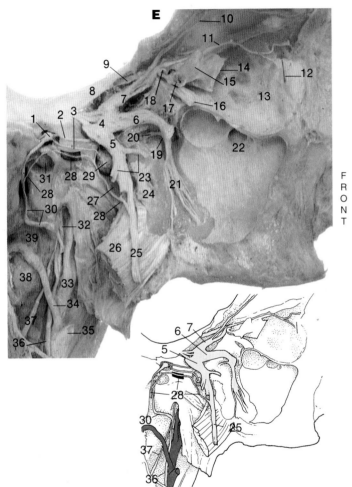

1	Genicular ganglion of facial nerve	22	Medial wall of maxillary sinus and opening
2	Greater ⎫ petrosal nerve	23	Muscular branches of mandibular nerve
3	Lesser ⎭	24	Lower head of lateral pterygoid and lateral pterygoid plate
4	Trigeminal ganglion		
5	Mandibular nerve	25	Lingual nerve
6	Maxillary nerve	26	Medial pterygoid
7	Ophthalmic nerve	27	Tensor veli palatini
8	Free margin of tentorium cerebelli	28	Chorda tympani
9	Oculomotor nerve	29	Otic ganglion
10	Frontal nerve	30	Facial nerve
11	Nasociliary nerve	31	Position of tympanic membrane
12	Bristle in lacrimal canaliculus	32	Glossopharyngeal nerve
13	Medial wall of orbit	33	Internal carotid artery
14	Medial rectus	34	Occipital artery
15	Optic nerve	35	External carotid artery
16	Inferior rectus	36	Hypoglossal nerve
17	Ciliary ganglion	37	Internal jugular vein and accessory nerve
18	Lacrimal nerve		
19	Pterygopalatine ganglion	38	Transverse process of atlas
20	Nerve of pterygoid canal	39	Rectus capitis lateralis
21	Greater and lesser palatine nerves		

• The greater petrosal nerve (2) is a branch of the facial (1) and can be remembered as the nerve of tear secretion (though it also supplies nasal glands). It carries preganglionic fibres from the superior salivary nucleus (in the pons), and runs in the groove on the floor of the middle cranial fossa (page 19, B44) to enter the foramen lacerum and become the nerve of the pterygoid canal (20) which joins the pterygopalatine ganglion (19). Postganglionic fibres leave the ganglion to join the maxillary nerve and enter the orbit by the zygomatic branch which communicates with the lacrimal nerve, supplying the gland (page 62, D2).

• The lesser petrosal nerve (3), although having a communication with the facial nerve, is a branch of the glossopharyngeal nerve, being derived from the tympanic branch which supplies the mucous membrane of the middle ear by the tympanic plexus (page 65, B21). Its fibres are derived from the inferior salivary nucleus in the pons, and after leaving the middle ear and running in its groove on the floor of the middle cranial fossa (3, and page 19, B45), the nerve reaches the otic ganglion (29) via the foramen ovale. From the ganglion secretomotor fibres join the mandibular nerve (5) to be distributed to the parotid gland by filaments from the auriculotemporal nerve.

• The chorda tympani (28) arises from the facial nerve before the latter leaves the stylomastoid foramen (30, upper leader line). It crosses the upper part of the tympanic membrane (31) underneath its mucosal covering

and runs through the temporal bone to emerge from the petrotympanic fissure (page 17, C19) and join the lingual nerve (25). It carries preganglionic fibres to the submandibular ganglion (page 47, B20) for the submandibular and sublingual salivary glands, and also taste fibres for the anterior part of the tongue.

• The otic ganglion (29), which normally adheres to the deep surface of the mandibular nerve (5), has been teased off from the nerve and a black marker has been placed behind it.

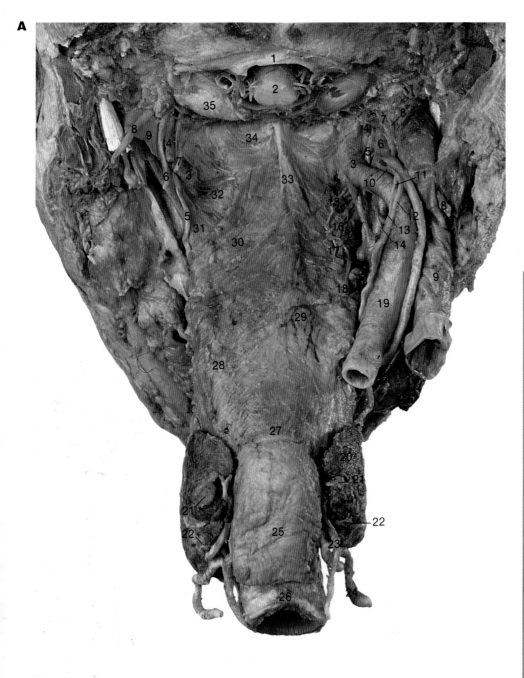

A

Pharynx, A from behind, B coronal MR image

The back of the pharynx has been exposed by removing the vertebral column and prevertebral muscles. On the left only the uppermost parts of the main vessels and nerves have been preserved; the glossopharyngeal nerve (5) is seen winding round stylopharyngeus (31). On the right the internal carotid artery (3) has been displaced slightly laterally to show the pharyngeal branches of the glossopharyngeal and vagus nerves (15 and 16) which form the pharyngeal nerve plexus on the surface of the middle constrictor (30). On the left the accessory nerve (8) passes behind the internal jugular vein (9)—its usual relationship; on the right it runs in front of the vein, a common variation. Both pairs of parathyroid glands (21 and 22) are seen behind the lateral lobes of the thyroid gland (20). Compare the dissection with the MR image in B

1   Margin of foramen magnum
2   Spinal cord
3   Internal carotid artery
4   Sympathetic trunk
5   Glossopharyngeal nerve
6   Vagus (inferior ganglion)
7   Hypoglossal nerve
8   Accessory nerve
9   Internal jugular vein
10 Superior laryngeal nerve
11 External laryngeal nerve
12 Internal laryngeal nerve
13 External carotid artery
14 Branches of glossopharyngeal and vagus nerves to carotid body and carotid sinus
15 Pharyngeal branch of glossopharyngeal nerve ⎫ pharyngeal
16 Pharyngeal branch of vagus nerve ⎭ plexus
17 Ascending pharyngeal artery
18 Tip of greater horn of hyoid bone ·
19 Common carotid artery
20 Lateral lobe of thyroid gland
21 Superior parathyroid gland
22 Inferior parathyroid gland
23 Recurrent laryngeal nerve
24 Inferior thyroid artery
25 Oesophagus
26 Trachea
27 Cricopharyngeal part ⎫ of inferior
28 Thyropharyngeal part ⎭ constrictor
29 Part of buccopharyngeal fascia and pharyngeal venous plexus
30 Middle constrictor
31 Stylopharyngeus
32 Superior constrictor
33 Pharyngeal raphe
34 Pharyngobasilar fascia
35 Occipital condyle

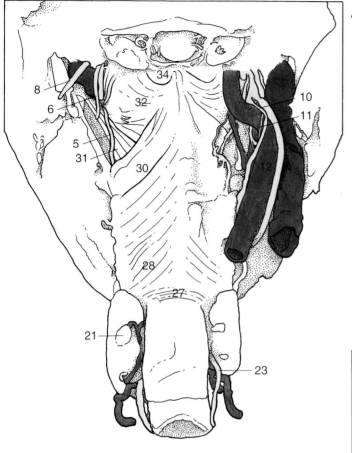

A

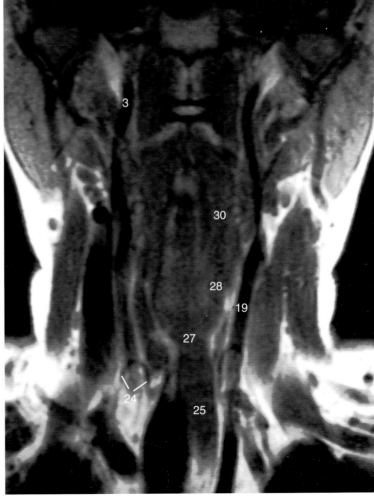

B

- The pharynx extends from the base of the skull to the level of the sixth cervical vertebra, and consists of nasal, oral and pharyngeal parts whose internal features (detailed below) are best seen in a sagittal section such as that on page 51, C.
- The nasal part (nasopharynx), as far down as the lower border of the soft palate, contains the openings of the auditory tubes, the pharyngeal tonsil and pharyngeal recesses, and opens anteriorly into the nasal cavity.
- The oral part, between the soft palate and the upper border of the epiglottis, contains the (palatine) tonsils and the palatopharyngeal arch, and opens anteriorly into the mouth. The palatoglossal arch is the boundary between the mouth and the oral pharynx.
- The laryngeal part, below the upper border of the epiglottis, contains the piriform recess on either side of the larynx, which bulges backwards into the pharynx with the laryngeal inlet below and behind the epiglottis.
- The lower end of the pharynx becomes continuous with the oesophagus, at the same level (opposite the sixth cervical vertebra) as the larynx continues as the trachea.

A

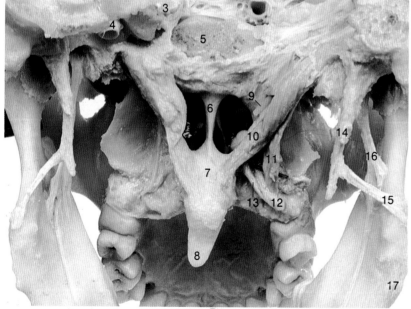

A Pharynx, from behind

By removing the upper part of the posterior pharyngeal wall, the posterior nasal apertures (6) can be seen above the back of the soft palate (8), while below it are the back of the tongue (40) and the tip of the epiglottis (39), seen through the arch formed by the two palatopharyngeus muscles (42) and the central uvula (41)

1	Sigmoid sinus	24	Angle of mandible
2	Jugular bulb	25	Hypoglossal nerve
3	Internal carotid artery	26	Nerve to thyrohyoid
4	Cartilaginous part of auditory tube (marker in opening)	27	Tip of greater horn of hyoid bone
5	Clivus	28	Middle constrictor (overlying red marker)
6	Posterior nasal aperture (choana)	29	Inferior constrictor (overlying blue marker)
7	Nasal septum (vomer)	30	Superior thyroid artery
8	Soft palate	31	Lateral lobe of thyroid gland
9	Levator veli palatini	32	Superior parathyroid gland
10	Salpingopharyngeus	33	Inferior thyroid artery
11	Superior constrictor (cut edge)	34	Recurrent laryngeal nerve
12	Medial pterygoid	35	Longitudinal ⎫ muscle of
13	Lingual nerve	36	Circular ⎭ oesophagus
14	Inferior alveolar nerve	37	Internal laryngeal nerve
15	Chorda tympani	38	Lingual artery
16	Glossopharyngeal nerve	39	Epiglottis
17	Stylopharyngeus	40	Foramen caecum in dorsum of tongue
18	Styloglossus	41	Uvula
19	Stylohyoid	42	Palatopharyngeus
20	Styloid process	43	Pterygoid hamulus
21	Posterior belly of digastric	44	Tensor veli palatini
22	Parotid gland		
23	Masseter		

● The palatopharyngeus (42) and salpingopharyngeus (10) pass downwards internal to the superior constrictor (11); the stylopharyngeus (17) passes downwards between the superior and middle constrictors (11 and 28).

B

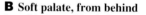

B Soft palate, from behind

Part of the base of the skull together with the pharynx and most other soft parts have been removed, leaving the central part of the soft palate (7)

1	Groove for sigmoid sinus	11	Tensor veli palatini
2	Tympanic membrane	12	Pterygoid hamulus
3	Apex of petrous part of temporal bone	13	Tendon of tensor veli palatini
4	Internal carotid artery	14	Styloid process
5	Clivus	15	Part of stylomandibular ligament
6	Vomer (nasal septum)	16	Sphenomandibular ligament
7	Soft palate	17	Angle of mandible
8	Uvula		
9	Marker in auditory tube		
10	Levator veli palatini		

● All the muscles of the pharynx and soft palate are supplied by the cranial part of the accessory nerve through the branches of the vagus that join the pharyngeal plexus, except for the stylopharyngeus which is supplied by the glossopharyngeal nerve and the tensor veli palatini by a branch from the nerve to the medial pterygoid muscle (mandibular nerve).
● Levator veli palatini (10), formerly called levator palati, is a short round muscle; tensor veli palatini (11), formerly called tensor palati, is a flat triangular muscle ending in a tendon (13) which hooks round the pterygoid hamulus (12) and then expands, to become with its fellow of the opposite side, the palatine aponeurosis.

Hyoid bone, A from above and in front, B with muscle attachments

1 Greater horn
2 Lesser horn
3 Body
4 Genioglossus
5 Geniohyoid
6 Stylohyoid ligament
7 Middle constrictor
8 Hyoglossus
9 Mylohyoid
10 Sternohyoid
11 Omohyoid
12 Thyrohyoid
13 Stylohyoid

C Cartilage of the epiglottis, from the front. D Thyroid cartilage from the front, E from the right with attachments

1 Superior horn
2 Lamina
3 Inferior horn
4 Thyroid notch
5 Laryngeal prominence (Adam's apple)
6 Superior ⎫ tubercle
7 Inferior ⎭
8 Inferior constrictor
9 Sternothyroid
10 Thyrohyoid
11 Cricothyroid

F Arytenoid cartilages, from behind

1 Apex
2 Muscular process
3 Articular surface for cricoid cartilage
4 Vocal process

Cricoid cartilage and muscle attachments, G from behind and below, H from the right

1 Lamina
2 Posterior crico-arytenoid
3 Tendon of oesophagus
4 Articular surface for arytenoid cartilage
5 Articular surface for inferior horn of thyroid cartilage
6 Arch
7 Inferior constrictor
8 Cricothyroid

J Larynx, from behind

The left lamina of the thyroid cartilage has been reflected forwards and a glass rod (seen below the label 1 on the epiglottis) holds the pharynx open. Black markers underlie filaments from the recurrent and internal laryngeal nerves (7 and 10)

1 Epiglottis
2 Posterior pharyngeal wall
3 Cuneiform ⎫ in
  cartilage ⎪ aryepi-
4 Corniculate ⎬ glottic
  cartilage ⎭ fold
5 Transverse arytenoid muscle
6 Branch of internal laryngeal nerve
7 Branches of recurrent laryngeal nerve
8 Tendon of oesophagus
9 Circular fibres of oesophagus
10 Anastomosis between internal and recurrent laryngeal nerves
11 Cricothyroid muscle (reflected forwards with lamina of thyroid cartilage)

K Tongue and the inlet of the larynx, from above

1 Posterior wall of pharynx
2 Corniculate ⎫ in
  cartilage ⎪ aryepi-
3 Cuneiform ⎬ glottic
  cartilage ⎭ fold
4 Epiglottis
5 Median glosso-epiglottic fold
6 Vallecula
7 Lateral glosso-epiglottic fold
8 Pharyngeal part of dorsum of tongue
9 Foramen caecum
10 Sulcus terminalis
11 Vallate papilla
12 Fungiform papilla
13 Vestibular fold
14 Vocal fold

● The V-shaped sulcus terminalis (10), behind the row of vallate papillae (11), is not well marked in this tongue.

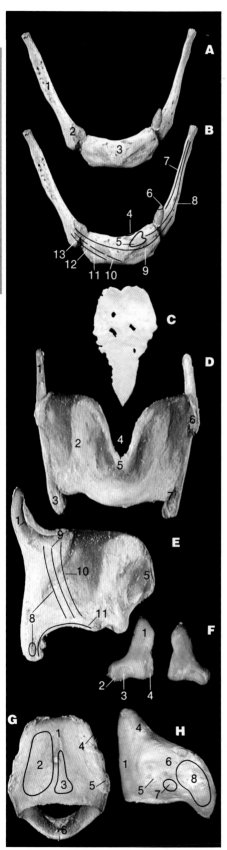

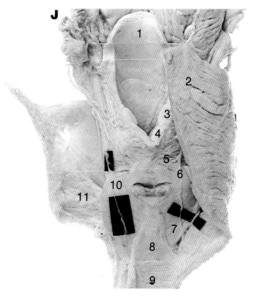

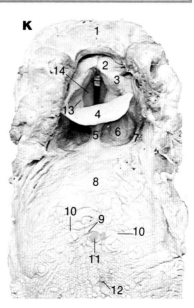

A

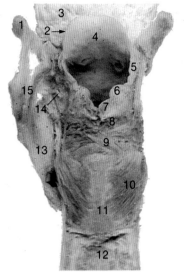

B

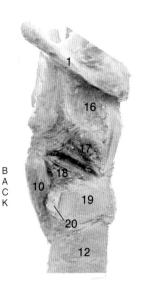

C

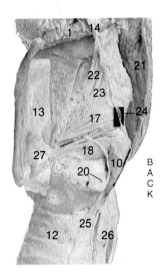

Intrinsic muscles of the larynx, A from behind, B from the right, C from the left

In B the right lamina of the thyroid cartilage has been removed, and in C part of the thyroid lamina has been turned forwards

D

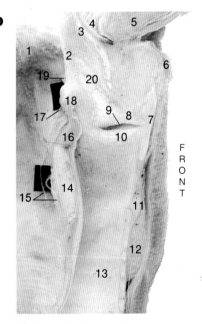

Larynx, in sagittal section, D left side from the right. E MR image of the neck

The vocal fold (vocal cord, 10) lies below the vestibular fold (false vocal cord, 8)

1 Greater horn of hyoid bone	15 Thyrohyoid membrane
2 Vallecula	16 Quadrangular membrane
3 Dorsum of tongue	17 Thyro-arytenoid muscle
4 Epiglottis	18 Lateral crico-arytenoid muscle
5 Aryepiglottic fold	19 Arch of cricoid cartilage
6 Cuneiform ⎫ cartilage	20 Cricothyroid joint
7 Corniculate ⎭	21 Posterior wall of pharynx
8 Transverse ⎫ arytenoid	22 Aryepiglottic ⎫ muscle
9 Oblique ⎭ muscle	23 Thyro-epiglottic ⎭
10 Posterior crico-arytenoid muscle	24 Anastomosis of internal and recurrent laryngeal nerves
11 Area on lamina of cricoid cartilage for tendon of oesophagus	25 Recurrent laryngeal nerve
12 Trachea	26 Oesophagus
13 Lamina of thyroid cartilage	27 Cricothyroid muscle (reflected from cricoid attachment)
14 Internal laryngeal nerve	

1 Pharyngeal wall	13 Trachea
2 Aryepiglottic fold and inlet of larynx	14 Lamina of cricoid cartilage
3 Epiglottis	15 Branches of recurrent laryngeal nerve
4 Vallecula	16 Transverse arytenoid muscle
5 Tongue	17 Branches of internal laryngeal nerve anastomosing with recurrent laryngeal nerve
6 Body of hyoid bone	
7 Lamina of thyroid cartilage	
8 Vestibular fold	18 Corniculate cartilage and apex of arytenoid cartilage
9 Sinus of larynx	
10 Vocal fold	19 Internal laryngeal nerve entering piriform recess
11 Arch of cricoid cartilage	
12 Isthmus of thyroid gland	20 Vestibule of larynx

• The space between the vestibular and vocal folds is the sinus of the larynx (D9), and this is continuous with the saccule, a small pouch that extends upwards for a few millimetres between the vestibular fold and the inner surface of the thyro-arytenoid muscle (B17).

• The fissure between the two vestibular folds (D8) is the rima of the vestibule. The fissure between the vocal folds (vocal cord, D10, E10) is the rima of the glottis (G5).

• The vestibular folds are sometimes called the false vocal cords.

• The intrinsic muscles of the larynx are supplied by the recurrent laryngeal nerve (C25), except the cricothyroid (page 42, A12) which is supplied by the external laryngeal nerve (page 42, A25).

E

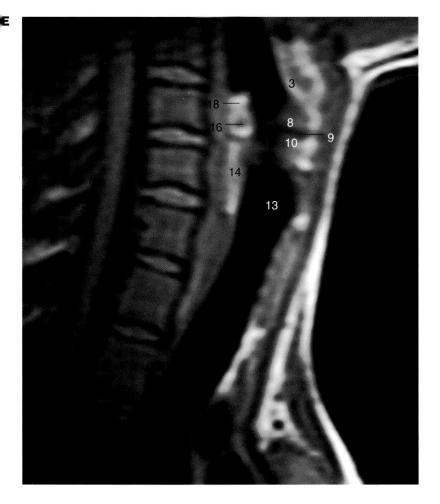

G

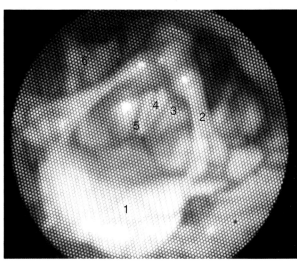

G Endoscopic view of the laryngeal inlet and vocal folds

1	Epiglottis
2	Aryepiglottic fold
3	Vestibular fold
4	Vocal fold
5	Rima of glottis
6	Piriform recess of pharynx

F Ligaments and membranes of the right side of the larynx, from the left

Most of the left side of the larynx has been removed but the whole of the cricoid cartilage remains intact

1	Hyoid bone
2	Hyo-epiglottic ligament
3	Epiglottis
4	Quadrangular membrane
5	Apex ⎫ of arytenoid
6	Vocal process ⎭ cartilage
7	Lamina ⎫ of cricoid
8	Arch ⎭ cartilage
9	Cricovocal membrane
10	Lamina of thyroid cartilage
11	Thyro-epiglottic ligament

F

FRONT

• The mucous membrane of the larynx above the level of the vocal folds is supplied by the internal laryngeal nerve, and below the vocal folds by the recurrent laryngeal nerve (D17 and 15).
• The recurrent laryngeal nerve (C25) enters the larynx by passing beneath the lower border of the inferior constrictor of the pharynx, and here it lies immediately behind the cricothyroid joint (C20).
• The anterior part of the vocal fold (D10, G4) is formed by the upper margin of the cricovocal membrane (F9), and the posterior part by the vocal process of the arytenoid cartilage (F6).
• The vestibular fold (false vocal cord, D8, G3) is formed by the lower margin of the quadrangular membrane (F4), whose upper margin forms the aryepiglottic fold (D2, A5, G2).
• The central (anterior) part of the cricothyroid membrane is usually known as the conus elasticus but sometimes this term is used for the cricovocal membrane.

59

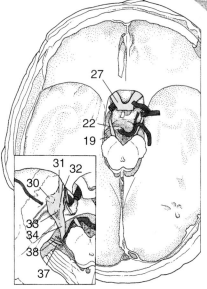

A Cerebral dura mater, outer surface
The right half of the cranial vault has been removed to show branches of the middle meningeal vessels on the outer surface of the dura, i.e. in the extradural space. These vessels do not supply the brain

A

FRONT

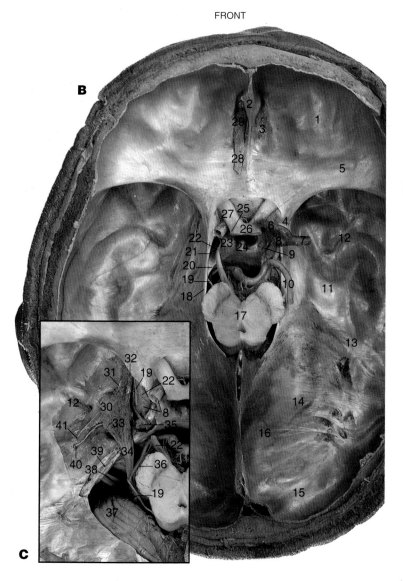

B

C

Cranial fossae, B with dura mater intact, C with some dura removed
On the right the anterior, middle and posterior cerebral arteries (6, 7 and 10) and the posterior communicating artery (9) have been preserved, but on the left they have been removed to give a clearer view of the trochlear nerve (19) piercing the dura mater at the junction of the free (18) and attached (20) margins of the tentorium cerebelli, and the oculomotor nerve (22) piercing the roof of the cavernous sinus (21). In C some dura on the left side has been removed, including the roof of the cavernous sinus (B21) and segments of the oculomotor (22) and trochlear (19) nerves. The trigeminal nerve and its branches (30 to 34) are exposed, together with the petrosal nerves (40 and 41). With part of the tentorium missing the vestibulocochlear and facial nerves (37 and 38) are on view in the posterior cranial fossa

1 Anterior cranial fossa	18 Free margin of tentorium cerebelli
2 Falx cerebri attached to crista galli	19 Trochlear nerve
3 Cribriform plate of ethmoid bone	20 Attached margin of tentorium cerebelli
4 Anterior clinoid process	21 Roof of cavernous sinus
5 Sphenoparietal sinus (at posterior border of lesser wing of sphenoid bone)	22 Oculomotor nerve
	23 Posterior clinoid process
	24 Pituitary stalk
6 Anterior cerebral artery	25 Optic tract
7 Middle cerebral artery	26 Optic chiasma
8 Internal carotid artery	27 Optic nerve
9 Posterior communicating artery	28 Olfactory tract
	29 Olfactory bulb
10 Posterior cerebral artery	30 Mandibular nerve
11 Lateral part of middle cranial fossa	31 Maxillary nerve
	32 Ophthalmic nerve
12 Middle meningeal vessels	33 Trigeminal ganglion
13 Superior petrosal sinus (at attached margin of tentorium cerebelli)	34 Trigeminal nerve
	35 Abducent nerve
14 Tentorium cerebelli	36 Superior cerebellar artery
15 Transverse sinus (at attached margin of tentorium cerebelli)	37 Vestibulocochlear nerve
	38 Facial nerve
	39 Superior petrosal sinus
16 Straight sinus (at junction of falx cerebri and tentorium cerebelli)	40 Hiatus for greater petrosal nerve
17 Midbrain (superior colliculus level)	41 Hiatus for lesser petrosal nerve

D Cerebral dura mater and cranial nerves

In this oblique view from the left and behind, the brain has been removed and a window has been cut in the posterior part of the falx cerebri (1) to show the upper surface of the tentorium cerebelli (7)

1 Falx cerebri
2 Sphenoparietal sinus
3 Inferior sagittal sinus
4 Arachnoid granulations
5 Superior sagittal sinus
6 Transverse sinus
7 Tentorium cerebelli
8 Straight sinus
9 Margin of foramen magnum
10 Posterior arch of atlas
11 Spinal cord
12 Dens of axis
13 Medulla oblongata
14 Rootlets of hypoglossal nerve
15 Spinal part of accessory nerve
16 Glossopharyngeal, vagus and accessory nerves
17 Vestibulocochlear nerve
18 Sensory root (nervus intermedius) } of facial nerve
19 Motor root }
20 Abducent nerve
21 Trigeminal nerve
22 Free margin of tentorium cerebelli
23 Trochlear nerve
24 Attached margin of tentorium cerebelli
25 Oculomotor nerve
26 Internal carotid artery
27 Optic nerve
28 Olfactory tract
29 Pituitary gland
30 Sphenoidal sinus
31 Choana (posterior nasal aperture)
32 Clivus
33 Nasal septum

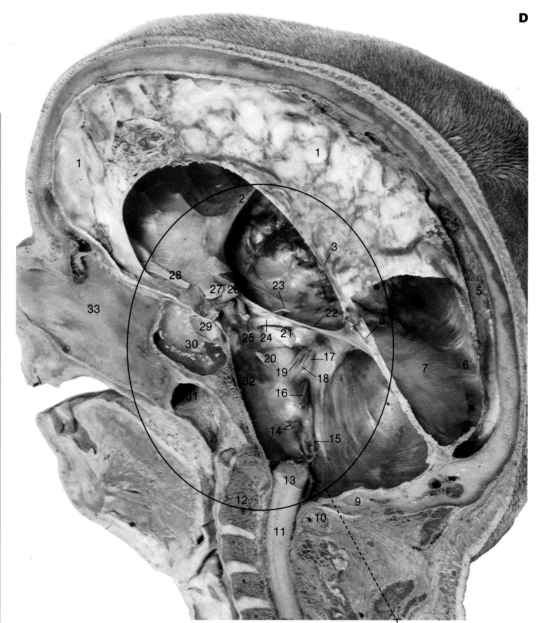

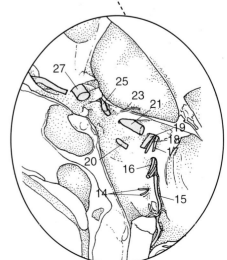

• The filaments of the olfactory (first cranial) nerve pierce the cribriform plate of the ethmoid to enter the olfactory bulb, at the front end of the olfactory tract (28) and just hidden by the curved edge of the falx cerebri (1).
• The optic (second cranial) nerve (27) emerges from the optic canal and passes medial to the internal carotid artery (26).
• The oculomotor (third cranial) nerve (25) pierces the dura mater of the roof of the cavernous sinus.
• The trochlear (fourth cranial) nerve (23) pierces the dura mater where the free margin of the tentorium cerebelli (22) crosses over the attached margin (24).
• The trigeminal (fifth cranial) nerve (21) crosses the apex of the petrous part of the temporal bone below the attached margin of the tentorium cerebelli (24).
• The abducent (sixth cranial) nerve (20) pierces the dura mater on the clivus (32).
• The facial (seventh cranial) nerve (18 and 19) and the vestibulocochlear (eighth cranial) nerve (17) enter the internal acoustic meatus.
• The filaments of the glossopharyngeal, vagus and accessory nerves (ninth, tenth and eleventh cranial nerves respectively, 16), and including the spinal part of the accessory nerve (15) which has entered the skull through the foramen magnum (9), enter the jugular foramen.
• The rootlets of the hypoglossal (twelfth cranial) nerve (14) enter the hypoglossal canal as two separate bundles.

A

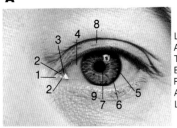

A Left eye. Surface features

With the eyelids in the normal open position, the lower margin of the upper lid (8) overlaps approximately the upper half of the iris (6); the margin of the lower lid (9) is level with the lower margin of the iris (6)

1	Lacrimal caruncle	6	Iris } behind cornea
2	Lacrimal papilla	7	Pupil } behind cornea
3	Plica semilunaris	8	Upper lid
4	Sclera	9	Lower lid
5	Limbus (corneoscleral junction)		

- The cornea is the transparent anterior part of the outer coat of the eyeball and is continuous with the sclera (4) at the limbus (5).
- The pupil (7) is the central aperture of the iris (6), the circular pigmented diaphragm that lies in front of the lens.
- Each lacrimal papilla (2) contains the lacrimal punctum, the minute opening of the lacrimal canaliculus (page 64, B6 and 7) which runs medially to open into the lacrimal sac, lying deep to the medial palpebral ligament (page 64, B3) and continuing downwards as the nasolacrimal duct (page 64, B4) within the nasolacrimal canal.

Right extra-ocular muscles, B from above, C from the right

The upper and lateral walls of the orbit have been removed, together with all fat, vessels and nerves, leaving only the muscles

1	Superior oblique	9	Tendinous ring
2	Trochlea	10	Optic nerve
3	Tendon of superior oblique	11	Optic canal
4	Levator palpebrae superioris	12	Anterior clinoid process
5	Eyeball	13	Pituitary fossa (sella turcica)
6	Inferior oblique	14	Posterior clinoid process
7	Lateral rectus	15	Ethmoidal air cells
8	Superior rectus	16	Inferior rectus

B

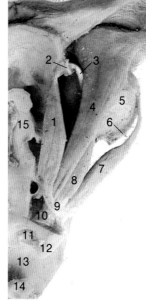

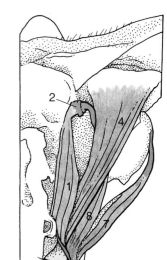

C

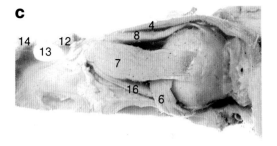

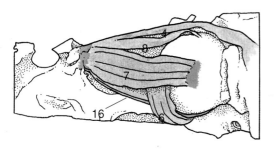

D

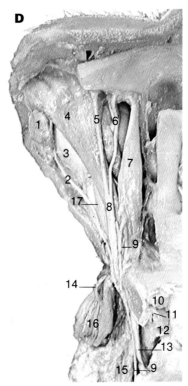

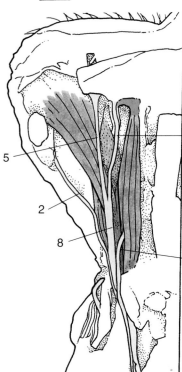

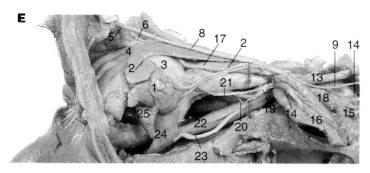

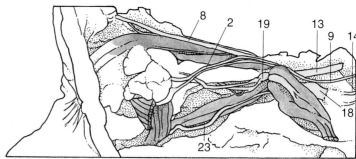

Left orbit, **D** from above, **E** from the left

The upper and lateral walls of the orbit have been removed, together with the blood vessels, leaving muscles and nerves. The lateral rectus (16) has been detached from the eyeball and turned backwards to show the abducent nerve (14) entering its deep (ocular) surface. In D the trochlear nerve (9) is seen entering the superficial (orbital) surface of the superior oblique (7). The frontal nerve (D8) divides on the upper surface of levator palpebrae superioris (4) into the supratrochlear (6) and supra-orbital (5) nerves. The levator muscle largely overlies the superior rectus (17), only a small part of which can be seen at the lateral border of the levator

- The lateral rectus (E16) is supplied by the abducent nerve (E14).
- The superior oblique (D7) is supplied by the trochlear nerve (D9).
- All the other muscles that move the eyeball (medial, superior and inferior recti and the inferior oblique) are supplied by the oculomotor nerve. The branch to the inferior oblique (E23) is surprisingly large and runs above the floor of the orbit lateral to the inferior rectus (E22), to enter the posterior border of the oblique muscle (E24). All the other branches enter the deep (ocular) surfaces of the respective muscles.
- Levator palpebrae superioris (D4) is also supplied by the oculomotor nerve, but some of its fibres consist of visceral muscle which receives a sympathetic supply.

1 Lacrimal gland	14 Abducent nerve
2 Lacrimal nerve	15 Trigeminal ganglion
3 Eyeball	16 Lateral rectus (reflected backwards)
4 Levator palpebrae superioris	17 Superior rectus
5 Supra-orbital nerve	18 Ophthalmic nerve
6 Supratrochlear nerve	19 Ciliary ganglion
7 Superior oblique	20 Short ciliary nerves (superficial to marker)
8 Frontal nerve	21 Nerve to medial rectus
9 Trochlear nerve	22 Inferior rectus
10 Optic nerve	23 Nerve to inferior oblique
11 Ophthalmic artery	24 Inferior oblique
12 Internal carotid artery	25 Lateral rectus
13 Oculomotor nerve	

F Orbits, from above

Both orbits have been exposed from above, and most of levator palpebrae superioris (2) and the superior rectus (3) have been removed. On the right, as is usual, the ophthalmic artery (11) and nasociliary nerve (9) cross above the optic nerve (16) from lateral to medial; on the left the artery has crossed below the nerve, which is uncommon. The supra-orbital artery (4) is unusually small on the left and is absent on the right

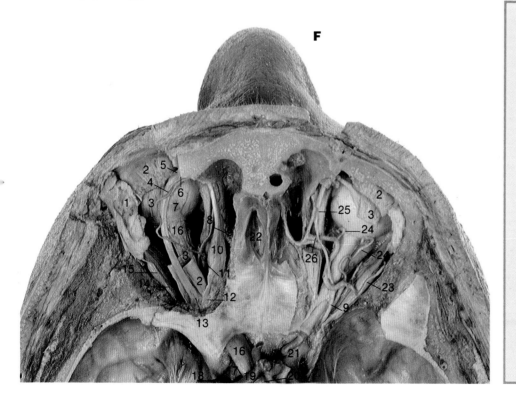

1	Lacrimal gland
2	Levator palpebrae superioris
3	Superior rectus
4	Supra-orbital artery
5	Supra-orbital nerve
6	Supratrochlear nerve
7	Eyeball
8	Medial rectus
9	Nasociliary nerve
10	Superior oblique
11	Ophthalmic artery
12	Trochlear nerve
13	Frontal nerve
14	Lacrimal nerve
15	Lateral rectus
16	Optic nerve (with overlying short ciliary nerves in left orbit)
17	Internal carotid artery
18	Middle cerebral artery
19	Anterior cerebral artery
20	Optic chiasma
21	Anterior communicating artery
22	Cribriform plate of ethmoid bone
23	Lacrimal artery
24	Posterior ciliary artery
25	Infratrochlear nerve and ophthalmic artery
26	Anterior ethmoidal artery and nerve

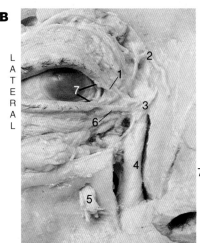

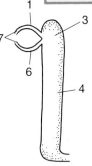

A Right orbit, from the front

The eye has been removed, leaving the cut end of the optic nerve (12) and the extra-ocular muscles

1	Supra-orbital nerve
2	Supratrochlear nerve
3	Trochlea
4	Tendon of superior oblique
5	Superior oblique
6	Anterior ethmoidal nerve
7	Infratrochlear nerve
8	Medial rectus
9	Attachment of medial palpebral ligament
10	Inferior oblique
11	Inferior rectus
12	Optic nerve
13	Lateral rectus
14	Part of orbital septum
15	Lacrimal gland
16	Superior rectus
17	Levator palpebrae superioris

Nasolacrimal duct, B dissected on the right side, C dacryocystogram

In B part of the maxilla has been dissected away to display the nasolacrimal duct (4). The upper end of the duct is continuous with the lacrimal sac (hidden behind the medial palpebral ligament, 3), into which the lacrimal canaliculi (1 and 6) open. Compare with the features outlined by contrast medium in C

1	Superior canaliculus
2	Dorsal nasal artery
3	Medial palpebral ligament overlying lacrimal sac
4	Nasolacrimal duct
5	Infra-orbital nerve
6	Inferior canaliculus
7	Bristles in puncta of lacrimal canaliculi

• The most important branch of the ophthalmic artery–the central artery of the retina– is hidden below the optic nerve. It runs within the dural sheath of the nerve and pierces the inferomedial surface of the nerve 1.25 cm behind the eyeball, passing forwards in the centre of the nerve to reach the retina where its branches can be observed with the ophthalmoscope.

• The two oblique muscles (superior and inferior) both pass below the corresponding rectus muscles.
• The lateral palpebral ligament (connected to the tarsal plates of both eyelids) is attached to a small tubercle on the zygomatic bone (immediately in front of the part of the orbital septum seen in this specimen, 14). The medial palpebral ligament is attached to the anterior lacrimal crest of the frontal process of the maxilla, and therefore lies anterior to the lacrimal sac.
• The orbital septum is the continuation into the eyelids of the orbital periosteum (properly called the orbital fascia).

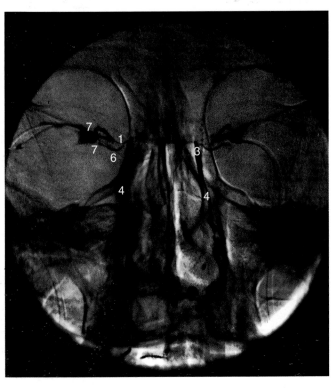

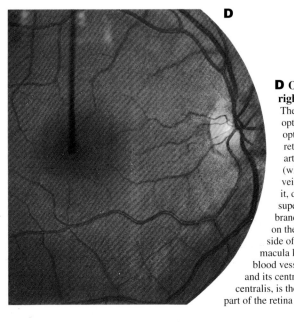

D Ophthalmoscopy, right eye

The pale area is the optic disc, where the optic nerve leaves the retina; the central artery of the retina (with accompanying veins) emerges from it, dividing into superior and inferior branches. The dark area on the lateral (temporal) side of the disc is the macula lutea. There are no blood vessels overlying it, and its central area, the fovea centralis, is the most sensitive part of the retina

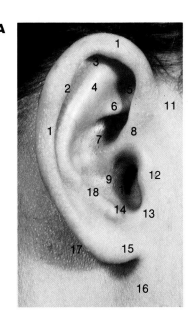

A Right external ear

1	Helix
2	Auricular tubercle
3	Scaphoid fossa
4	Upper crus of antihelix
5	Triangular fossa
6	Lower crus of antihelix
7	Upper part of concha
8	Crus of helix
9	Lower part of concha
10	External acoustic meatus
11	Superficial temporal vessels and auriculotemporal nerve
12	Tragus
13	Intertragic notch
14	Antitragus
15	Lobule
16	Transverse process of atlas
17	Mastoid process
18	Antihelix

• The external ear consists of the auricle (pinna) and external acoustic meatus (10).
• The concha (7 and 9) is the deepest part of the external ear. The lower part of the concha leads into the external acoustic meatus; the suprameatal triangle and mastoid antrum lie behind the upper part.
• For enlarged diagrams of the ear see page 68.
• The middle ear or tympanic cavity is an irregular space within the temporal bone, containing the auditory ossicles and filled with air that communicates with the nasopharynx through the auditory tube.

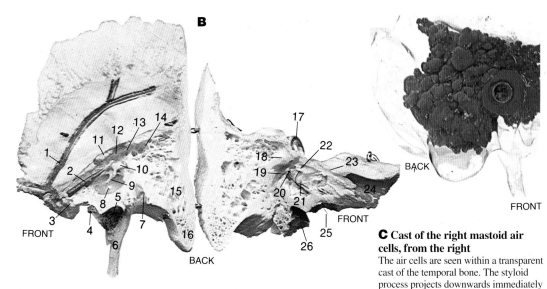

B Right temporal bone and ear

The bone has been bisected and opened out like opening a book, with some removal of the upper part of the petrous part. The section has opened up the tympanic (middle ear) cavity. On the left side of the figure the lateral wall of the middle ear, which includes the tympanic membrane (8), is seen from the medial side, while on the right the main features of the medial wall are in view

1	Groove for middle meningeal vessels	16	Mastoid process
2	Tensor tympani muscle in its canal	17	Anterior ⎫ semicircular canal
		18	Lateral ⎭
3	Bony part of auditory tube	19	Canal for facial nerve (yelllow)
4	Part of carotid canal (red)	20	Stapes in oval window and stapedius muscle
5	Part of jugular bulb (blue)	
6	Styloid process	21	Promontory with overlying tympanic plexus
7	Stylomastoid foramen	
8	Tympanic membrane	22	Lesser petrosal nerve
9	Malleus	23	Groove for greater petrosal nerve (yellow)
10	Incus	
11	Tegmen tympani	24	Carotid canal (red)
12	Epitympanic recess	25	Tympanic branch of glossopharyngeal nerve entering its canaliculus
13	Aditus to mastoid antrum	
14	Mastoid antrum	
15	Mastoid air cells	26	Jugular bulb (blue)

• The epitympanic recess (12) is the part of the tympanic cavity that lies above the tympanic membrane (8), and lodges the head of the malleus (9) and the body of the incus (10). It leads backwards through the aditus (13) into the mastoid antrum (14), which is an enlarged mastoid air cell.
• The medial wall of the middle ear contains (from below upwards) the promontory (21, due to the first turn of the cochlea), the canal for the facial nerve (19) and the prominence due to the lateral semicircular canal (18). Below and behind the promontory (and just hidden by it in this view) is the round window (fenestra cochleae, closed by the secondary tympanic membrane), and above and behind it is the oval window (fenestra vestibuli, closed by the footplate of the stapes, 20).
• The roof of the middle ear is the tegmen tympani (11); the jugular bulb (5) lies below the floor, and the carotid canal (4) in the anterior wall.

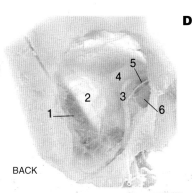

C Cast of the right mastoid air cells, from the right

The air cells are seen within a transparent cast of the temporal bone. The styloid process projects downwards immediately below the external acoustic meatus, with the mastoid process behind

D Mastoid region of the right temporal bone, from the right

The mastoid air cells have been removed and the canal for the facial nerve (3) has been opened up to show the origin of the chorda tympani (5)

1	Sigmoid sinus
2	Dura mater of posterior cranial fossa
3	Facial nerve
4	Lateral semicircular canal
5	Chorda tympani
6	Tympanic membrane (upper part removed)

•The mastoid air cells are closely related to the sigmoid sinus (1) and posterior cranial fossa (2) posteromedially; above is the temporal lobe of the brain in the middle cranial fossa. The mastoid antrum and air cells can be approached surgically by opening up the bone through the suprameatal triangle (page 31, A13).

A

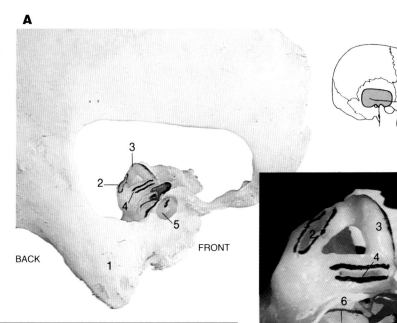

Dissections of the middle and inner ear in the right temporal bone. A and B from the right and above. C and D from the left, above and in front. B and D are enlarged views of A and C respectively

Auditory ossicles: dark blue = malleus; red = incus; green = stapes. Margins of opened semicircular canals and cochlea: black.

A and B are viewed as when looking slightly downwards at the right side of the skull from the outside, through a window cut in the temporal bone, with the back of the skull (and mastoid process, 1) towards the left (see the adjacent diagram). C and D are of the same specimen, viewed as when looking at the inside of the skull from the left, above and in front, with the back of the skull towards the right (see the adjacent diagram). Note the depth of the middle ear in relation to the mastoid process

BACK

FRONT

B

1 Mastoid process	9 Margins of auditory tube (mauve)
2 Posterior ⎫	10 Tensor tympani muscle
3 Anterior ⎬ semicircular canal	11 Cochleariform process
4 Lateral ⎭	12 Tendon of tensor tympani
5 Tympanic membrane and (dark blue) handle of	13 Cochlea
malleus	14 Cochlear part ⎫ of vestibulocochlear nerve
6 Facial nerve (yellow)	15 Vestibular part ⎭
7 Stapedius muscle	16 Internal acoustic meatus
8 Chorda tympani (purple)	17 Genicular ganglion of facial nerve

• The handle of the malleus is attached to the tympanic membrane (5).
• The chorda tympani (B8) passes between the fibrous and mucous layers of the tympanic membrane and crosses the handle of the malleus
• From the genicular ganglion (D17) the facial nerve passes backwards in its canal (at label 6 in B) above the promontory (page 65, B21) and then downwards (page 65, B19) in the medial wall of the aditus to reach the stylomastoid foramen.
• Distinguish between semicircular and cochlear canals, and semicircular and cochlear ducts: the canals are the spaces within bone and contain perilymph, while the ducts (containing endolymph) are membranous structures inside the canals and therefore surrounded by perilymph.

C

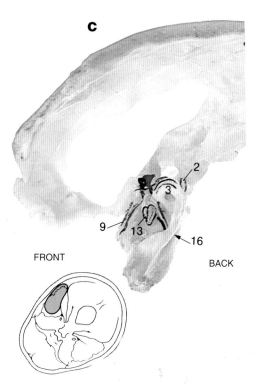

FRONT

BACK

D

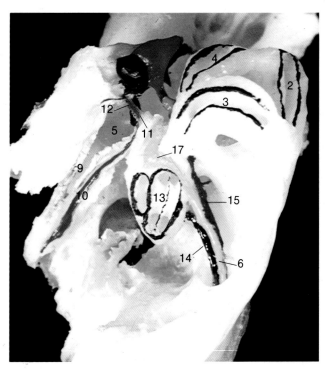

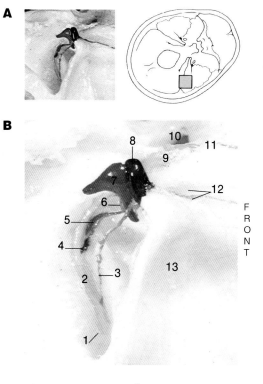

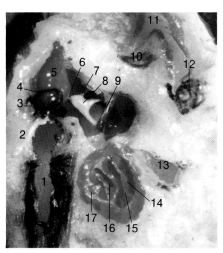

FRONT

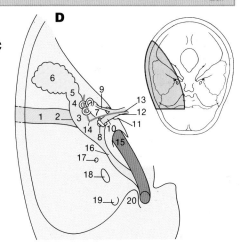

D

Right temporal bone. A Middle ear and the facial nerve and branches, B enlarged view of A

This dissection is seen from the right and above, looking forwards and medially. Bone has been removed to show the upper parts of the malleus (8) and incus (7), which normally project up into the epitympanic recess. The upper part of the facial canal (1) has been opened to show the facial nerve (2) giving off the chorda tympani (3) and the nerve to stapedius (4). The genicular ganglion of the facial nerve (9) is seen giving off the greater petrosal nerve (11)

1	Facial canal leading to stylomastoid foramen
2	Facial nerve
3	Chorda tympani
4	Nerve to stapedius
5	Stapedius
6	Stapes
7	Incus
8	Malleus
9	Genicular ganglion of facial nerve
10	Internal acoustic meatus
11	Greater petrosal nerve
12	Margin of auditory tube
13	Paraffin wax (for support) overlying tympanic membrane

• The stapedius (5) tendon emerges from a small conical projection on the posterior wall of the tympanic cavity, the pyramid (here dissected away).

C Right temporal bone. Middle ear and inner ear, enlarged

This dissection is viewed from above, looking slightly backwards and laterally. Within the cavity of the middle ear are the three auditory ossicles—malleus (3), incus (5) and stapes (8). The tympanic membrane and external acoustic meatus are not seen but lie below the label 4. The cochlea has been opened up to show its internal bony structure (14 to 17)

1	Auditory tube
2	Chorda tympani
3	Malleus
4	Incudomallear joint
5	Incus
6	Incudostapedial joint
7	Stapedius muscle
8	Stapes
9	Footplate of stapes in oval window of vestibule
10	Lateral ⎫
11	Posterior ⎬ semicircular canal
12	Anterior ⎭
13	Internal acoustic meatus
14	Bony canal ⎫
15	Osseous spiral lamina ⎬ of
16	Modiolus ⎬ cochlea
17	Cupola ⎭

• The spiral organ (the end organ of hearing) lies on the basilar membrane, which stretches between the free edge of the osseous spiral lamina (15) and the side of the bony cochlear canal.
• The modiolus (16) is the central axis of the cochlea, and the cupola (17) is its apex.

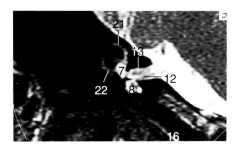

Right ear, from above, D diagram of parts, E MR image–high resolution

The schematic diagram of part of the right side of the base of the skull (D) indicates the position of the parts of the ear within the temporal bone. (The auditory ossicles have been omitted from the middle ear cavity, 3.) The external acoustic meatus (1) is at a right angle to the side of the skull, and the internal acoustic meatus (11) is level with it on the inner side of the temporal bone. The line (from front to back) of the auditory tube (16), middle ear cavity (3), mastoid antrum (4 and 5) and mastoid air cells (6) lies at about 60° to the line of the external meatus. The cochlear part of the inner ear (8) is in front of the vestibular part (7). The facial nerve (13) runs immediately above the vestibulocochlear nerve (12) and takes a right-angled turn backwards at the genicular ganglion (14) to pass below the lateral semicircular canal in the medial wall of the middle ear and then turns downwards in the medial wall of the aditus to the antrum (4) to reach the stylomastoid foramen. In the MR image note two of the semicircular canals (21, 22)

1	External acoustic meatus
2	Tympanic membrane
3	Middle ear
4	Aditus to mastoid antrum
5	Mastoid antrum
6	Mastoid air cells
7	Vestibular part of inner ear
8	Cochlear part of inner ear
9	Vestibular nerve
10	Cochlear nerve
11	Internal acoustic meatus
12	Vestibulocochlear nerve
13	Facial nerve
14	Genicular ganglion of facial nerve
15	Internal carotid artery emerging from foramen lacerum
16	Auditory tube
17	Foramen spinosum
18	Foramen ovale
19	Foramen rotundum
20	Anterior clinoid process
21	Anterior semicircular canal
22	Lateral semicircular canal

A Right ear, from the front

This schematic diagram shows a vertical section through the ear to indicate how the three auditory ossicles (malleus, incus and stapes—6, 7 and 8) bridge the tympanic cavity (4) so that vibrations of the tympanic membrane (2) are transmitted to the footplate of the stapes (9) in the oval window of the vestibule

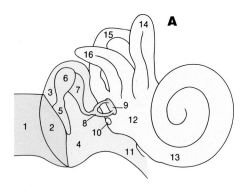

1	External acoustic meatus
2	Tympanic membrane
3	Epitympanic recess
4	Middle ear cavity
5	Handle of malleus
6	Body of malleus
7	Incus
8	Stapes
9	Footplate of stapes in oval window
10	Round window
11	Auditory tube
12	Vestibule
13	Cochlea
14	Anterior
15	Posterior } semicircular canal
16	Lateral

- The internal ear consists of the bony labyrinth and the membranous labyrinth
- The bony labyrinth is a space within the temporal bone (B) and consists of the vestibule, semicircular canals and cochlea (cochlear canal).
- The membranous labyrinth (C) is inside the bony labyrinth and consists of the utricle and saccule (within the vestibule), the semicircular ducts (within the semicircular canals) and the cochlear duct (within the cochlea).
- The membranous labyrinth contains endolymph and is separated from the walls of the bony labyrinth by perilymph. These two fluids do not communicate with one another, but the perilymph probably communicates with the subarachnoid space via the cochlear canaliculus (page 31, D23).

- The cochlear part of the ear is concerned with hearing.
- The vestibular part of the ear is concerned with balance (equilibrium).
- Vibrations of the footplate of the stapes in the oval window (A9, B9) cause vibrations in the perilymph of the cochlear canal (D1 and 2). This causes movement of the basilar membrane (D5) and stimulation of the hair cells on the surface of the spiral organ (D6), so causing impulses that proceed along the cochlear nerve (D9) to the brain for the sense of hearing.
- The round window (A10, B11) is closed by the secondary tympanic membrane, to prevent perilymph escaping from the cochlear canal. When the footplate of the stapes moves inwards, the secondary tympanic membrane moves outwards (to compensate for the increase of pressure in the perilymph) because the scala vestibuli and scala tympani parts of the cochlear canal (D1 and 2) are in continuity with one another at the apex of the cochlea.
- In the ampullae of the semicircular ducts (C1, 2 and 3) and in specialized areas (maculae) of the utricle and saccule (C4 and 8) there are receptors innervated by the vestibular nerve which respond to the movement of endolymph, so providing the basis for the sense of balance.

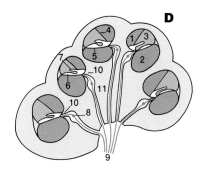

D Diagram of the cochlea

The basilar membrane (5) supports the spiral organ (6), which is supplied by fibres of the cochlear nerve (9) whose ganglion cells (8) lie within the petrous bone adjacent to the osseous spiral lamina (10)—the part of the cochlea that looks like the thread of a short fat screw (page 67, C15). For diagrammatic purposes, only one nerve fibre and ganglion cell is shown in each of the representative canals passing through the central part (modiolus, 11) of the osseous labyrinth. The basilar membrane (5) and the vestibular membrane (4) are part of the cochlear duct (3) of the membranous labyrinth, and the roughly triangular space between those two membranes is filled with endolymph. The outer wall of the cochlear duct (the third side of the triangle) lies against the wall of the osseous labyrinth without an intervening space, but there are spaces above and below the cochlear duct; these are the parts of the cochlear canal called the scala vestibuli (1) and scala tympani (2), and are filled with perilymph

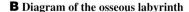

B Diagram of the osseous labyrinth

The drawing represents a cast of the space within the temporal bone. The central part is the vestibule (8) with the cochlea (12) at the front and the semicircular canals (2, 4 and 6) at the back. The beginning of the first turn of the cochlea (10) forms the promontory, between the oval window above and behind it (9) and the round window below and behind it (11). The promontory is one of the main features of the medial wall of the middle ear (see page 65, B21)

1	Ampulla of 2
2	Anterior semicircular canal
3	Common limb of 2 and 4
4	Posterior semicircular canal
5	Ampulla of 4
6	Lateral semicircular canal
7	Ampulla of 6
8	Vestibule
9	Oval window (fenestra vestibuli)
10	Promontory at base of first turn of cochlea
11	Round window (fenestra cochleae)
12	Cochlea (cochlear canal)

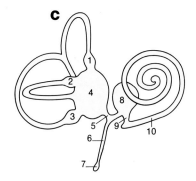

C Diagram of the membranous labyrinth

The utricle (4) and saccule (8) lie within the vestibule of the osseous labyrinth (B8), the cochlear duct (10) within the cochlea (B12), and the semicircular ducts (1, 2 and 3) within the semicircular canals (B2, 4 and 6). The endolymphatic duct (6) from the saccule (8) is joined by the utriculosaccular duct (5) from the utricle (4), and then runs in the aqueduct of the vestibule in the petrous part of the temporal bone (page 31, B21) to end under the dura mater there as the endolymphatic sac (7). The saccule (8) is connected to the cochlear duct (10) by the ductus reuniens (9)

1	Ampulla of anterior
2	Ampulla of lateral } semicircular duct
3	Ampulla of posterior
4	Utricle
5	Utriculosaccular duct
6	Endolymphatic duct
7	Endolymphatic sac
8	Saccule
9	Ductus reuniens
10	Cochlear duct

1	Scala vestibuli } of cochlear canal
2	Scala tympani } containing perilymph
3	Cochlear duct, containing endolymph
4	Vestibular membrane
5	Basilar membrane
6	Spiral organ
7	Tectorial membrane
8	Spiral (cochlear) ganglion
9	Filaments of cochlear nerve
10	Osseous spiral lamina
11	Modiolus

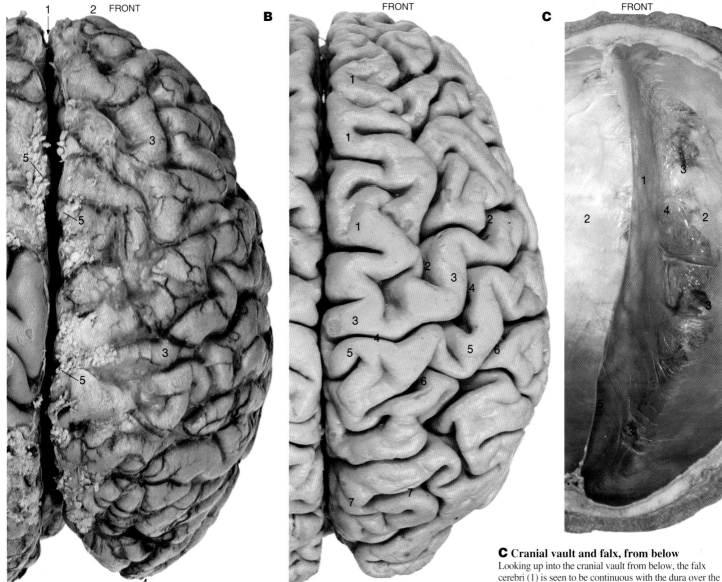

A
FRONT
1   2

B
FRONT

C
FRONT

A Brain, from above

The right cerebral hemisphere is seen with the overlying arachnoid mater and arachnoid granulations (5) adjacent to the longitudinal fissure (1). Over the small part of the left hemisphere shown, a window has been cut in the arachnoid

1	Longitudinal fissure	4	Occipital pole
2	Frontal pole	5	Arachnoid granulations
3	Superolateral surface		

- When removed from the cranial cavity the brain remains covered by the arachnoid mater, which collapses on to most of the brain surface. In life the arachnoid is slightly separated from the brain surface by the cerebrospinal fluid in the subarachnoid space. In some areas the gap is larger, forming the cerebrospinal cisterns, e.g. the cerebellomedullary cistern

B Right cerebral hemisphere, from above

Removal of the arachnoid and the underlying vessels displays the gyri and sulci. Only a small number are named here; the most important are the central sulcus (4) and the precentral and postcentral gyri (3 and 5)

1	Superior frontal gyrus	5	Postcentral gyrus
2	Precentral sulcus	6	Postcentral sulcus
3	Precentral gyrus	7	Parieto-occipital sulcus
4	Central sulcus		

(cisterna magna) between the cerebellum and medulla oblongata (as shown on page 50, A18).

- The cerebral arteries and veins that appear to be on the brain surface are within the subarachnoid space, i.e. between the arachnoid and the pia mater which adheres intimately to the brain surface.

C Cranial vault and falx, from below

Looking up into the cranial vault from below, the falx cerebri (1) is seen to be continuous with the dura over the vault (2), and has been cut off at the back (5) from the tentorium cerebelli. With the brain in place, the falx lies in the longitudinal fissure (A1) between the cerebral hemispheres (page 50), and the superior sagittal sinus (4) is within the dura at the top of the falx. The sinus receives superior cerebral veins (3 and page 70, A3) and is penetrated by the arachnoid granulations (A5) which make impressions on the bone (page 16, B2)

1	Falx cerebri	4	Superior sagittal sinus
2	Dura mater over cranial vault	5	Cut edge of falx cerebri
3	Superior cerebral veins		

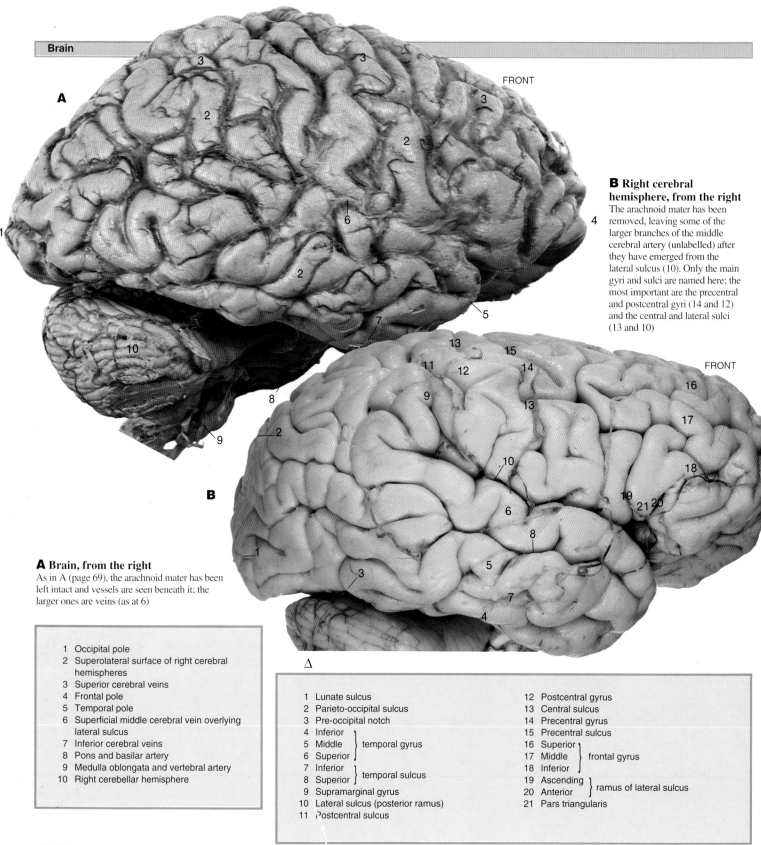

A

B

B Right cerebral hemisphere, from the right
The arachnoid mater has been removed, leaving some of the larger branches of the middle cerebral artery (unlabelled) after they have emerged from the lateral sulcus (10). Only the main gyri and sulci are named here; the most important are the precentral and postcentral gyri (14 and 12) and the central and lateral sulci (13 and 10)

FRONT

A Brain, from the right
As in A (page 69), the arachnoid mater has been left intact and vessels are seen beneath it; the larger ones are veins (as at 6)

1 Occipital pole
2 Superolateral surface of right cerebral hemispheres
3 Superior cerebral veins
4 Frontal pole
5 Temporal pole
6 Superficial middle cerebral vein overlying lateral sulcus
7 Inferior cerebral veins
8 Pons and basilar artery
9 Medulla oblongata and vertebral artery
10 Right cerebellar hemisphere

1 Lunate sulcus	12 Postcentral gyrus	
2 Parieto-occipital sulcus	13 Central sulcus	
3 Pre-occipital notch	14 Precentral gyrus	
4 Inferior ⎫	15 Precentral sulcus	
5 Middle ⎬ temporal gyrus	16 Superior ⎫	
6 Superior ⎭	17 Middle ⎬ frontal gyrus	
7 Inferior ⎫ temporal sulcus	18 Inferior ⎭	
8 Superior ⎭	19 Ascending ⎫ ramus of lateral sulcus	
9 Supramarginal gyrus	20 Anterior ⎭	
10 Lateral sulcus (posterior ramus)	21 Pars triangularis	
11 Postcentral sulcus		

• The brain consists of the forebrain (cerebrum, comprising the two cerebral hemispheres), the midbrain, and the hindbrain (comprising the pons, medulla oblongata and cerebellum).
• The midbrain, pons and medulla oblongata constitute the brainstem.
• The central sulcus (B4 (page 69) and B13 (above)) marks the boundary between the frontal and parietal lobes.
• An arbitrary line from the pre-occipital notch (B3) to the parieto-occipital sulcus (B2) marks the boundary between the

parietal and occipital lobes, and the part of the hemisphere in front of this line and below the lateral sulcus (strictly, the posterior ramus of the lateral sulcus, B10) forms the temporal lobe.
• The precentral and postcentral gyri (B14 and 12) contain the classically described 'motor' and 'sensory' areas of the cortex.
• The motor speech areas (usually in the left cerebral hemisphere)

are in the region of the ascending and anterior rami of the lateral sulcus and the pars triangularis (B19 to 21).
• The auditory areas of the cortex probably comprise parts of the superior temporal gyrus (B6), especially the upper surface of it within the lateral sulcus (B10).

C Brain, from below

This is the view of the under-surface of the brain as typically seen when first removed from the skull, without any dissection. Arachnoid mater, torn in places and with blood vessels beneath it, remains on the outer surface

1 Inferior surface of frontal lobe
2 Frontal pole
3 Longitudinal fissure
4 Gyrus rectus
5 Olfactory bulb
6 Olfactory tract
7 Anterior perforated substance
8 Optic nerve
9 Optic chiasma
10 Pituitary stalk (infundibulum)
11 Internal carotid artery
12 Posterior communicating artery
13 Oculomotor nerve
14 Crus of cerebral peduncle (midbrain)
15 Basilar artery
16 Pons
17 Trigeminal nerve
18 Abducent nerve
19 Facial nerve
20 Vestibulocochlear nerve
21 Vertebral artery
22 Medulla oblongata
23 Spinal part of accessory nerve
24 Cerebellar hemisphere
25 Inferior surface of temporal lobe
26 Uncus
27 Arachnoid mater overlying mamillary bodies
28 Temporal pole

D Optic tract and geniculate bodies, from below

The brainstem has been mostly removed, leaving only the upper part of the midbrain. The most medial parts of each cerebral hemisphere have also been dissected away. To find the geniculate bodies (15 and 16), which are on the under-surface of the posterior part (pulvinar, 17) of the thalamus, identify the optic chiasma (4) and then follow the optic tract (9) backwards round the side of the midbrain (10)

1 Olfactory tract
2 Anterior perforated substance
3 Optic nerve
4 Optic chiasma
5 Pituitary stalk (infundibulum)
6 Tuber cinereum
7 Mamillary body
8 Posterior perforated substance
9 Optic tract
10 Crus ⎫
11 Substantia nigra ⎪
12 Tegmentum ⎬ of midbrain
13 Tectum ⎪
14 Aqueduct ⎭
15 Lateral ⎫ geniculate body
16 Medial ⎭
17 Pulvinar of thalamus
18 Splenium of corpus callosum

• The lateral geniculate body is part of the visual pathway.
• The medial geniculate body is part of the acoustic pathway.

FRONT

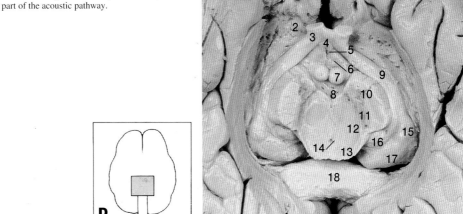

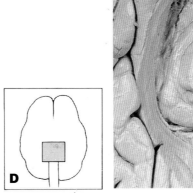

FRONT

A

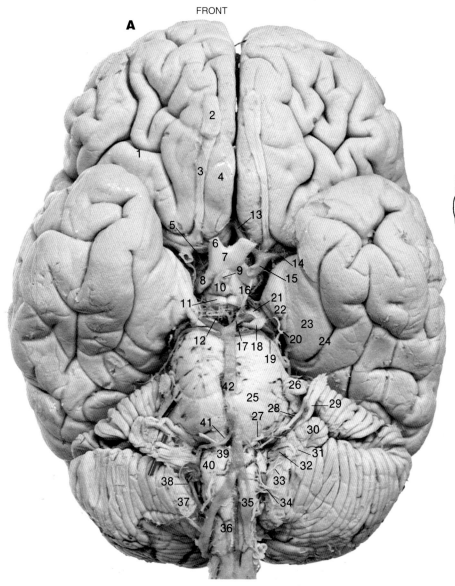

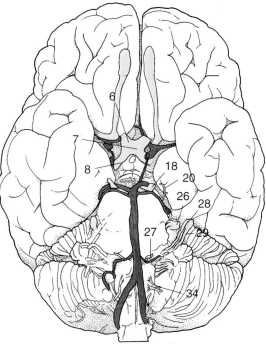

A Brain, from below

After removal of the arachnoid mater the cranial nerves and the major blood vessels can be identified. The basilar artery (42) overlies the pons (25), and its terminal branches (the posterior cerebral arteries, 17) take part in the formation of the arterial circle (see page 75, E), whose other components are derived from the internal carotid arteries (15). The olfactory bulb (2) leads backwards into the olfactory tract (3), behind which is the anterior perforated substance (5). The pituitary stalk (9) is behind the optic chiasma (7), and the posterior perforated substance (12) is behind the mamillary bodies (11). For further details of the cranial nerves see page 74, B, and the notes on page 61

1 Orbital sulcus	17 Posterior cerebral artery
2 Olfactory bulb	18 Oculomotor nerve
3 Olfactory tract	19 Superior cerebellar artery
4 Gyrus rectus	20 Trochlear nerve
5 Anterior perforated substance	21 Crus of cerebral peduncle
6 Optic nerve	22 Uncus
7 Optic chiasma	23 Parahippocampal gyrus
8 Optic tract	24 Collateral sulcus
9 Pituitary stalk (infundibulum)	25 Pons
10 Tuber cinereum and median eminence	26 Trigeminal nerve
11 Mamillary body	27 Abducent nerve
12 Posterior perforated substance	28 Facial nerve
13 Anterior cerebral artery	29 Vestibulocochlear nerve
14 Middle cerebral artery	30 Flocculus of cerebellum
15 Internal carotid artery	31 Choroid plexus from lateral recess of fourth
16 Posterior communicating artery	ventricle

32 Roots of glossopharyngeal, vagus and accessory nerves
33 Spinal part of accessory nerve
34 Rootlets of hypoglossal nerve (superficial to marker)
35 Vertebral artery
36 Medulla oblongata
37 Tonsil of cerebellum
38 Posterior inferior cerebellar artery
39 Pyramid } of medulla oblongata
40 Olive
41 Anterior inferior cerebellar artery
42 Basilar artery

• A blue marker has been placed behind the right flocculus and the overlying facial and vestibulocochlear nerves (labelled 30, 28 and 29 on the left side).

• A red marker has been placed behind the roots of the right glossopharyngeal, vagus and accessory nerves (labelled 32 on the left side).

B Right half of the brain, in a midline sagittal section, from the left

In this typical half-section of the brain, the medial surface of the right cerebral hemisphere is seen, together with the sectioned brainstem (midbrain, 18 to 21, pons, 16, and medulla oblongata, 13). The septum pellucidum, which is a midline structure and whose cut edge (28) is seen below the body of the corpus callosum (4), has been removed to show the interior of the body of the lateral ventricle (29). The third ventricle has the thalamus (30) and hypothalamus (33) in its lateral wall, while in its floor from front to back are the optic chiasma (38), the base of the pituitary stalk (37), the median eminence (36), the mamillary bodies (35), and the posterior perforated substance (34)

FRONT

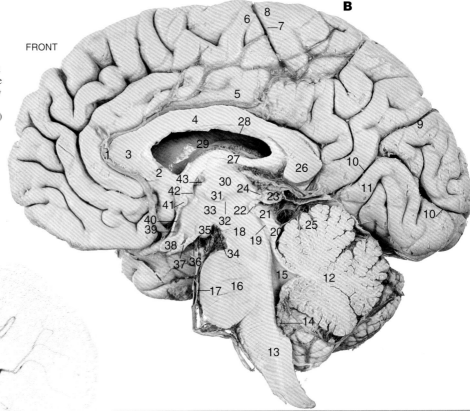

C Digitally subtracted arterial phase of carotid arteriogram, lateral projection

1	Anterior cerebral artery
2	Pericallosal artery
3	Middle cerebral artery
4	Ophthalmic artery
5	Internal carotid artery
6	Frontopolar artery
7	Posterior communicating artery

1	Anterior cerebral artery	24	Suprapineal recess
2	Rostrum	25	Great cerebral vein
3	Genu } of corpus callosum	26	Splenium of corpus callosum
4	Body	27	Fornix
5	Cingulate gyrus	28	Cut edge of septum pellucidum
6	Precentral gyrus	29	Body of lateral ventricle
7	Central sulcus	30	Thalamus
8	Postcentral gyrus	31	Interthalamic connexion
9	Parieto-occipital sulcus	32	Hypothalamic sulcus
10	Calcarine sulcus	33	Hypothalamus
11	Lingual gyrus	34	Posterior perforated substance
12	Cerebellum	35	Mamillary body
13	Medulla oblongata	36	Tuber cinereum and median eminence
14	Median aperture of fourth ventricle	37	Infundibular recess (base of pituitary stalk)
15	Fourth ventricle	38	Optic chiasma
16	Pons	39	Supra-optic recess
17	Basilar artery	40	Lamina terminalis
18	Tegmentum	41	Anterior commissure
19	Aqueduct } of midbrain	42	Anterior column of fornix
20	Inferior colliculus	43	Interventricular foramen and choroid plexus
21	Superior colliculus		
22	Posterior commissure		
23	Pineal body		

- The third ventricle is the cavity which has in its lateral wall the thalamus (B30) and hypothalamus (B33).
- The fourth ventricle (B15) is largely between the pons (B16) and cerebellum (B12), although its lower end is behind the upper part of the medulla oblongata (B13) (see page 76, A).
- The aqueduct of the midbrain (B19) connects the third and fourth ventricles; cerebrospinal fluid normally flows through it from the third to the fourth ventricle.

- The interventricular foramen (B43) connects the third to the lateral ventricle, and is bounded in front by the anterior column of the fornix (B42) and behind by the thalamus (B30).
- The median eminence (B36) in the floor of the third ventricle is of great importance as the site of the neurosecretory cells whose products are released into the portal system of pituitary blood vessels (hypophysial portal system) and which control the secretion of anterior pituitary hormones.

- Posterior pituitary hormones are manufactured by cells of the supra-optic and paraventricular nuclei in the lateral wall of the hypothalamus (B33). The axons of these cells pass down the whole length of the pituitary stalk into the posterior part of the gland; the hormones are stored within the axons.

73

FRONT

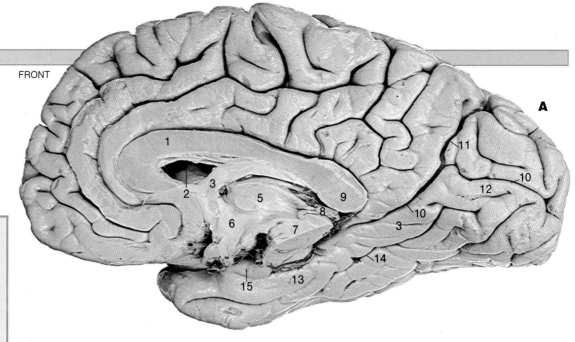

A Medial surface of the right cerebral hemisphere
The brainstem has been removed through the midbrain (7) so that the lower part of the hemisphere can be seen; in B, on page 73, the brainstem hides this part

1 Corpus callosum
2 Anterior horn of lateral ventricle
3 Anterior column of fornix
4 Interventricular foramen
5 Thalamus ⎫ in lateral wall
6 Hypo- ⎬ of third
   thalamus ⎭ ventricle
7 Midbrain
8 Pineal body
9 Splenium of corpus callosum
10 Calcarine sulcus
11 Parieto-occipital sulcus
12 Lingual gyrus
13 Parahippocampal gyrus
14 Collateral sulcus
15 Uncus

B Cranial nerves
In this ventral view of the central part of the brain, the right vertebral artery (on the left of the picture) has been removed almost at the junction with its fellow (21). The twelve cranial nerves on the right side are identified by their official numbers, although of course the filaments of the first nerve (olfactory) are not seen entering the olfactory bulb (1) as they are torn off when removing the brain. The roots forming the glossopharyngeal, vagus and accessory nerves (9, 10 and 11) cannot be clearly identified from one another, but the spinal part of the accessory nerve (11) is seen running up beside the medulla to join the cranial part (see the note on page 43)

1 Olfactory bulb	13 Pituitary stalk
2 Optic nerve	14 Internal carotid artery
3 Oculomotor nerve	15 Posterior communicating artery
4 Trochlear nerve	16 Posterior cerebral artery
5 Trigeminal nerve	17 Crus of cerebral peduncle
6 Abducent nerve	18 Superior cerebellar artery
7 Facial nerve	19 Basilar artery
8 Vestibulocochlear nerve	20 Pons
9 Glossopharyngeal nerve	21 Vertebral artery
10 Vagus nerve	22 Pyramid ⎫ of medulla
11 Accessory nerve	23 Olive ⎬ oblongata
12 Hypoglossal nerve	

B

FRONT

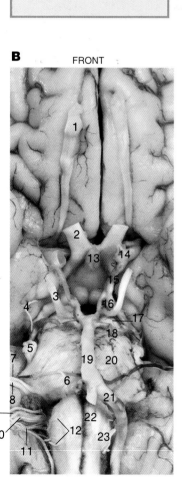

• The oculomotor nerve (B3) emerges on the *medial* side of the crus of the cerebral peduncle (B17), and the trochlear nerve (B4) winds round the *lateral* side of the peduncle. Both nerves pass between the posterior cerebral and superior cerebellar arteries (B16 and 18).
• The trochlear nerve (C4) is the only cranial nerve to emerge from the *dorsal* surface of the brainstem (from the midbrain, behind the inferior colliculus, C3).
• The trigeminal nerve (B5) emerges from the lateral side of the pons (B20).
• The abducent nerve (B6) emerges between the pons and the pyramid (B20 and 22).
• The facial and vestibulocochlear nerves (B7 and 8) emerge from the lateral pontomedullary angle.
• The glossopharyngeal and vagus nerves and the cranial root of the accessory nerve (B9, 10, 11) emerge from the medulla oblongata lateral to the olive (B23).
• The hypoglossal nerve (B12) emerges as two series of rootlets from the medulla oblongata between the pyramid (B22) and the olive (B23).
• The spinal part of the accessory nerve emerges from the lateral surface of the upper five or six cervical segments of the spinal cord, dorsal to the denticulate ligament (page 76, B5).

C Roof of the fourth ventricle
In this dorsal view of the brainstem, the cerebellum has been removed by cutting through the cerebellar peduncles (6 to 8), but the pia mater and ependyma (10) forming the posterior part of the roof of the fourth ventricle have been preserved. The anterior part of the roof is the superior medullary velum (5)

1 Pulvinar of thalamus
2 Superior colliculus
3 Inferior colliculus
4 Trochlear nerve
5 Superior medullary velum and lingula of cerebellum
6 Superior ⎫ cerebellar
7 Middle ⎬ peduncle
8 Inferior ⎭
9 Nodule of cerebellum
10 Pia mater and ependyma of roof of fourth ventricle
11 Median aperture
12 Lateral recess

• The median aperture (C11) in the posterior part of the roof of the fourth ventricle and the two lateral apertures (in the lateral recess of each side, C12) are the only sites of communication between the ventricular system and the subarachnoid space.

FRONT **C**

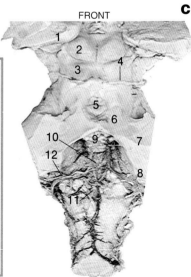

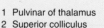

1 Anterior choroidal
2 Middle cerebral
3 Internal carotid
4 Anterior cerebral
5 Anterior communicating
6 Optic nerve
7 Olfactory tract
8 Posterior communicating
9 Posterior cerebral
10 Oculomotor nerve
11 Superior cerebellar
12 Basilar with pontine branches
13 Pons
14 Trigeminal nerve
15 Anterior inferior cerebellar
16 Abducent nerve
17 Pyramid
18 Olive
19 Unusually large branch of 15 overlying facial and vestibulocochlear nerves
20 Filaments of glossopharyngeal, vagus and accessory nerves
21 Vertebral
22 Posterior inferior cerebellar
23 Spinal cord
24 Spinal part of accessory nerve
25 Rootlets of first cervical nerve
26 Anterior spinal
27 Medulla oblongata

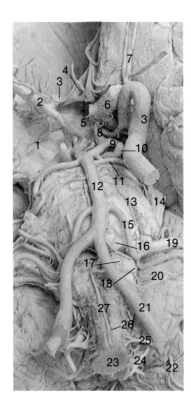

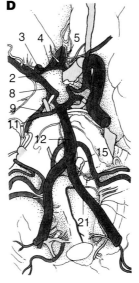

D

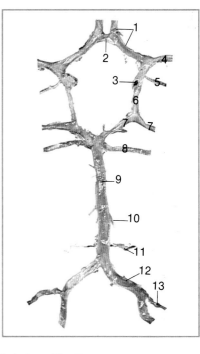

D Injected arteries of the base of the brain
Part of the right cerebral hemisphere (on the left of the picture) has been removed to show the right middle cerebral artery (2)

E

E Arterial circle and basilar artery
The anastomosing vessels have been removed from the base of the brain and spread out in their relative positions

1 Anterior cerebral	8 Superior cerebellar
2 Anterior communicating	9 Basilar
3 Internal carotid	10 Labyrinthine
4 Middle cerebral	11 Anterior inferior cerebellar
5 Anterior choroidal	12 Vertebral
6 Posterior communicating	13 Posterior inferior cerebellar
7 Posterior cerebral	

• The internal carotid artery (E3) gives off the anterior cerebral (E1) which passes forwards and medially to join its fellow by the anterior communicating artery (E2). The middle cerebral (E4) passes laterally from the carotid and the posterior communicating (E6) passes backwards to join the posterior cerebral (E7) which is the terminal branch of the basilar artery (E9).
• The basilar artery (E9) is formed by the union of the two vertebrals (E12).

F

F Brainstem and cerebellum in sagittal section, from the left
The left half of the cerebellum has been removed by sagittal section in the midline and by transecting the left cerebellar peduncles (9 to 11)

BACK

• The central part of the cerebellum constitutes the vermis (nodule, uvula and pyramid—F20, 19 and 17), which is continuous laterally with the hemispheres.
• The folia of the cerebellar cortex are considerably narrower than the gyri of the cerebral cortex.
• The largest of the subcortical nuclei of the cerebellar hemisphere is the dentate nucleus, whose axons constitute the main efferent pathway from the cerebellum and leave in the superior peduncle.

1 Pons	9 Superior ⎫	17 Pyramid of vermis	25 Roots of glossopharyngeal, vagus and accessory nerves
2 Trigeminal nerve	10 Middle ⎬ cerebellar peduncle	18 Postpyramidal fissure	
3 Superior cerebellar artery	11 Inferior ⎭	19 Uvula	26 Olive
4 Trochlear nerve	12 Superior medullary velum	20 Nodule	27 Rootlets of hypoglossal nerve
5 Basal cerebral vein	13 Lingula	21 Tonsil	28 Pyramid of medulla oblongata
6 Crus of cerebral peduncle	14 Anterior lobe	22 Fourth ventricle	29 Abducent nerve
7 Posterior cerebral artery	15 Primary fissure	23 Choroid plexus in lateral recess	30 Facial and vestibulocochlear nerves
8 Inferior colliculus	16 Prepyramidal fissure	24 Medulla oblongata	

A Brainstem and floor of the fourth ventricle

In this view of the dorsal surface of the brainstem, it has been cut off from the rest of the brain at the top of the midbrain, just above the superior colliculi (1). The cerebellum has been removed by transecting the superior (17), middle (16) and inferior (15) cerebellar peduncles

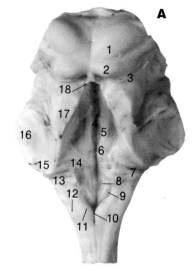

A

1 Superior colliculus	8 Hypoglossal triangle	15 Inferior
2 Inferior colliculus	9 Vagal triangle	16 Middle } cerebellar peduncle
3 Trochlear nerve	10 Obex	17 Superior
4 Median sulcus	11 Gracile tubercle	18 Cut edge of superior medullary
5 Medial eminence	12 Cuneate tubercle	velum
6 Facial colliculus	13 Lateral recess	
7 Medullary striae	14 Vestibular area	

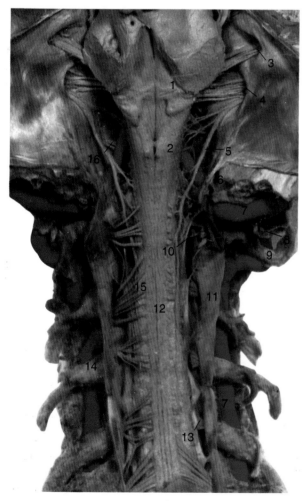

B Brainstem and upper part of the spinal cord, from behind

The posterior part of the skull, the cerebellum and vertebral arches have been removed, and the meninges have been dissected away to show the medulla oblongata (2) passing through the foramen magnum to become continuous with the spinal cord (12). The vertebral artery (7), after passing up through the foramina in the transverse processes of the cervical vertebrae, runs horizontally on the posterior arch of the atlas before entering the foramen magnum (6). In the skull the spinal part of the accessory nerve (5) is behind the artery; at the side of the spinal cord it lies between cervical nerve dorsal rootlets (as at 15; many of which have been removed on the right) and the denticulate ligament (10)

1	Pons	9 Lateral part of axis
2	Medulla oblongata	10 Denticulate ligament
3	Facial and vestibulocochlear nerves and internal acoustic meatus	11 Dura and arachnoid mater (turned laterally)
4	Glossopharyngeal, vagus and accessory nerves and jugular foramen	12 Spinal cord
		13 Ventral root of fifth cervical nerve
5	Spinal part of accessory nerve	14 Dorsal root ganglion of fourth cervical nerve in meningeal sheath
6	Margin of foramen magnum	15 Dorsal rootlets of third cervical nerve
7	Vertebral artery	16 Roots of hypoglossal nerve
8	Dorsal ramus of first cervical nerve	

● The medulla oblongata passes through the foramen magnum of the skull (B6); the spinal cord begins at the level of the atlas vertebra, i.e. where the first cervical nerve rootlets emerge from the side of the cord.

● The lower part of the diamond-shaped floor of the fourth ventricle containing the hypoglossal and vagal triangles (A8 and 9) is part of the medulla oblongata; the rest of the floor is part of the pons.

● The gracile and cuneate tubercles (A11 and 12) are caused by the underlying gracile and cuneate nuclei, where the fibres of the gracile and cuneate tracts (posterior white columns) end by synapsing with the cells of the nuclei. The fibres from these cells form the medial lemniscus which runs through the brainstem to the thalamus.

● The facial colliculus (A6), at the lower end of the medial eminence (A5) in the floor of the fourth ventricle, is caused by fibres of the facial nerve overlying the abducent nerve nucleus; it is not produced by the facial nerve nucleus, which lies at a deeper level in the pons.

● After emerging from the foramen in the transverse process of the atlas the vertebral artery (B7) winds backwards round the lateral mass of the atlas on its posterior arch before turning upwards to enter the skull.

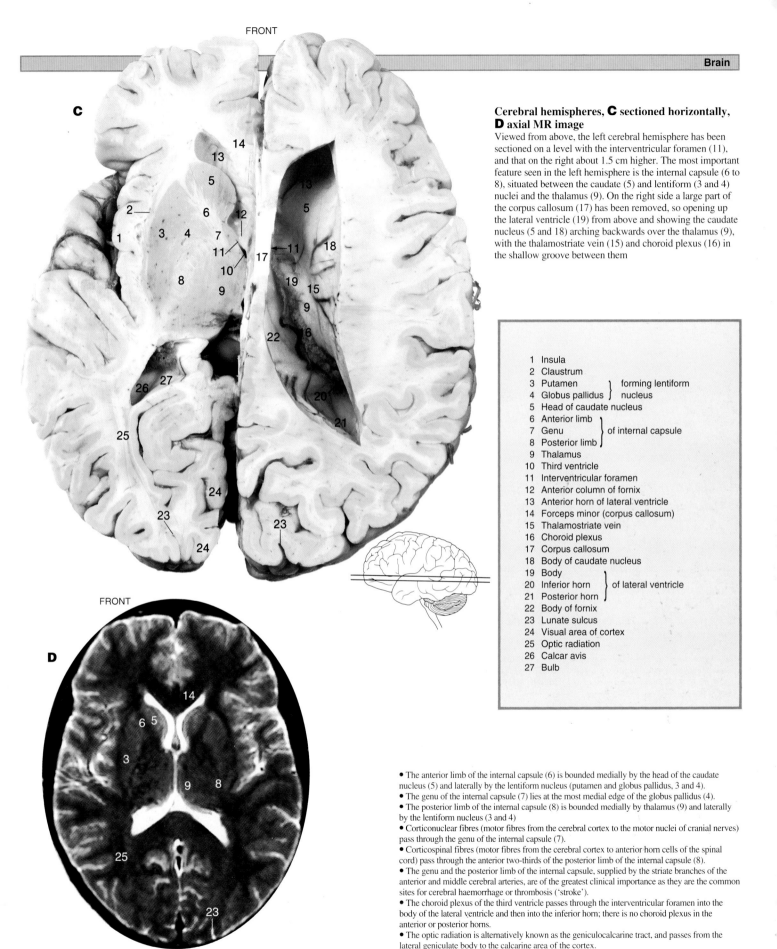

C

14
13
5
2
6
1 12
3 4 7
11
10
8
9

13
5
18
11
17
19
15
9
6
22
20
21

26 27
25
24
23
24
23
24

Cerebral hemispheres, C sectioned horizontally, D axial MR image

Viewed from above, the left cerebral hemisphere has been sectioned on a level with the interventricular foramen (11), and that on the right about 1.5 cm higher. The most important feature seen in the left hemisphere is the internal capsule (6 to 8), situated between the caudate (5) and lentiform (3 and 4) nuclei and the thalamus (9). On the right side a large part of the corpus callosum (17) has been removed, so opening up the lateral ventricle (19) from above and showing the caudate nucleus (5 and 18) arching backwards over the thalamus (9), with the thalamostriate vein (15) and choroid plexus (16) in the shallow groove between them

1	Insula
2	Claustrum
3	Putamen ⎫ forming lentiform
4	Globus pallidus ⎬ nucleus
5	Head of caudate nucleus
6	Anterior limb ⎫
7	Genu ⎬ of internal capsule
8	Posterior limb ⎭
9	Thalamus
10	Third ventricle
11	Interventricular foramen
12	Anterior column of fornix
13	Anterior horn of lateral ventricle
14	Forceps minor (corpus callosum)
15	Thalamostriate vein
16	Choroid plexus
17	Corpus callosum
18	Body of caudate nucleus
19	Body ⎫
20	Inferior horn ⎬ of lateral ventricle
21	Posterior horn ⎭
22	Body of fornix
23	Lunate sulcus
24	Visual area of cortex
25	Optic radiation
26	Calcar avis
27	Bulb

FRONT

D

14
6 5
3
9 8
25
23

• The anterior limb of the internal capsule (6) is bounded medially by the head of the caudate nucleus (5) and laterally by the lentiform nucleus (putamen and globus pallidus, 3 and 4).
• The genu of the internal capsule (7) lies at the most medial edge of the globus pallidus (4).
• The posterior limb of the internal capsule (8) is bounded medially by thalamus (9) and laterally by the lentiform nucleus (3 and 4)
• Corticonuclear fibres (motor fibres from the cerebral cortex to the motor nuclei of cranial nerves) pass through the genu of the internal capsule (7).
• Corticospinal fibres (motor fibres from the cerebral cortex to anterior horn cells of the spinal cord) pass through the anterior two-thirds of the posterior limb of the internal capsule (8).
• The genu and the posterior limb of the internal capsule, supplied by the striate branches of the anterior and middle cerebral arteries, are of the greatest clinical importance as they are the common sites for cerebral haemorrhage or thrombosis ('stroke').
• The choroid plexus of the third ventricle passes through the interventricular foramen into the body of the lateral ventricle and then into the inferior horn; there is no choroid plexus in the anterior or posterior horns.
• The optic radiation is alternatively known as the geniculocalcarine tract, and passes from the lateral geniculate body to the calcarine area of the cortex.

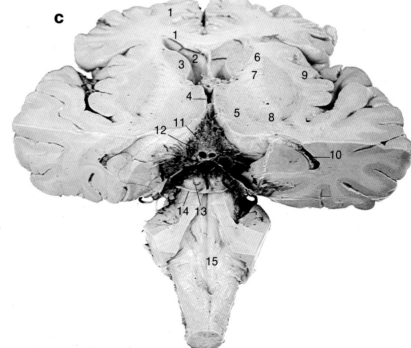

Brain, A coronal section, from the front, B coronal MR image

This coronal section is not quite vertical but passes slightly backwards, through the third ventricle (14) and bodies of the lateral ventricles (7) from a level about 0.5 cm behind the interventricular foramina, and down through the pons (22) and the pyramid of the medulla (23). It has been cut in this way to show the path of the important corticospinal (motor) fibres passing down through the internal capsule (4) and pons (22) to form the pyramid of the the medulla (23). Compare with features in the MR image

1 Insula
2 Putamen ⎫
3 Globus pallidus ⎬ lentiform nucleus
4 Internal capsule
5 Body of caudate nucleus
6 Corpus callosum
7 Body of lateral ventricle
8 Septum pellucidum
9 Body of fornix
10 Choroid plexus of lateral ventricle
11 Choroid plexus of third ventricle
12 Thalamostriate vein
13 Thalamus
14 Third ventricle
15 Interpeduncular cistern
16 Choroidal fissure
17 Optic tract
18 Choroid plexus of inferior horn of lateral ventricle
19 Tail of caudate nucleus
20 Hippocampus
21 Posterior cerebral artery
22 Pons
23 Pyramid ⎫
24 Olive ⎬ of medulla oblongata
25 Substantia nigra

C Sectioned cerebral hemispheres and the brainstem, from above and behind

The cerebral hemispheres have been sectioned horizontally just above the level of the interventricular foramina, and the posterior parts of the hemispheres have been removed, together with the whole of the cerebellum, to show the tela choroidea (11) of the posterior part of the roof of the third ventricle and the underlying internal cerebral veins (12)

1 Forceps minor
2 Anterior horn of lateral ventricle
3 Head of caudate nucleus
4 Third ventricle
5 Thalamus
6 Anterior limb ⎫
7 Genu ⎬ of internal capsule
8 Posterior limb ⎭
9 Insula
10 Choroid plexus and junction of inferior and posterior horn of lateral ventricle
11 Tela choroidea of roof of third ventricle
12 Internal cerebral vein
13 Inferior colliculus
14 Trochlear nerve
15 Floor of fourth ventricle

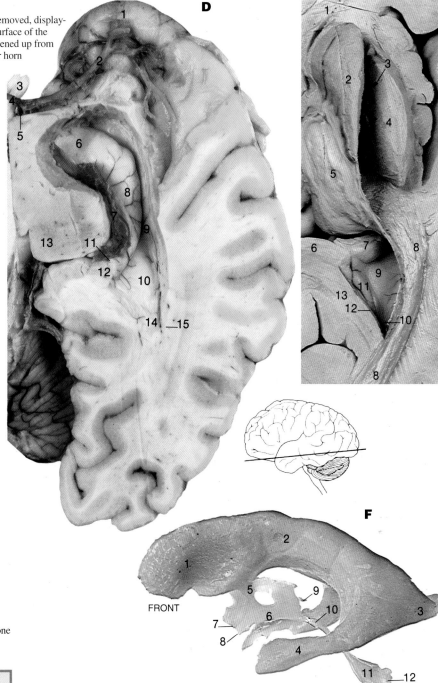

D Inferior horn of right lateral ventricle

Brain substance above the front part of the lateral sulcus has been removed, displaying the middle cerebral artery (2) running laterally over the upper surface of the front of the temporal lobe (1). Part of the temporal lobe has been opened up from above to show the hippocampus (6 and 8) in the floor of the inferior horn

1 Temporal pole of temporal lobe	7 Choroid plexus
2 Middle cerebral artery	8 Hippocampus
	9 Collateral eminence
3 Optic nerve	10 Collateral trigone
4 Anterior cerebral artery	11 Fimbria
	12 Fornix
5 Anterior choroidal artery	13 Thalamus
	14 Posterior horn
6 Pes hippocampi	15 Tapetum

E Dissection of the right cerebral hemisphere, from above

Much of the cerebral substance has been dissected away to show the caudate nucleus (2), thalamus (5) and lentiform nucleus (4). The intervening gap (3) is occupied by the internal capsule. The optic radiation (8) has also been dissected out; it runs backwards lateral to the posterior horn of the lateral ventricle. Compare this three-dimensional view of these structures with the brain sections on page 78

1 Forceps minor	8 Optic radiation
2 Caudate nucleus	9 Collateral trigone
3 Internal capsule	10 Posterior horn of lateral ventricle
4 Lentiform nucleus	
5 Thalamus	11 Calcar avis
6 Splenium of corpus callosum	12 Bulb
	13 Forceps major
7 Fornix	

F Cast of the cerebral ventricles, from the left

In this side view the left lateral ventricle largely overlaps the right one

1 Anterior horn	
2 Body	of lateral ventricle
3 Posterior horn	
4 Inferior horn	
5 Interventricular foramen	
6 Third ventricle (with gap for interthalamic connexion)	
7 Supra-optic	
8 Infundibular	recess of third ventricle
9 Suprapineal	
10 Aqueduct of midbrain	
11 Fourth ventricle	
12 Lateral recess	

● The third ventricle (F6) communicates at its upper front end with each lateral ventricle through the interventricular foramen (F5).
● The main part of the lateral ventricle is the body (F2). The part in front of the interventricular foramen (F5) is the anterior horn (F1) which extends into the frontal lobe of the brain. At its posterior end the body divides into the posterior horn (F3, D14 and E10) which extends backwards into the occipital lobe, and the inferior horn (F4) which passes downwards and forwards into the temporal lobe.
● The lower posterior part of the third ventricle (F6) communicates with the fourth ventricle (F11) through the aqueduct of the midbrain (F10).
● The floor of the inferior horn consists of the hippocampus (D6 and 8) medially and the collateral eminence (D9) laterally. At its junction with the posterior horn (D14 and E10) the eminence broadens into the collateral trigone (D10, E9).
● The collateral eminence (D9) is produced by the inward projection of the collateral sulcus (page 74, A14).
● In the medial wall of the posterior horn, the bulb (E12) is produced by fibres of the corpus callosum, and the calcar avis (E11) by the inward projection of the calcarine sulcus (page 74, A10).

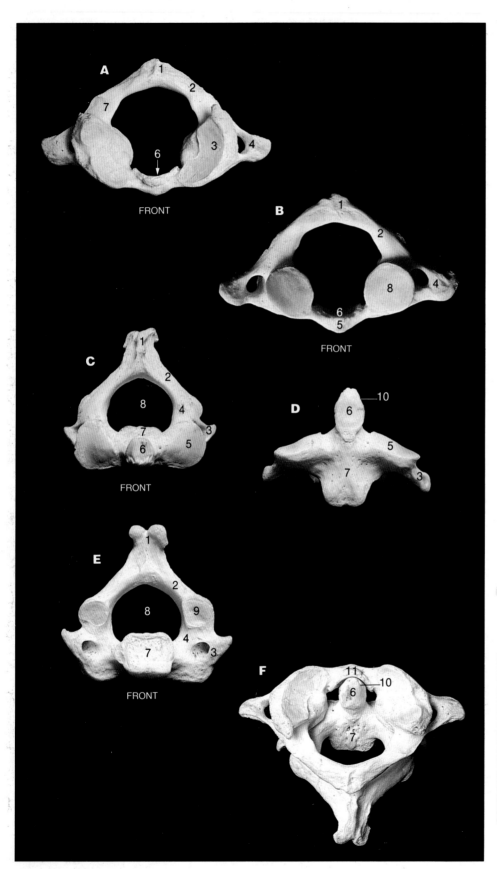

FRONT

FRONT

FRONT

FRONT

Atlas (first cervical vertebra), A from above, B from below

1	Posterior tubercle
2	Posterior arch
3	Lateral mass with superior articular facet
4	Transverse process and foramen
5	Anterior arch and tubercle
6	Facet for dens of axis
7	Groove for vertebral artery
8	Lateral mass with inferior articular facet

- The superior articular facets (3) are concave and kidney-shaped.
- The inferior articular facets (8) are round and almost flat.
- The anterior arch (5) is straighter and shorter than the posterior arch (2), and contains on its posterior surface the facet for the dens of the axis (6).
- The atlas is the only vertebra that has no body.

Axis (second cervical vertebra), C from above, D from the front, E from below, F articulated with the atlas, from above and behind

1	Bifid spinous process
2	Lamina
3	Transverse process and foramen
4	Pedicle
5	Superior articular surface
6	Dens
7	Body
8	Vertebral foramen
9	Inferior articular process
10	Impression for alar ligament
11	Anterior arch of atlas

- The axis is unique in having the dens (6) which projects upwards from the body, and represents the body of the atlas.

Fifth cervical vertebra (a typical cervical vertebra), **A** from above, **B** from the front, **C** from the left

1   Bifid spinous process
2   Lamina
3   Superior articular process
4   Posterior tubercle
5   Intertubercular lamella ⎫
6   Anterior tubercle   ⎬ of transverse process
7   Foramen   ⎭
8   Body
9   Posterolateral lip (uncus)
10 Pedicle
11 Vertebral foramen
12 Inferior articular process

D Seventh cervical vertebra (vertebra prominens), from above

1   Spinous process with tubercle
2   Lamina
3   Superior articular process
4   Posterior tubercle
5   Intertubercular lamella ⎫
6   Anterior tubercle   ⎬ of transverse process
7   Foramen   ⎭
8   Posterolateral lip (uncus)
9   Body
10 Pedicle
11 Vertebral foramen

• All cervical vertebrae (first to seventh) have a foramen in each transverse process (as A7).
• Typical cervical vertebrae (third to sixth) have superior articular processes that face backwards and upwards (A3, C3), posterolateral lips on the upper surface of the body (A9), a triangular vertebral foramen (A11) and a bifid spinous process (A1).
• The anterior tubercle of the transverse process of the sixth cervical vertebra is large and known as the carotid tubercle.
• The seventh cervical vertebra (vertebra prominens) has a spinous process that ends in a single tubercle (D1).
• The rib element of a cervical vertebra is represented by the anterior root of the transverse process, the anterior tubercle, the intertubercular lamella (with groove for the ventral ramus of a spinal nerve), and the anterior part of the posterior tubercle (as at D6, 5 and 4).

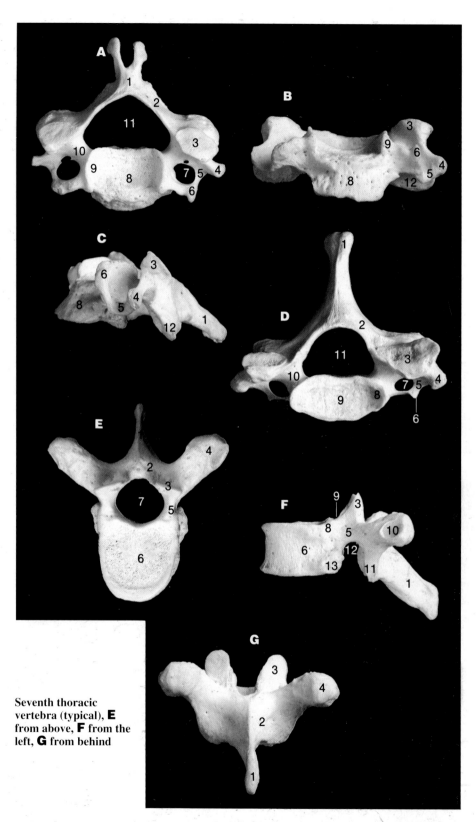

1 Spinous process	9	Superior vertebral notch
2 Lamina	10	Costal facet of transverse process
3 Superior articular process	11	Inferior articular process
4 Transverse process	12	Inferior vertebral notch
5 Pedicle	13	Inferior costal facet
6 Body		
7 Vertebral foramen		
8 Superior costal facet		

Seventh thoracic vertebra (typical), **E** from above, **F** from the left, **G** from behind

• Typical thoracic vertebrae (second to ninth) are characterized by costal facets on the bodies (F8, 13), costal facets on the transverse processes (F10), a round vertebral foramen (E7), a spinous process that points downwards as well as backwards (F1, G1), and superior articular processes that are vertical, flat and face backwards and laterally (E3, F3, G3).

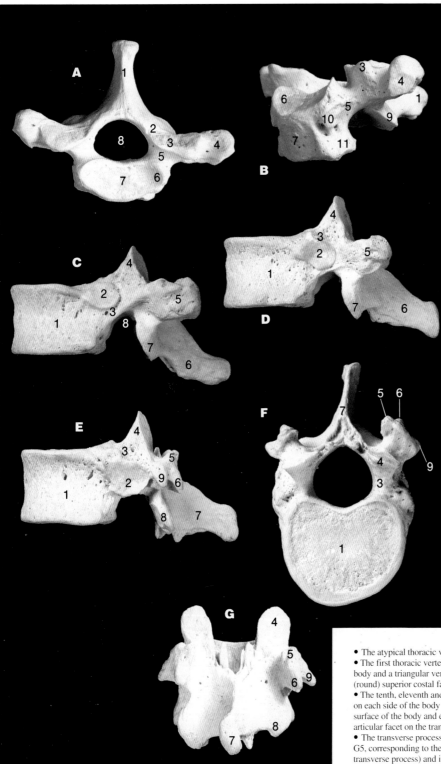

First thoracic vertebra, **A** from above, **B** from the front and the left

 1 Spinous process
 2 Lamina
 3 Superior articular process
 4 Transverse process with costal facet
 5 Pedicle
 6 Posterolateral lip (uncus)
 7 Body
 8 Vertebral foramen
 9 Inferior articular process
10 Superior costal facet
11 Inferior costal facet

Tenth thoracic vertebra, **C,** and eleventh thoracic vertebra, **D**, from the left

1 Body
2 Costal facet
3 Pedicle
4 Superior articular process
5 Transverse process
6 Spinous process
7 Inferior articular process
8 Inferior vertebral notch

Twelfth thoracic vertebra, **E** from the left, **F** from above, **G** from behind

1 Body
2 Costal facet
3 Pedicle
4 Superior articular process
5 Superior tubercle
6 Inferior tubercle
7 Spinous process
8 Inferior articular process
9 Lateral tubercle

• The atypical thoracic vertebrae are the first, tenth, eleventh and twelfth.
• The first thoracic vertebra has a posterolateral lip (A6, B6) on each side of the upper surface of the body and a triangular vertebral foramen (features like typical cervical vertebrae), and complete (round) superior costal facets (B10) on the sides of the body.
• The tenth, eleventh and twelfth thoracic vertebrae are characterized by a single complete costal facet on each side of the body that in the successive vertebrae comes to lie increasingly far from the upper surface of the body and encroaches increasingly on to the pedicle (C2, D2 and E2). There is also no articular facet on the transverse process.
• The transverse process of the twelfth thoracic vertebra is replaced by three tubercles—superior (E5, G5, corresponding to the mamillary process of a lumbar vertebra), lateral (F9, corresponding to a true transverse process) and inferior (E6, G6, corresponding to the accessory process of a lumbar vertebra).
• The inferior articular processes of the twelfth thoracic vertebra (E8) are curved to articulate with the curved superior processes of the first lumbar vertebra.

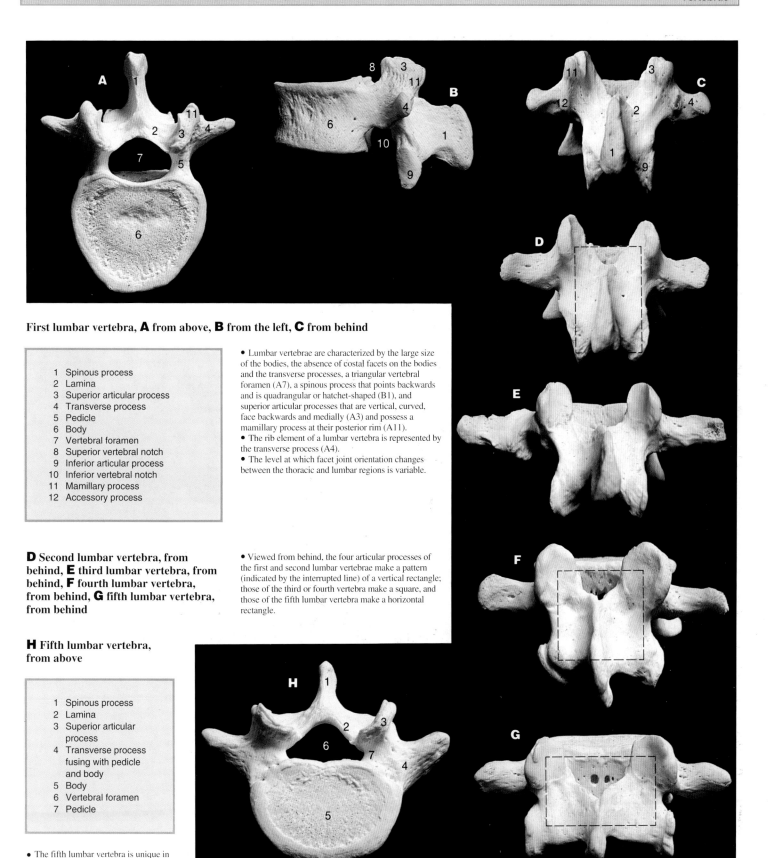

First lumbar vertebra, A from above, B from the left, C from behind

1 Spinous process
2 Lamina
3 Superior articular process
4 Transverse process
5 Pedicle
6 Body
7 Vertebral foramen
8 Superior vertebral notch
9 Inferior articular process
10 Inferior vertebral notch
11 Mamillary process
12 Accessory process

• Lumbar vertebrae are characterized by the large size of the bodies, the absence of costal facets on the bodies and the transverse processes, a triangular vertebral foramen (A7), a spinous process that points backwards and is quadrangular or hatchet-shaped (B1), and superior articular processes that are vertical, curved, face backwards and medially (A3) and possess a mamillary process at their posterior rim (A11).
• The rib element of a lumbar vertebra is represented by the transverse process (A4).
• The level at which facet joint orientation changes between the thoracic and lumbar regions is variable.

D Second lumbar vertebra, from behind, **E** third lumbar vertebra, from behind, **F** fourth lumbar vertebra, from behind, **G** fifth lumbar vertebra, from behind

• Viewed from behind, the four articular processes of the first and second lumbar vertebrae make a pattern (indicated by the interrupted line) of a vertical rectangle; those of the third or fourth vertebra make a square, and those of the fifth lumbar vertebra make a horizontal rectangle.

H Fifth lumbar vertebra, from above

1 Spinous process
2 Lamina
3 Superior articular process
4 Transverse process fusing with pedicle and body
5 Body
6 Vertebral foramen
7 Pedicle

• The fifth lumbar vertebra is unique in that the transverse process (H4) unites directly with the side of the body (H5) as well as with the pedicle (H7).

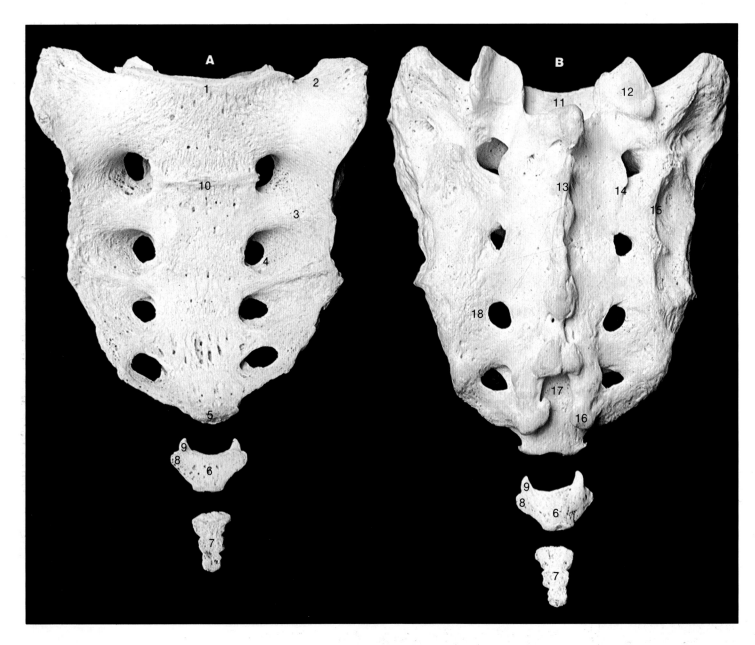

Sacrum and coccyx, A pelvic surface, B dorsal surface

1 Promontory	11 Sacral canal
2 Upper surface of lateral part (ala)	12 Superior articular process
3 Lateral part	13 Median sacral crest
4 Second pelvic sacral foramen	14 Intermediate sacral crest
5 Facet for coccyx	15 Lateral sacral crest
6 First coccygeal vertebra	16 Sacral cornu
7 Fused second to fourth vertebrae	17 Sacral hiatus
8 Transverse process	18 Third dorsal sacral foramen
9 Coccygeal cornu	
10 Site of fusion of first and second sacral vertebrae	

- The sacrum is formed by the fusion of the five sacral vertebrae. The median sacral crest (B13) represents the fused spinous processes, the intermediate crest (B14) the fused articular processes, and the lateral crest (B15) the fused transverse processes.
- The sacral hiatus (B17) is the lower opening of the sacral canal (B11).
- The coccyx is usually formed by the fusion of four rudimentary vertebrae but the number varies from three to five. In this specimen the first piece of the coccyx (6) is not fused with the remainder (7).

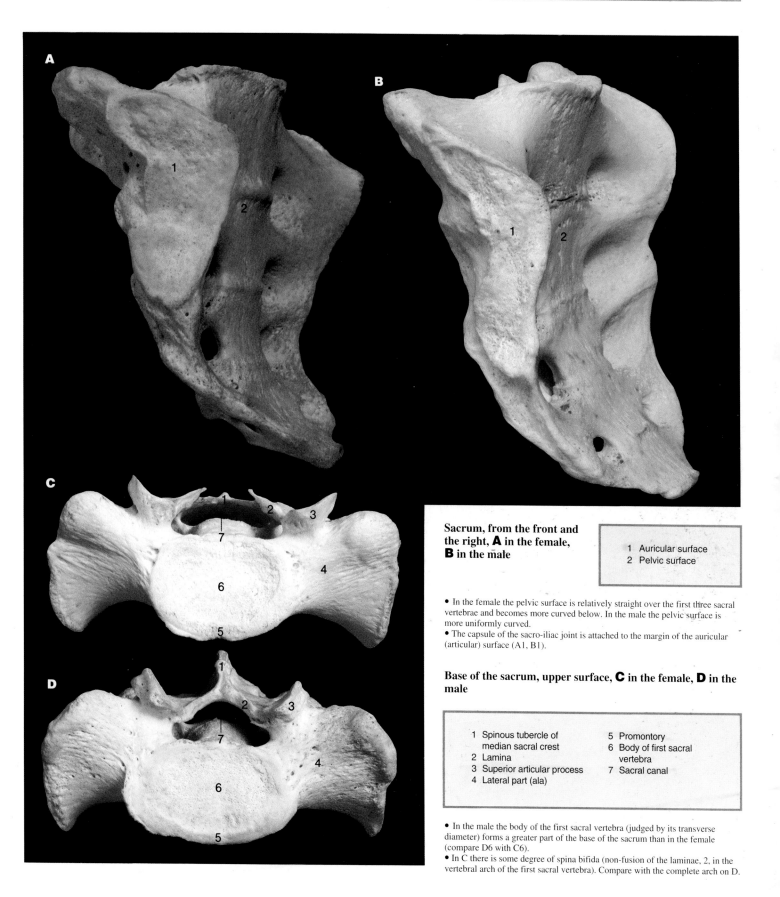

Sacrum, from the front and the right, **A** in the female, **B** in the male

1	Auricular surface
2	Pelvic surface

• In the female the pelvic surface is relatively straight over the first three sacral vertebrae and becomes more curved below. In the male the pelvic surface is more uniformly curved.

• The capsule of the sacro-iliac joint is attached to the margin of the auricular (articular) surface (A1, B1).

Base of the sacrum, upper surface, **C** in the female, **D** in the male

1	Spinous tubercle of median sacral crest	5	Promontory
2	Lamina	6	Body of first sacral vertebra
3	Superior articular process	7	Sacral canal
4	Lateral part (ala)		

• In the male the body of the first sacral vertebra (judged by its transverse diameter) forms a greater part of the base of the sacrum than in the female (compare D6 with C6).

• In C there is some degree of spina bifida (non-fusion of the laminae, 2, in the vertebral arch of the first sacral vertebra). Compare with the complete arch on D.

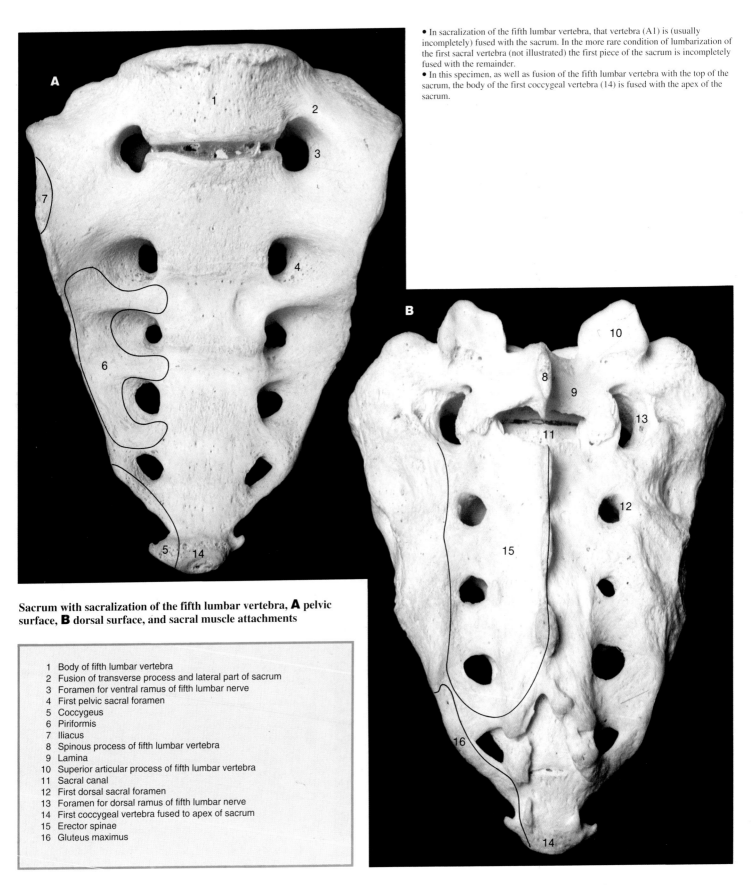

• In sacralization of the fifth lumbar vertebra, that vertebra (A1) is (usually incompletely) fused with the sacrum. In the more rare condition of lumbarization of the first sacral vertebra (not illustrated) the first piece of the sacrum is incompletely fused with the remainder.

• In this specimen, as well as fusion of the fifth lumbar vertebra with the top of the sacrum, the body of the first coccygeal vertebra (14) is fused with the apex of the sacrum.

Sacrum with sacralization of the fifth lumbar vertebra, A pelvic surface, B dorsal surface, and sacral muscle attachments

1 Body of fifth lumbar vertebra
2 Fusion of transverse process and lateral part of sacrum
3 Foramen for ventral ramus of fifth lumbar nerve
4 First pelvic sacral foramen
5 Coccygeus
6 Piriformis
7 Iliacus
8 Spinous process of fifth lumbar vertebra
9 Lamina
10 Superior articular process of fifth lumbar vertebra
11 Sacral canal
12 First dorsal sacral foramen
13 Foramen for dorsal ramus of fifth lumbar nerve
14 First coccygeal vertebra fused to apex of sacrum
15 Erector spinae
16 Gluteus maximus

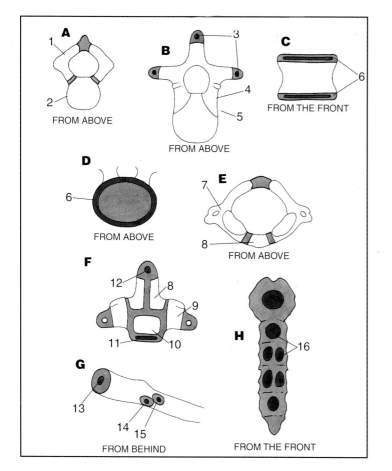

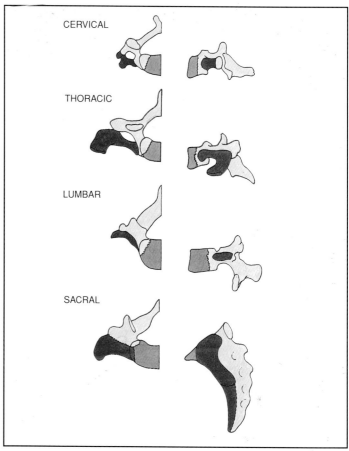

Ossification of vertebrae, ribs and sternum, **A** typical vertebra in a 6-month fetus, **B** at 4 years, **C** and **D** during puberty, **E** atlas at 4 years, **F** axis, primary and secondary centres, **G**, typical rib, secondary centres, **H** sternum at birth, with primary centres

A typical vertebra, which is first cartilaginous, ossifies in early fetal life from three primary centres – one for most of the body (the centrum, A2) and one for each half of the neural arch (A1). The part of the adult body to which the pedicle is attached (B4) is part of the centre for the arch; the site in the developing vertebra where they meet is the neurocentral junction (B5). The two halves of the arch and the neurocentral junctions unite at variable times between birth and 6 years. Ossification spreads into the transverse processes and spine which grow out from the arch, but secondary centres (B3) appear at their tips during puberty and become fused at about 25 years. (Lumbar vertebrae have similar additional secondary centres for the mamillary processes.) There are also ring-like epiphyses on the periphery of the upper and lower surfaces of the vertebral bodies (C6 and D6).

The atlas has a primary centre (E7) for each lateral mass and the adjacent half of the posterior arch, and one for the anterior arch (E8). Fusion is complete by about 8 years.

The axis has five primary centres – one for most of the body (F10), one for each lateral mass (F9), and one for each half of the dens and adjacent part of the body (F8). They should all fuse by about 3 years. There are secondary centres for the tip of the dens (F12, appearing by about 2 years and fusing at 12) and the lower surface of the body (F11, puberty, fusing about 25 years).

The seventh cervical vertebra, in addition to the typical vertebral centres, has additional centres for the costal elements, appearing during the first year and fusing at about 5 years.

The sacrum, representing five fused sacral vertebrae, has many ossification centres, corresponding to the centrum, neural arch halves and costal elements of each vertebra, as well as ring epiphyses for the vertebral bodies and for the auricular surfaces. Most have fused by about 20 years, but some not until middle age or later.

A typical rib has a primary centre for the body with secondary centres for the head (G13) and the articular and non-articular parts of the tubercle (G14 and 15), appearing during puberty and uniting at about 20 years.

The sternum has a variable number of primary centres (H16), one or two in the manubrium and in each of the four pieces of the body. Fusion occurs between puberty and 25 years. 'Bullet holes' in the sternum (sternal foramina) may occur when fusion is incomplete.

- The nucleus pulposus of an intervertebral disc represents the remains of the notochord.
- The annulus fibrosus of an intervertebral disc is derived from the mesenchyme between adjacent vertebral bodies.

Costal elements of vertebrae

Red: costal elements
Green: centrum
Yellow: neural arch

Parts of the cervical, lumbar and sacral vertebrae represent the ribs that articulate with thoracic vertebrae. These costal elements are indicated here in red.

Cervical: anterior and posterior tubercles and the inter-tubercular lamella.

Thoracic: the true rib articulates with the vertebra.

Lumbar: the anterior part of the transverse process.

Sacral: the lateral part, including the auricular surface.

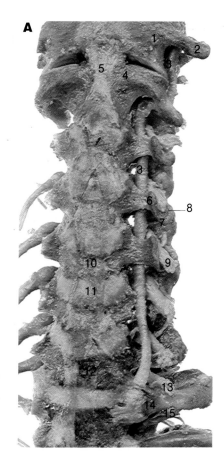

A

A Vertebral column, cervical region, from the front

The left vertebral artery (3) is seen within foramina of cervical transverse processes, which are partly removed from the sixth and seventh (12) cervical vertebrae. On the right side (left of the picture, unlabelled) all transverse processes have been removed and some dorsal root ganglia and nerve rami are displayed

1	Lateral mass ⎫ of atlas
2	Transverse process ⎭
3	Vertebral artery
4	Axis
5	Anterior longitudinal ligament
6	Anterior tubercle ⎫ of transverse
7	Intertubercular lamella ⎬ process
8	Posterior tubercle ⎭
9	Ventral ramus of fifth cervical nerve
10	Body of fifth cervical vertebra
11	Intervertebral disc
12	Body of seventh cervical vertebra
13	Ventral ramus of eighth cervical nerve
14	Joint of head of first rib
15	Ventral ramus of first thoracic nerve

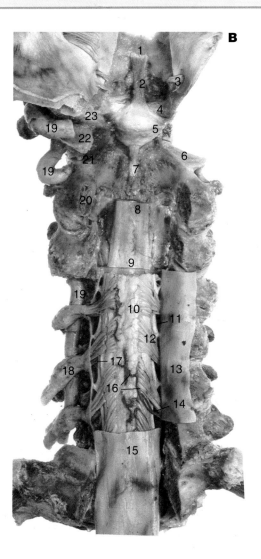

B

B Vertebral column, cervical region, from behind

Much of the skull, the vertebral arches, brainstem and the upper part of the spinal cord have been removed to show the cruciform, transverse and alar ligaments (2, 7, 5 and 4). Lower down, the arachnoid and dura mater (13) have been reflected to show dorsal and ventral nerve roots (as at 12 and 17)

1 Basilar part of occipital bone and position of attachment of tectorial membrane
2 Superior longitudinal band of cruciform ligament
3 Hypoglossal nerve and canal
4 Alar ligament
5 Transverse ligament of atlas (transverse part of cruciform ligament)
6 Superior articular surface of axis
7 Inferior longitudinal band of cruciform ligament
8 Tectorial membrane
9 Posterior longitudinal ligament
10 Spinal cord
11 Denticulate ligament
12 Dorsal rootlets of spinal nerve
13 Arachnoid and dura mater (reflected)
14 Radicular artery
15 Dura mater
16 Posterior spinal arteries
17 Ventral rootlets of spinal nerve
18 Dural sheath over dorsal root ganglion
19 Vertebral artery
20 Pedicle of axis
21 Lateral atlanto-axial joint
22 Posterior arch of atlas
23 Atlanto-occipital joint

C

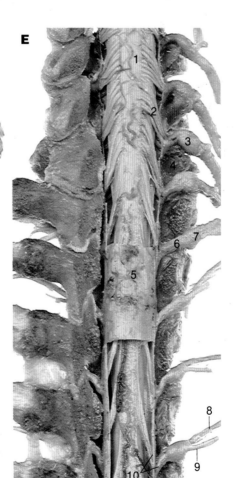

D Vertebral column, cervical region, from the left

Soft tissue has been removed to show the boundaries of intervertebral foramina (as at 4). Compare with the cleared specimens of thoracic and lumbar vertebrae on page 92, A and B

1	Body of third cervical vertebra		5	Zygapophysial joint	
2	Intervertebral disc		6	Posterior tubercle	} of transverse
3	Pedicle		7	Intertubercular lamella	} process of fifth
4	Intervertebral foramen		8	Anterior tubercle	} cervical vertebra

- Each intervertebral foramen (as at D4) is bounded in front by a vertebral body and intervertebral disc (D1 and 2), above and below by pedicles (D3), and behind by a zygapophysial joint (D5).
- In the thoracic and lumbar regions there are the same number of pairs of spinal nerves as there are vertebrae (twelve thoracic and five lumbar), and spinal nerves are numbered from the vertebra beneath whose pedicles they emerge. In the cervical region there are seven cervical

vertebrae and eight cervical nerves. The first nerve emerges between the occipital bone of the skull and the atlas, and the eighth (A13) below the pedicle of the seventh cervical vertebra (A12).
- The zygapophysial joints between the articular processes of adjacent vertebrae are commonly called facet joints (between the articular facets of those processes).
- For further details of spinal nerves see the notes on the following page.

D

E Vertebral column and spinal cord, lower cervical and upper thoracic regions, from behind

The vertebral arches and most of the dura mater and arachnoid have been removed, to show dorsal nerve rootlets (2) emerging from the spinal cord (1) to unite as a dorsal nerve root and enter the dural sheath (as at 6). Ventral nerve roots do the same from the ventral aspect of the cord but are not seen in this view as they are obscured by the dorsal roots

C Vertebral column, cervical and upper thoracic regions, from the left

Ventral and dorsal rami of spinal nerves (as at 10 and 11) are seen emerging from intervertebral foramina (as at 9)

1	Lateral mass	}
2	Transverse process	} of atlas
3	Posterior arch	}
4	Vertebral artery	
5	First cervical nerve	
6	Dorsal root ganglion and rami of second cervical nerve	
7	Lateral atlanto-axial joint	
8	Zygapophysial joint	
9	Intervertebral foramen	
10	Ventral	} ramus of fifth cervical nerve
11	Dorsal	}
12	Anterior tubercle	} of transverse process
13	Posterior tubercle	} of fifth cervical vertebra
14	Body of seventh cervical vertebra	
15	Ventral ramus of eighth cervical nerve	
16	Head of first rib	
17	Body of first thoracic vertebra	
18	Ventral	} ramus of first thoracic nerve
19	Dorsal	}

1	Spinal cord and posterior spinal vessels	
2	Dorsal rootlets	} of eighth
3	Dorsal root ganglion	} cervical nerve
4	Pedicle of first thoracic vertebra	
5	Dura mater	
6	Dural sheath	} of second
7	Dorsal root ganglion	} thoracic nerve
8	Ventral	} ramus of fifth
9	Dorsal	} thoracic nerve
10	Angulation of nerve roots entering dural sheath	

- The first and second cervical nerves pass respectively above and below the posterior arch of the atlas.
- On its upward course from the subclavian artery the vertebral artery enters the foramen of the transverse process of the sixth cervical vertebra.
- For the joints of the ribs with thoracic vertebrae see page 195.

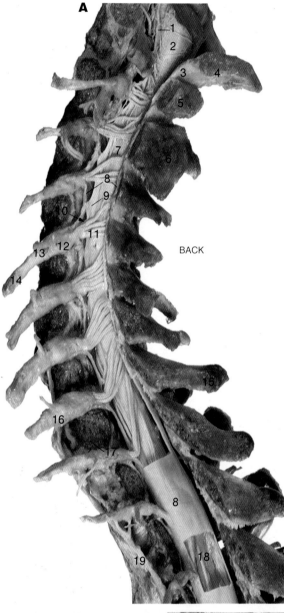

A

BACK

A Vertebral column and spinal cord, cervical and upper thoracic regions, from the left

Parts of the vertebral arches and meninges have been removed, to show the denticulate ligament (9). Dorsal nerve rootlets lie behind it (as at 11) and ventral nerve roots in front of it (as at 10 but largely hidden in this view)

1	Spinal part of accessory nerve	15	Spinous process of seventh cervical vertebra
2	Medulla oblongata		
3	Foramen magnum	16	Dorsal root ganglion of eighth cervical nerve
4	Occipital bone		
5	Posterior arch of atlas	17	Body of first thoracic vertebra
6	Spinous process of axis (abnormally large)	18	Arachnoid mater
		19	Sympathetic trunk
7	Spinal cord		
8	Dura mater		
9	Denticulate ligament		
10	Ventral rootlets		
11	Dorsal rootlets		of fifth cervical nerve
12	Dorsal root ganglion		
13	Dorsal ramus		
14	Ventral ramus		

- The spinal cord is properly called the spinal medulla (not to be confused with medulla oblongata, the lowest part of the brainstem, which continues as the spinal medulla).
- Each spinal nerve is formed by the union of ventral and dorsal nerve roots.
- Each nerve root is formed by the union of several rootlets (as at A11).
- The union of ventral and dorsal nerve roots to form a spinal nerve occurs immediately distal to the ganglion on the dorsal root (as at A12), within the intervertebral foramen, and the nerve at once divides into a ventral and a dorsal ramus (formerly called ventral and dorsal primary rami) (as at A13 and 14). The spinal nerve proper is thus only a millimetre or two in length, but is often so short that the rami appear to be branches of the ganglion itself.
- The lowest cervical and upper thoracic nerve roots become acutely angled in order to enter their dural sheaths.

B

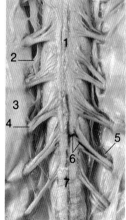

B Cervical region of the spinal cord, from the front

For this ventral view of the upper part of the spinal cord (1), the dura and arachnoid mater have been incised longitudinally and turned aside (3) to show the ventral nerve rootlets and roots (as at 4) passing laterally in front of the denticulate ligament (2) to enter meningeal nerve sheaths with dorsal roots (as at 5) and form a spinal nerve. On some roots branches of radicular vessels (as at 6) are seen anastomosing with anterior spinal vessels (7)

1	Spinal cord
2	Denticulate ligament
3	Arachnoid and dura mater
4	Ventral root of fifth cervical nerve entering dural sheath
5	Dorsal root of sixth cervical nerve
6	Radicular vessels
7	Anterior spinal vessels

- The denticulate ligament (B2) is composed of pia mater. The ventral and dorsal nerve roots pass respectively ventral and dorsal to the ligament, which extends laterally from the side of the cord and is attached by its spiky denticulations (as at B2) to the arachnoid and dura mater in the intervals between dural nerve sheaths. The highest denticulation is above the first cervical nerve and the lowest below the twelfth thoracic nerve.
- For the continuity of the spinal cord with the brainstem see page 76, B.

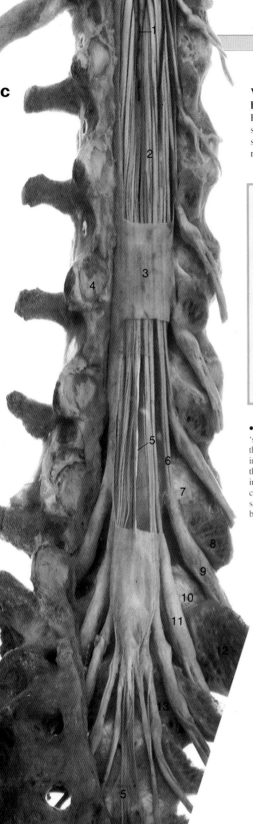

C

Vertebral column, **C** lumbar and sacral regions, from behind, **D** lumbar radiculogram

Parts of the vertebral arches and meninges have been removed, to show the cauda equina (2) and nerve roots entering their meningeal sheaths (as at 6), outlined as linear bands by contrast medium in the radiculogram

1   Conus medullaris of spinal cord
2   Cauda equina
3   Dura mater
4   Superior articular process of third lumbar vertebra
5   Filum terminale
6   Roots of fifth lumbar nerve
7   Fourth lumbar intervertebral disc
8   Pedicle of fifth lumbar vertebra
9   Dorsal root ganglion of fifth lumbar nerve
10 Fifth lumbar (lumbosacral) intervertebral disc
11 Dural sheath of first sacral nerve roots
12 Lateral part of sacrum
13 Second sacral vertebra

• If the fifth lumbar intervertebral disc protrudes backwards (the commonest 'slipped disc') it may irritate the roots of the first sacral nerve (C11). This is the general rule for any part of the vertebral column—a protruded disc may irritate the roots of the nerve numbered one below the disc. Note for example that the fifth lumbar nerve roots (C6) within their dural sheath pass laterally immediately below the pedicle of the fifth lumbar vertebra (C8) and so do not come to lie immediately behind the fifth lumbar disc (C10); it is the first sacral roots (C11) which lie in this position. The fifth nerve roots (C6) lie behind the fourth disc (C7).

E Vertebral column and spinal cord, lower thoracic and upper lumbar regions

The specimen is seen from the left with parts of the vertebral arches and meninges removed, to show (at the front) part of the sympathetic trunk (2) on the vertebral bodies and (at the back) the spinous ligaments (9 and 10)

1   Greater splanchnic nerve
2   Sympathetic trunk
3   Sympathetic ganglion
4   Rami communicantes
5   Dorsal root ganglion of tenth thoracic nerve
6   Spinal cord
7   Dura mater
8   Spinous process of tenth thoracic vertebra
9   Interspinous ligament
10 Supraspinous ligament
11 Cauda equina
12 Body of first lumbar vertebra
13 First lumbar intervertebral disc

• The spinal cord ends at the level of the first lumbar vertebra.
• The subarachnoid space ends at the level of the second sacral vertebra.
• The conus medullaris (1) is the lower, pointed end of the spinal cord.
• The cauda equina (2) consists of the dorsal and ventral roots of the lumbar, sacral and coccygeal nerves. Note that it is nerve *roots* which form the cauda, not the spinal nerves themselves; these are not formed until ventral and dorsal roots unite at the level of an intervertebral foramen, immediately distal to the dorsal root ganglion (as at C9).

D

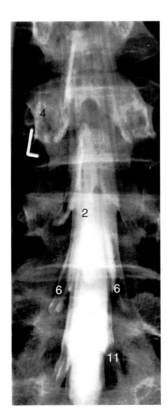

E

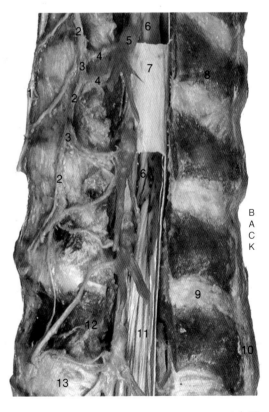

BACK

A

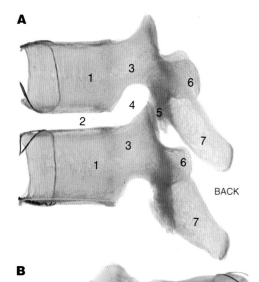

BACK

Cleared specimens, **A** thoracic vertebrae, **B** lumbar vertebrae

The pairs of vertebrae are seen from the side and articulated to show the boundaries of an intervertebral foramen (4)

```
1  Body
2  Space for intervertebral disc
3  Pedicle
4  Intervertebral foramen
5  Zygapophysial joint
6  Transverse process
7  Spinous process
```

• The intervertebral foramen (4) is bounded in front by the lower part of the vertebral body (1) and the intervertebral disc (2), above and below by the pedicles (3), and behind by the zygapophysial joint (5).

B

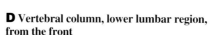

BACK

D Vertebral column, lower lumbar region, from the front

At the top the anterior longitudinal ligament (1) has a marker behind it, and part of it lower down has been reflected off an intervertebral disc (3) and vertebral bodies (2 and 4)

```
1  Anterior longitudinal ligament
2  Body of fourth lumbar vertebra
3  Fourth lumbar intervertebral disc
4  Body of fifth lumbar vertebra
5  Ventral ramus of fifth lumbar nerve
6  Lateral part of sacrum
```

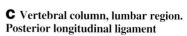

C Vertebral column, lumbar region. Posterior longitudinal ligament

The vertebral arches of the three upper lumbar vertebrae have been cut away through their pedicles (as at 1) and the meninges have been removed to show the posterior longitudinal ligament. Part of the internal vertebral venous plexus has been preserved

```
1  Pedicle of first lumbar vertebra
2  Posterior longitudinal ligament
3  Intervertebral disc
4  Intervertebral foramen
5  Internal vertebral venous plexus
```

• The posterior longitudinal ligament (C2) is broad where it is firmly attached to the intervertebral discs (C3), but narrow and less firmly attached to the vertebral bodies, leaving vascular foramina patent and allowing the basivertebral veins which emerge from them to enter the internal vertebral venous plexus (C5).

• The anterior longitudinal ligament (D1) is uniformly broad and firmly attached to discs and vertebral bodies.

D

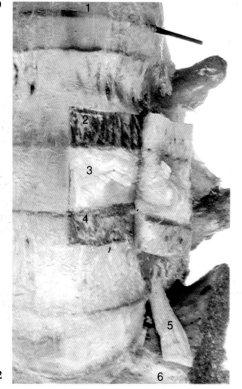

E Vertebral column, upper lumbar region, from the right

This side view shows lumbar nerves emerging from intervertebral foramina (as at 6)

```
1   Twelfth rib
2   Sympathetic trunk ganglion
3   Anterior longitudinal
    ligament
4   First lumbar vertebra
5   Rami communicantes
6   First lumbar nerve
    emerging from
    intervertebral foramen
7   Ventral ⎱ ramus of first
8   Dorsal  ⎰ lumbar nerve
9   First lumbar intervertebral
    disc
10  Ventral ⎱ ramus of second
11  Dorsal  ⎰ lumbar nerve
12  Zygapophysial joint
13  Spinous process of second
    lumbar vertebra
14  Interspinous ligament
15  Supraspinous ligament
```

BACK

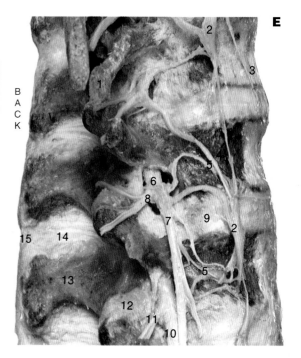

E

A

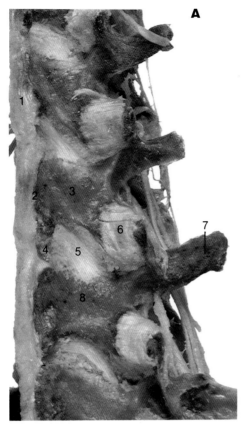

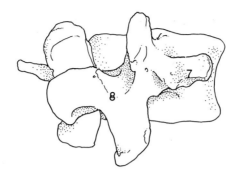

B **C**

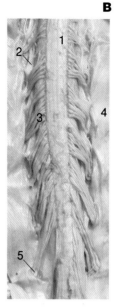

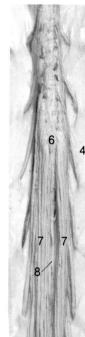

A Vertebral column, lumbar region, from the right and behind

This posterolateral view of the right side of some lumbar vertebrae shows ligamenta flava (as at 5), which pass between the laminae of adjacent vertebrae (as at 3 and 8)

1	Supraspinous ligament
2	Spinous process ⎫ of second lumbar
3	Lamina ⎭ vertebra
4	Interspinous ligament
5	Ligamentum flavum
6	Zygapophysial joint
7	Transverse process ⎫ of third lumbar
8	Lamina ⎭ vertebra

E Intervertebral disc

This disc, on the upper surface of the body of a lumbar vertebra, has been cut horizontally to show the central nucleus pulposus (1) and the concentric fibrocartilaginous laminae of the surrounding annulus fibrosus (2). At the back the annulus has been shaved off to reveal part of the plate of hyaline cartilage (3) on the surface of the vertebra.

• The nucleus pulposus of an intervertebral disc represents the remains of the notochord.
• The annulus fibrosus of an intervertebral disc is derived from the mesenchyme between adjacent vertebral bodies.
• 'Bullet holes' that may be found in a sternum are the result of incomplete fusion of ossification centres.

Spinal cord and cauda equina, B dorsal surface of upper end, C dorsal surface of lower end with cauda, D axial MR image of cauda

The dura and arachnoid mater have been incised longitudinally and turned outwards (B4 and C4) to show the nerve roots entering their dural sheaths (as at B5 and C9). Below the level of the conus medullaris (the lower end of the spinal cord, C6) the nerve roots constitute the cauda equina (C7). Compare B with the ventral surface of the cervical part of the cord (page 90, B)

1	Nucleus pulposus
2	Annulus fibrosus
3	Plate of hyaline cartilage

E

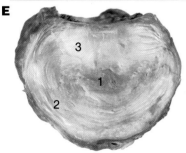

FRONT

1	Spinal cord
2	Denticulate ligament
3	Dorsal rootlets of fifth cervical nerve
4	Arachnoid overlying dura mater
5	Eighth cervical nerve roots entering dural sheath
6	Conus medullaris
7	Cauda equina
8	Filum terminale
9	Fifth lumbar nerve roots entering dural sheath

• The filum terminale (C8), which consists of connective tissue, not neural elements, extends from the tip of the conus medullaris (C6) through the subarachnoid space to the level of the second sacral vertebra where it fuses with the dura mater and continues downwards to become attached to the first piece of the coccyx.

D

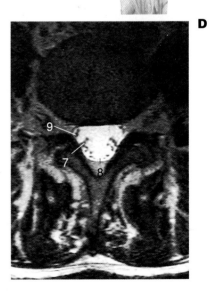

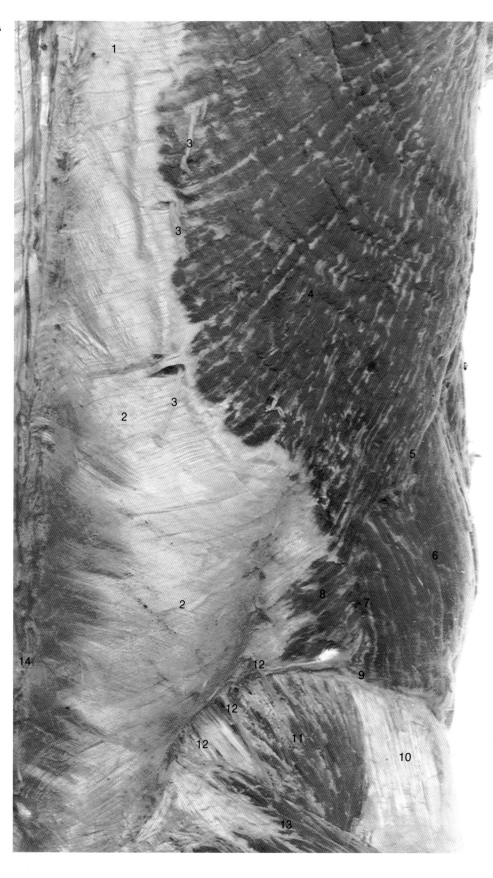

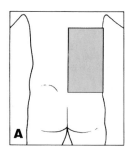

A Muscles of the vertebral column. Right erector spinae and thoracolumbar fascia
The thoracolumbar fascia (1 and 2) covers erector spinae and laterally gives origin to latissimus dorsi (4, a muscle of the upper limb) and internal oblique (8, a muscle of the anterolateral abdominal wall)

1 Thoracic part of thoracolumbar fascia overlying erector spinae
2 Posterior layer of lumbar part of thoracolumbar fascia overlying erector spinae
3 Branches of dorsal rami of thoracic nerves
4 Latissimus dorsi
5 Free lateral border of 4
6 External oblique
7 Free posterior border of 6
8 Internal oblique
9 Iliac crest
10 Gluteal fascia
11 Gluteus medius
12 Cutaneous branches of dorsal rami of first three lumbar nerves
13 Gluteus maximus
14 Level of fourth lumbar spinous process

• The thoracolumbar fascia consists of a thoracic part, single-layered, covering the thoracic part of the erector spinae (1), and a lumbar part (where there are no ribs) which is commonly called simply the lumbar fascia and which consists of three layers.
• The posterior layer (2) is continuous with the thoracic part (1). The middle and anterior layers are usually studied with the posterior abdominal wall; the quadratus lumborum muscle lies between them, and psoas major is in front of the anterior layer. The lumbar part of erector spinae is between the posterior and middle layers. The three layers come together approximately at the lateral border of erector spinae (see the transverse section on page 238, B8 to 10).
• For other parts of erector spinae see opposite and page 96.

B

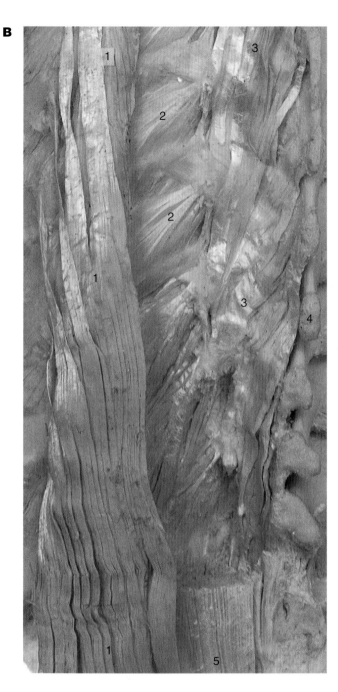

C

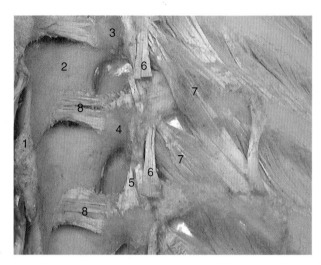

B

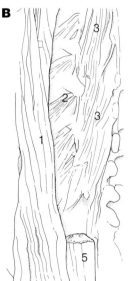

C

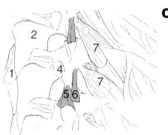

C Muscles of the vertebral column, right midthoracic region
All parts of erector spinae have been removed to show some rotator muscles (8) and intertransverse muscles and ligaments (5)

B Muscles of the vertebral column, left thoracolumbar region
Some of the iliocostalis (1), longissimus (5) and spinalis (3) parts of erector spinae are shown, together with levator costae muscles (2)

1 Iliocostalis	4 Spine of eighth thoracic
2 Levator costae	vertebra
3 Parts of spinalis	5 Lower part of longissimus

1 Spinous process	⎫
2 Lamina	⎬ of fourth thoracic vertebra
3 Transverse process	⎭
4 Transverse process of fifth thoracic vertebra
5 Intertransverse muscle and ligament
6 Tendons of longissimus
7 Levator costae
8 Rotator muscle

• The rotator muscles (8) pass from the transverse process of one vertebra (4) to the lamina of the vertebra above (2). They are prominent only in the thoracic region.
• The intertransverse muscles and ligaments (5) pass between adjacent transverse processes. The muscles are best developed in the cervical region and are usually absent over most of the thorax.

• In the upper lumbar region, erector spinae divides into three muscle masses: iliocostalis (1) laterally, an intermediate longissimus (5, mostly removed in this specimen), and spinalis (3) medially.
• The levator costae muscles (2) are classified as muscles of the thorax, not of the vertebral column. They are revealed here because much of the longissimus part of the erector spinae (5) has been removed.

95

Muscles of the back and thorax, **A** left erector spinae and serratus posterior inferior, from behind, **B** surface anatomy

In the view (A) of the lower left thorax and lumbar region from behind, latissimus dorsi has been removed to display serratus posterior inferior (4), part of whose aponeurotic origin from vertebral spines has also been removed to uncover part of erector spinae (6, 7 and 8) (which belongs to the vertebral column group of muscles—pages 94 and 95). The surface view in B, with the arms abducted, shows well-developed erector spinae muscles

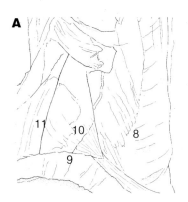

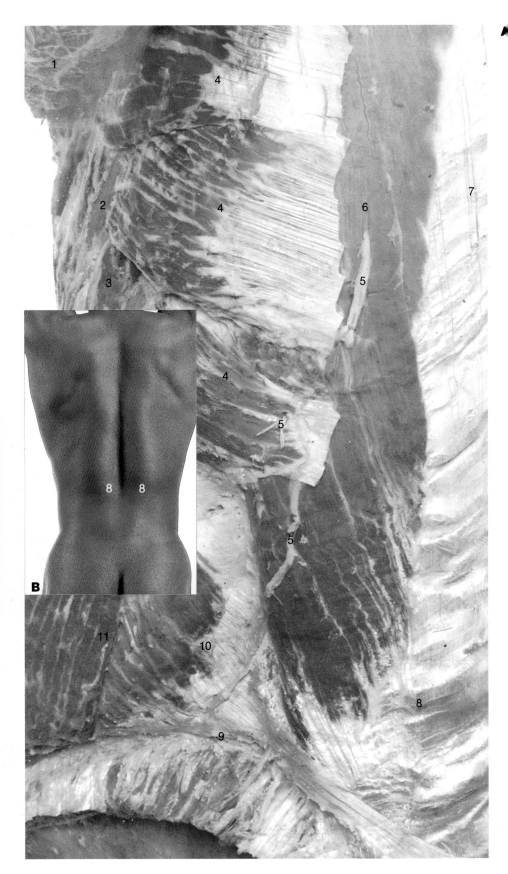

1	Latissimus dorsi
2	Tenth rib
3	External intercostal
4	Serratus posterior inferior
5	Dorsal rami of lower thoracic and upper lumbar nerves
6	Longissimus part of erector spinae
7	Spinalis part of erector spinae
8	Erector spinae
9	Iliac crest
10	Internal oblique
11	Posterior (free) border of external oblique

• The medial part of serratus posterior *inferior* (4) (arising from the last two thoracic and upper two lumbar spinous processes and the supraspinous ligament, and blending with the underlying lumbar part of the thoracolumbar fascia) has been removed, so displaying the medial and intermediate parts of erector spinae (6 and 7) which belongs to the muscles of the vertebral column (page 94). The lateral (iliocostalis) part of erector spinae is under cover of the lateral part of the serratus muscle, which becomes attached to the lower four ribs lateral to their angles.

• The serratus posterior *superior* muscle (not illustrated) passes to the second to fifth ribs lateral to their angles, under cover of the rhomboid muscles (page 120), having arisen from the lower part of the ligamentum nuchae and the spinous processes of the seventh cervical and upper two or three thoracic vertebrae and the supraspinous ligament.

• On each side there is one serratus *anterior* muscle (belonging to the group connecting the upper limb to the trunk) and two serratus *posterior* muscles (belonging to the muscles of the thorax).

C Radiograph of upper cervical vertebrae

This is a standard radiographic view of the axis and its dens (1). The correct angle must be chosen with the mouth open to avoid overlying shadows of the teeth and jaws. The surfaces of the lateral atlanto-axial joints (2 and 4) do not appear congruent because the hyaline cartilage which covers the bony surfaces is not radio-opaque (this applies to any synovial joint). The outlines of the arches of the atlas are seen faintly between the sides of the shadow of the dens (1) and the lateral masses of the atlas (2)

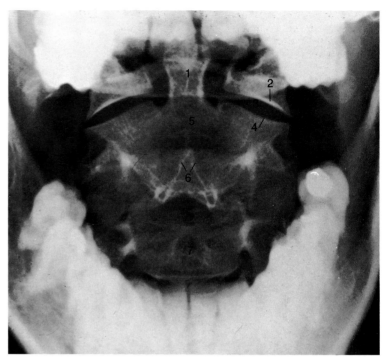

1 Dens of axis
2 Inferior articular surface of lateral mass of atlas
3 Lateral atlanto-axial joint
4 Superior articular surface of axis
5 Body of axis
6 Bifid spinous process of axis
7 Body of third cervical vertebra

D Radiograph of lower cervical and upper thoracic vertebrae, from the front

Note the tracheal shadow produced by the translucency of its contained air

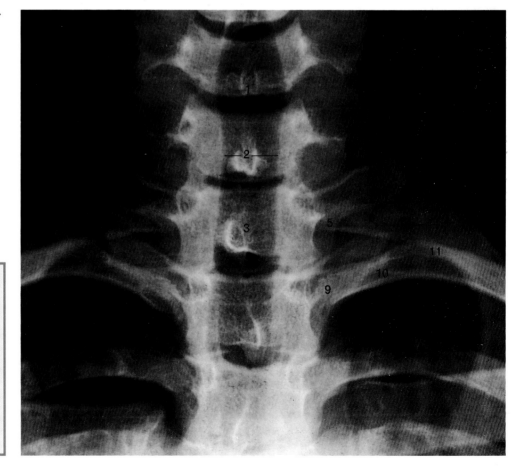

1 Body of sixth cervical vertebra
2 Margin of tracheal shadow
3 Body ⎫ of first thoracic
4 Transverse process ⎬ vertebra
5 Head
6 Neck ⎫
7 Tubercle ⎬ of first rib
8 Shaft ⎭
9 Head
10 Neck ⎬ of second rib
11 Tubercle ⎭

A

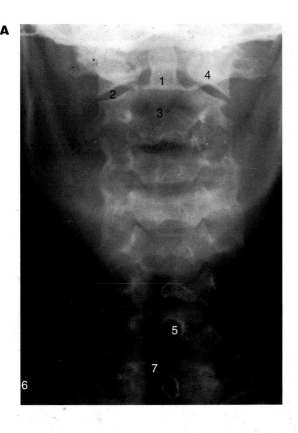

B

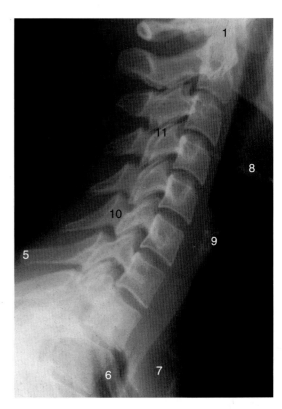

Vertebral radiographs, **A** cervical spine, anteroposterior projection, **B** cervical spine, lateral projection, **C** lumbar spine, anteroposterior projection, **D** lumbar spine, oblique projection

1 Dens of axis
2 Lateral atlanto-axial joint
3 Body of axis
4 Lateral mass of atlas
5 Spinous process of seventh cervical vertebra
6 First rib
7 Trachea
8 Hyoid bone
9 Larynx
10 Lamina of sixth cervical vertebra
11 Zygapophysial joint
12 Inferior articular process of first lumbar vertebra
13 Superior articular process of second lumbar vertebra
14 Spinous process of second lumbar vertebra
15 Intervertebral disc space L2/3 level
16 Pedicles of third lumbar vertebra
17 Transverse process of third lumbar vertebra
18 Pars interarticularis of second lumbar vetebra

C

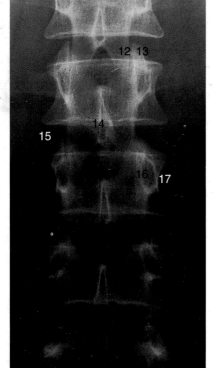

D

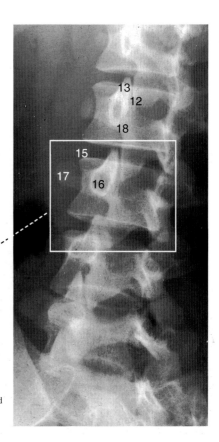

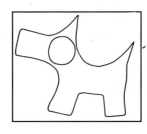

• The Scottie dog is seen on the oblique projection lumbar spine. The nose (17) is the transverse process, the ear (13) is the superior articular process, the eye (16) is the pedicle and the neck (18) is the pars interarticularis which may be fractured in spondylolisthesis.

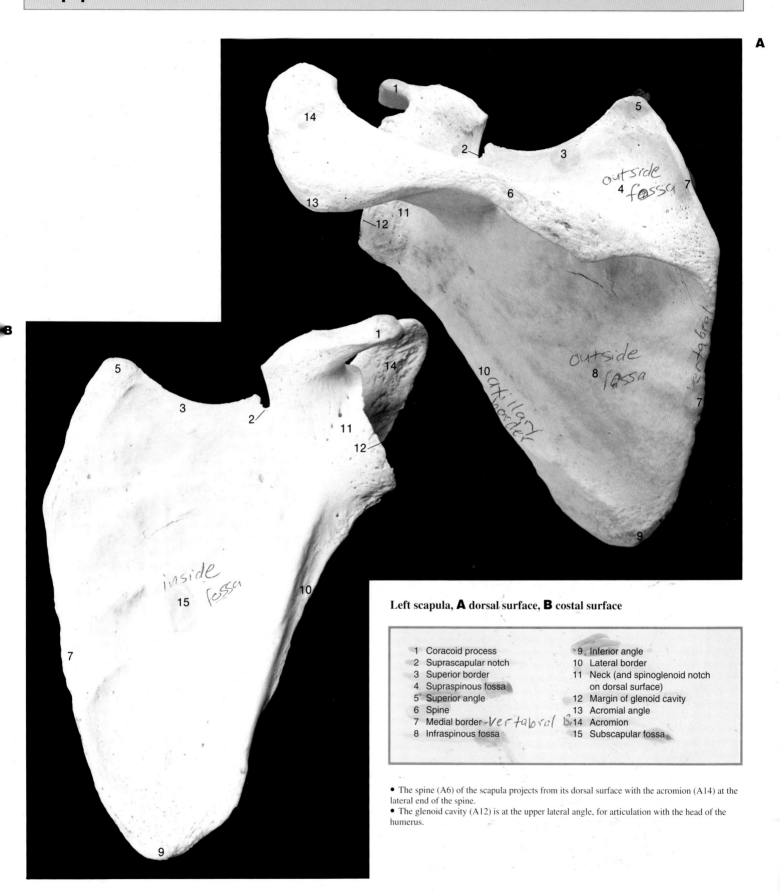

A

B

Left scapula, A dorsal surface, B costal surface

1 Coracoid process	9 Inferior angle
2 Suprascapular notch	10 Lateral border
3 Superior border	11 Neck (and spinoglenoid notch
4 Supraspinous fossa	on dorsal surface)
5 Superior angle	12 Margin of glenoid cavity
6 Spine	13 Acromial angle
7 Medial border—Vertabral B	14 Acromion
8 Infraspinous fossa	15 Subscapular fossa

• The spine (A6) of the scapula projects from its dorsal surface with the acromion (A14) at the lateral end of the spine.
• The glenoid cavity (A12) is at the upper lateral angle, for articulation with the head of the humerus.

99

• The shoulder joint is the glenohumeral joint, and is the articulation between the glenoid cavity of the scapula and the head of the humerus.

• The suprascapular notch is bridged by the superior transverse scapular ligament (16).

• The conoid (15) and trapezoid (14) ligaments together form the coracoclavicular ligament, which attaches the coracoid process of the scapula to the under-surface of the lateral end of the clavicle (C4 and C5, opposite).

• The coracohumeral ligament (page 102, A3) reinforces the upper part of the capsule of the shoulder joint.

• The coraco-acromial ligament (13) passes between the coracoid process and the acromion, forming with these bony processes an arch above the shoulder joint.

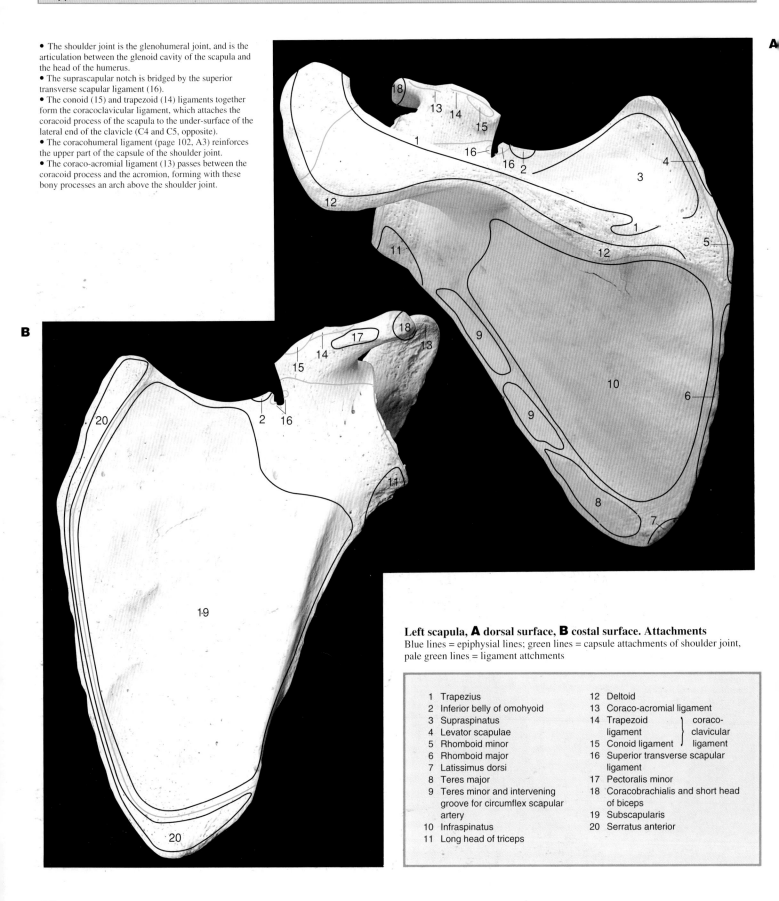

Left scapula, A dorsal surface, B costal surface. Attachments
Blue lines = epiphysial lines; green lines = capsule attachments of shoulder joint, pale green lines = ligament attchments

1 Trapezius	12 Deltoid
2 Inferior belly of omohyoid	13 Coraco-acromial ligament
3 Supraspinatus	14 Trapezoid ligament } coraco-clavicular ligament
4 Levator scapulae	
5 Rhomboid minor	15 Conoid ligament }
6 Rhomboid major	16 Superior transverse scapular ligament
7 Latissimus dorsi	
8 Teres major	17 Pectoralis minor
9 Teres minor and intervening groove for circumflex scapular artery	18 Coracobrachialis and short head of biceps
10 Infraspinatus	19 Subscapularis
11 Long head of triceps	20 Serratus anterior

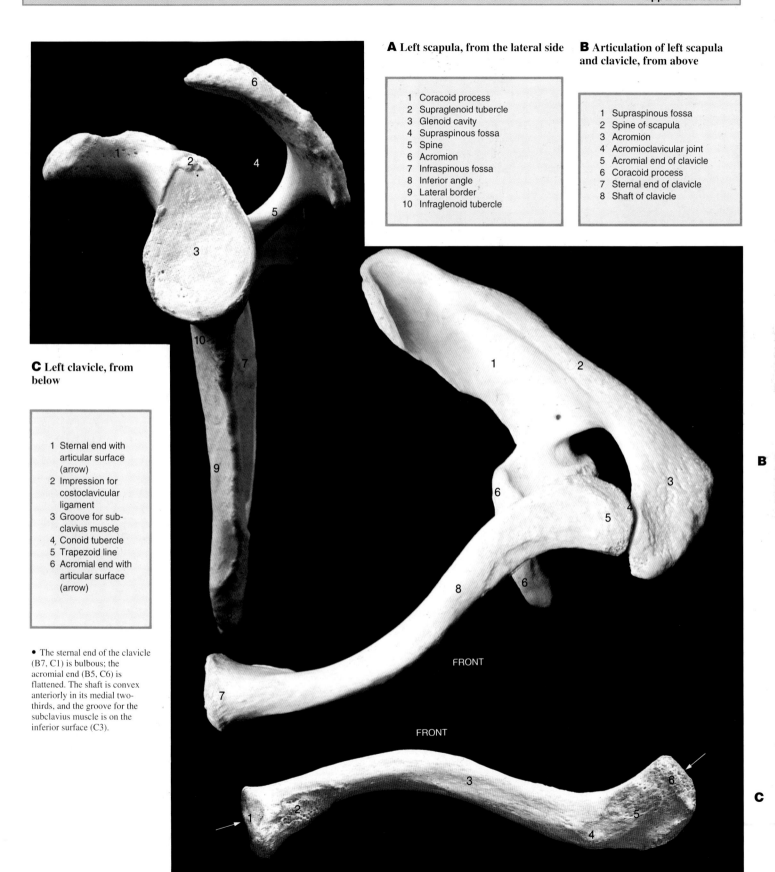

A Left scapula, from the lateral side

1	Coracoid process
2	Supraglenoid tubercle
3	Glenoid cavity
4	Supraspinous fossa
5	Spine
6	Acromion
7	Infraspinous fossa
8	Inferior angle
9	Lateral border
10	Infraglenoid tubercle

B Articulation of left scapula and clavicle, from above

1	Supraspinous fossa
2	Spine of scapula
3	Acromion
4	Acromioclavicular joint
5	Acromial end of clavicle
6	Coracoid process
7	Sternal end of clavicle
8	Shaft of clavicle

C Left clavicle, from below

1	Sternal end with articular surface (arrow)
2	Impression for costoclavicular ligament
3	Groove for sub-clavius muscle
4	Conoid tubercle
5	Trapezoid line
6	Acromial end with articular surface (arrow)

• The sternal end of the clavicle (B7, C1) is bulbous; the acromial end (B5, C6) is flattened. The shaft is convex anteriorly in its medial two-thirds, and the groove for the subclavius muscle is on the inferior surface (C3).

FRONT

FRONT

B

C

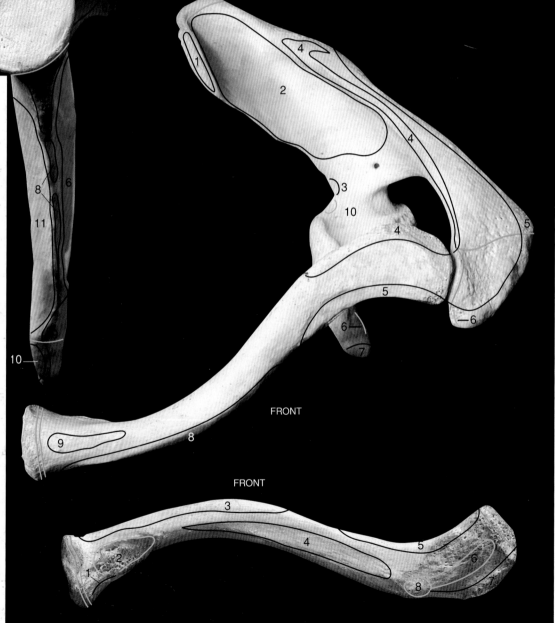

A Left scapula, from the lateral side. Attachments

Blue lines = epiphysial lines; green lines = capsule attachment of shoulder joint; pale green lines = ligament attachments

1	Coracobrachialis and short head of biceps	7	Long head of triceps
2	Coraco-acromial ligament	8	Teres minor (with intervening groove for circumflex scapular artery)
3	Coracohumeral ligament	9	Teres major
4	Long head of biceps	10	Serratus anterior
5	Deltoid	11	Subscapularis
6	Infraspinatus		

B Articulation of left scapula and clavicle, from above

Blue lines = epiphysial lines; green lines = capsule attachments of sternoclavicular and acromioclavicular joints; pale green lines = ligament attachments

1 Levator scapulae
2 Supraspinatus
3 Inferior belly of omohyoid
4 Trapezius
5 Deltoid
6 Coraco-acromial ligament
7 Coracobrachialis and short head of biceps
8 Pectoralis major
9 Sternocleidomastoid
10 Superior transverse scapular ligament

C Left clavicle, from below. Attachments

Blue lines = epiphysial lines; green lines = capsule attachments of sternoclavicular and acromio-clavicular joints; pale green lines = ligament attachments

1 Sternohyoid
2 Costoclavicular ligament
3 Pectoralis major
4 Subclavius and clavipectoral fascia
5 Deltoid
6 Trapezoid ligament
7 Trapezius
8 Conoid ligamont

FRONT

FRONT

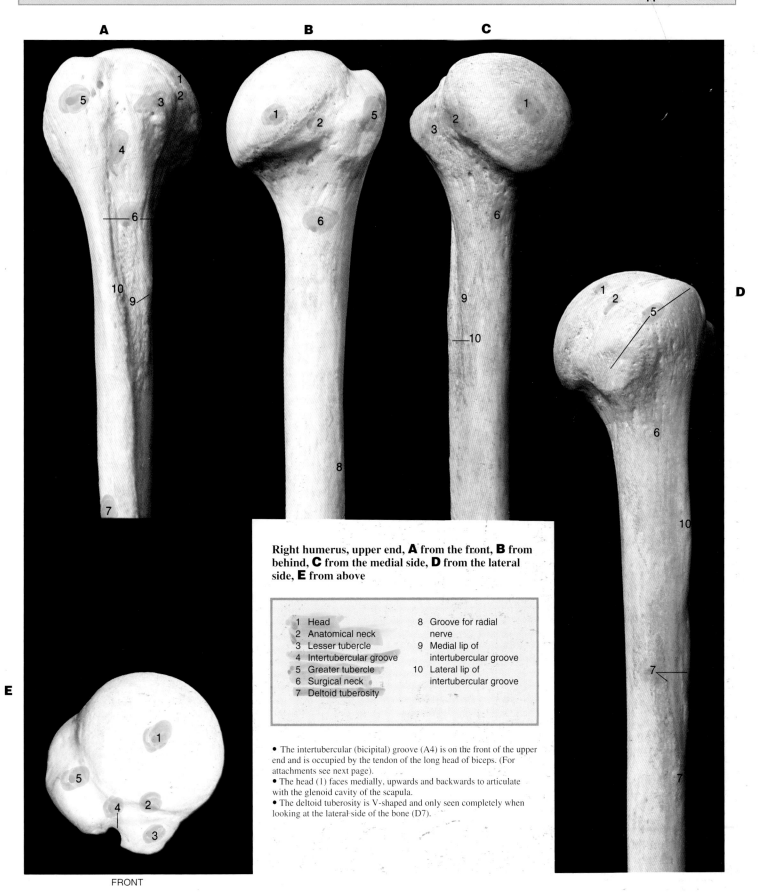

A   **B**   **C**

D

E

FRONT

Right humerus, upper end, A from the front, B from behind, C from the medial side, D from the lateral side, E from above

1	Head	8	Groove for radial nerve
2	Anatomical neck	9	Medial lip of intertubercular groove
3	Lesser tubercle		
4	Intertubercular groove		
5	Greater tubercle	10	Lateral lip of intertubercular groove
6	Surgical neck		
7	Deltoid tuberosity		

• The intertubercular (bicipital) groove (A4) is on the front of the upper end and is occupied by the tendon of the long head of biceps. (For attachments see next page).

• The head (1) faces medially, upwards and backwards to articulate with the glenoid cavity of the scapula.

• The deltoid tuberosity is V-shaped and only seen completely when looking at the lateral side of the bone (D7).

103

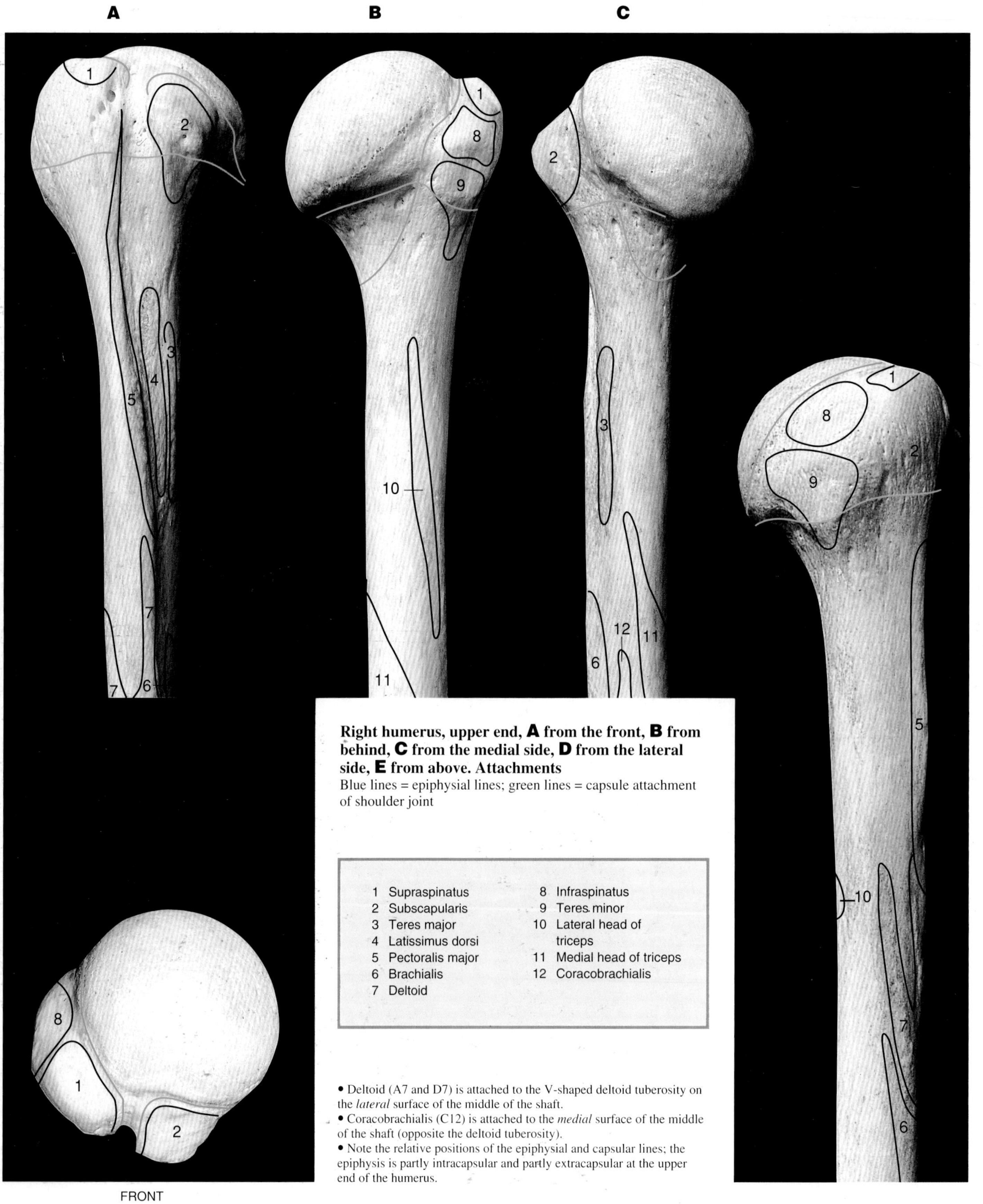

A B C

D

E

Right humerus, upper end, A from the front, B from behind, C from the medial side, D from the lateral side, E from above. Attachments

Blue lines = epiphysial lines; green lines = capsule attachment of shoulder joint

1 Supraspinatus	8 Infraspinatus
2 Subscapularis	9 Teres minor
3 Teres major	10 Lateral head of
4 Latissimus dorsi	triceps
5 Pectoralis major	11 Medial head of triceps
6 Brachialis	12 Coracobrachialis
7 Deltoid	

• Deltoid (A7 and D7) is attached to the V-shaped deltoid tuberosity on the *lateral* surface of the middle of the shaft.

• Coracobrachialis (C12) is attached to the *medial* surface of the middle of the shaft (opposite the deltoid tuberosity).

• Note the relative positions of the epiphysial and capsular lines; the epiphysis is partly intracapsular and partly extracapsular at the upper end of the humerus.

FRONT

Right humerus, lower end, A from the front, **B** from behind, **C** from below, **D** from the medial side, **E** from the lateral side

1   Lateral supracondylar ridge
2   Lateral epicondyle
3   Capitulum
4   Radial fossa
5   Trochlea
6   Coronoid fossa
7   Medial epicondyle
8   Medial supracondylar ridge
9   Anterior surface
10 Posterior surface
11 Olecranon fossa
12 Medial surface of trochlea
13 Lateral edge of capitulum

● The medial epicondyle (7) is more prominent than the lateral (2).
● The medial part of the trochlea (5) is more prominent than the lateral part.
● The olecranon fossa (11) on the posterior surface is deeper than the radial and coronoid fossae on the anterior surface (4 and 6).

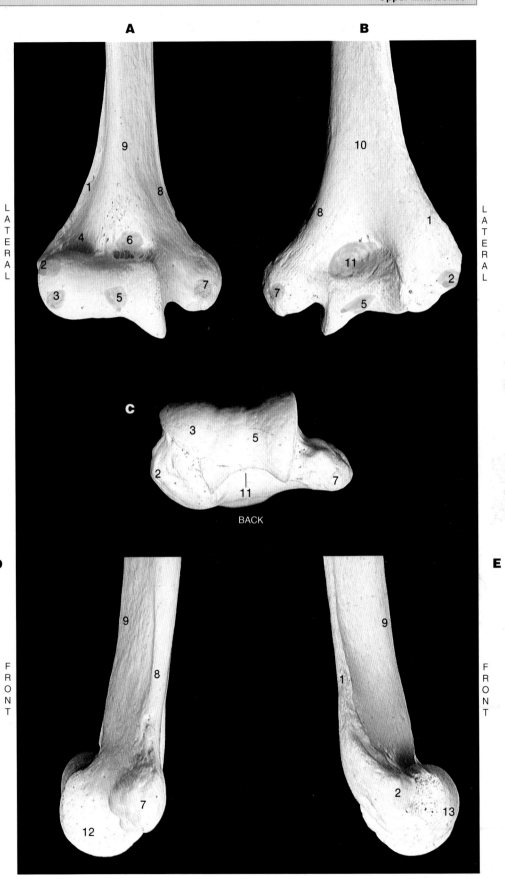

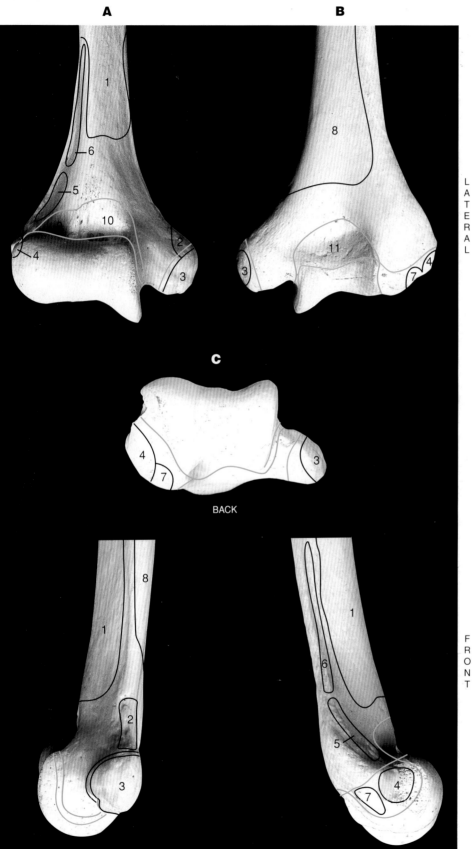

A **B**

C

BACK

D **E**

LATERAL

FRONT

Right humerus, lower end, A from the front, B from behind, C from below, D from the medial side, E from the lateral side. Attachments
Blue lines = epiphysial lines; green lines = capsule attachment of elbow joint

1 Brachialis
2 Pronator teres
3 Common flexor origin
4 Common extensor origin
5 Extensor carpi radialis longus
6 Brachioradialis
7 Anconeus
8 Medial head of triceps
9 Radial fossa
10 Coronoid fossa
11 Olecranon fossa

● The ulnar and radial collateral ligaments of the elbow joint are attached to the medial and lateral epicondyles respectively (beneath the common flexor and extensor origins, 3 and 4).
● Pain from a tear of the common extensor origin at 4 is known as 'tennis elbow'. Note that extensor carpi radialis longus (5) and brachioradialis (6) arise from the humeral shaft above the common extensor origin.
● Note that the capsular attachment runs above the radial, coronoid and olecranon fossae (9, 10 and 11) which therefore lie within the joint. The fossae house fat pads which are intracapsular and extrasynovial in position.

Right radius, upper end, A from the front, **B** from behind, **C** from the medial side, **D** from the lateral side

1 Head
2 Neck
3 Tuberosity
4 Anterior oblique line
5 Interosseous border
6 Anterior surface
7 Anterior border
8 Lateral surface
9 Posterior border
10 Posterior surface
11 Rough area for pronator teres

• The head of the radius (1) is at its upper end; the head of the ulna is at its lower end (page 108, E3).
• The tuberosity (3) is rough posteriorly for the attachment of the biceps tendon, and smooth anteriorly where it is covered by the intervening bursa.
• The shaft is triangular in cross section, and its surfaces are anterior (6), posterior (10) and lateral (8); its borders are interosseous (5), anterior (7) and posterior (9) (compare with the ulna, page 108).

Right radius, lower end, E from the front, **F** from behind, **G** from the medial side, **H** from the lateral side

1 Anterior surface
2 Interosseous border
3 Ulnar notch
4 Styloid process
5 Lateral surface
6 Posterior surface
7 Groove for extensor digitorum and extensor indicis
8 Groove for extensor pollicis longus
9 Dorsal tubercle
10 Groove for extensor carpi radialis brevis
11 Groove for extensor carpi radialis longus
12 Groove for extensor pollicis brevis
13 Groove for abductor pollicis longus

• The lower end of the radius is concave anteriorly (at the lower label 1 in E), with the ulnar notch medially (G3) and the dorsal tubercle on the posterior surface (F9).

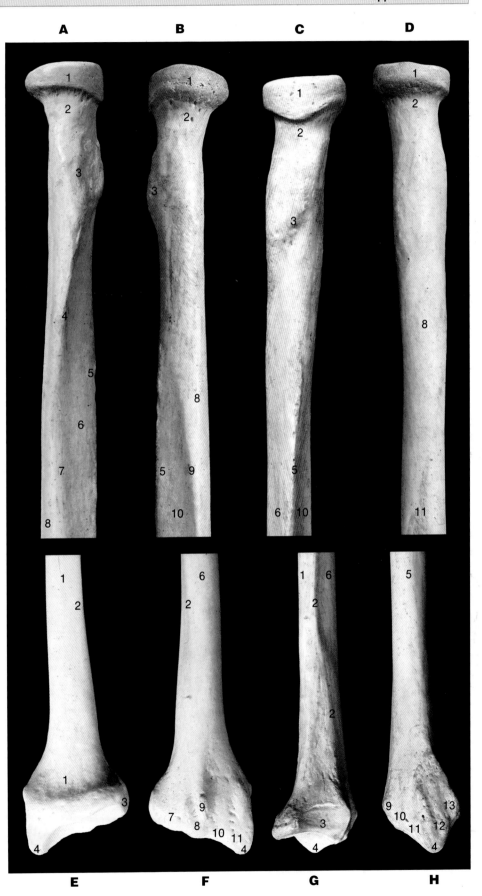

A B C D

E F G H

trocheolar

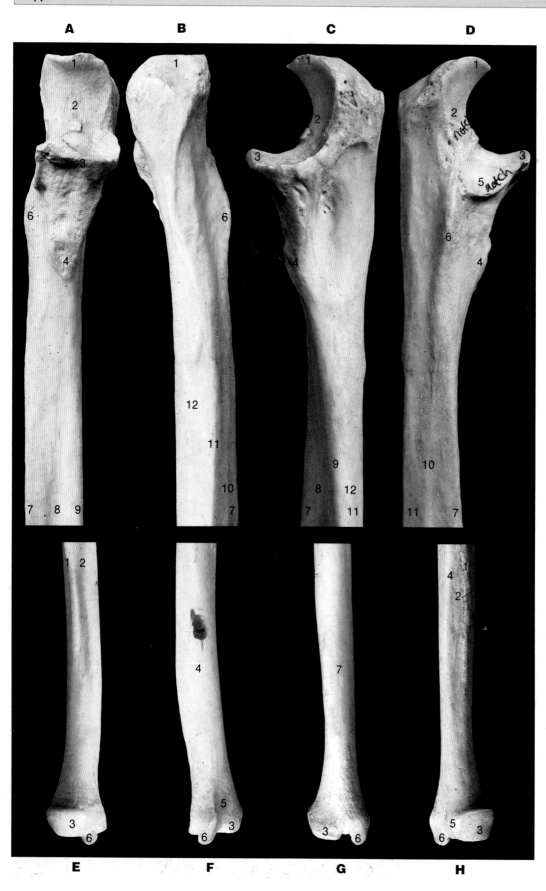

A   B   C   D

Right ulna, upper end, A from the front, B from behind, C from the medial side, D from the lateral side

1	Olecranon
2	Trochlear notch
3	Coronoid process
4	Tuberosity
5	Radial notch
6	Supinator crest
7	Interosseous border
8	Anterior surface
9	Anterior border
10	Posterior surface
11	Posterior border
12	Medial surface

• The trochlear notch (2) faces forwards, with the radial notch (5) on the lateral side.
• The upper part of the shaft is triangular in cross section but the lower quarter is almost cylindrical. The surfaces of the shaft are anterior (8), posterior (10) and medial (12); the borders are interosseous (7), anterior (9) and posterior (11) (compare with the radius, page 107).

Right ulna, lower end, E from the front, F from behind, G from the medial side, H from the lateral side

1	Interosseous border
2	Anterior surface
3	Head
4	Posterior surface
5	Groove for extensor carpi ulnaris
6	Styloid process
7	Medial surface

• The head of the ulna (3) is at its lower end, with the styloid process (6) situated posteromedially. The head of the radius is at its upper end (page 107).

E   F   G   H

108

A Right radius and ulna, upper ends, from above and in front

1 Olecranon	
2 Trochlear notch	
3 Coronoid process	of ulna
4 Tuberosity	
5 Tuberosity	
6 Neck	of radius
7 Head	

B Right radius and ulna, lower ends, from below

1 Styloid process of radius
2 Surface for scaphoid
3 Surface for lunate
4 Attachment of articular disc
5 Surface for disc
6 Styloid process of ulna
7 Groove for extensor carpi ulnaris
8 Groove for extensor digitorum and extensor indicis
9 Groove for extensor pollicis longus
10 Dorsal tubercle
11 Groove for extensor carpi radialis brevis
12 Groove for extensor carpi radialis longus

Articulation of right humerus, radius and ulna, **C** from the front, **D** from behind

1 Lateral epicondyle	
2 Capitulum	
3 Trochlea	of humerus
4 Medial epicondyle	
5 Coronoid process of ulna	
6 Head of radius	
7 Olecranon	of ulna
8 Radial notch	

• The elbow joint is the articulation of the humerus with the radius and ulna — the capitulum of the humerus (2) with the head of the radius (6), and the trochlea of the humerus (3) with the trochlear notch of the ulna.
• The head of the radius (6) also articulates with the radial notch of the ulna (8), forming the proximal radio-ulnar joint.
• The elbow joint and the proximal radio-ulnar joint share a common synovial cavity.

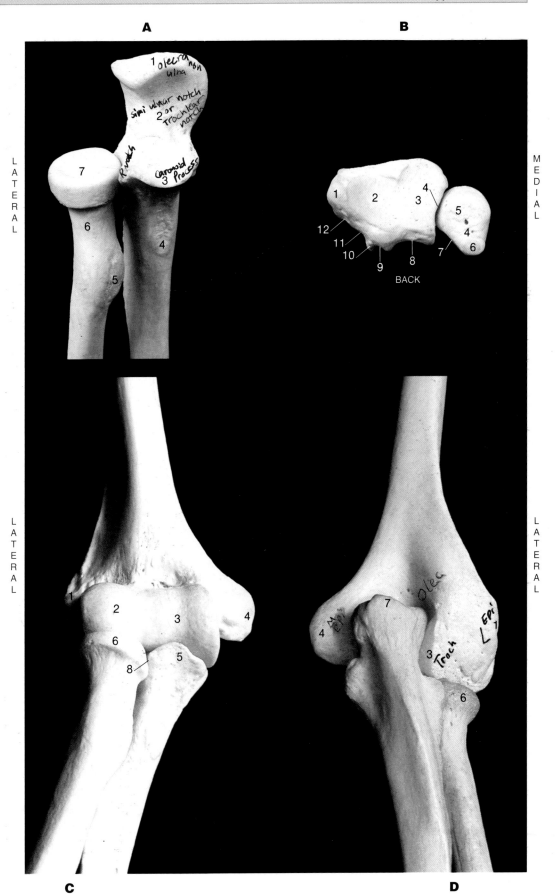

A

B

BACK

C

D

A   **B**

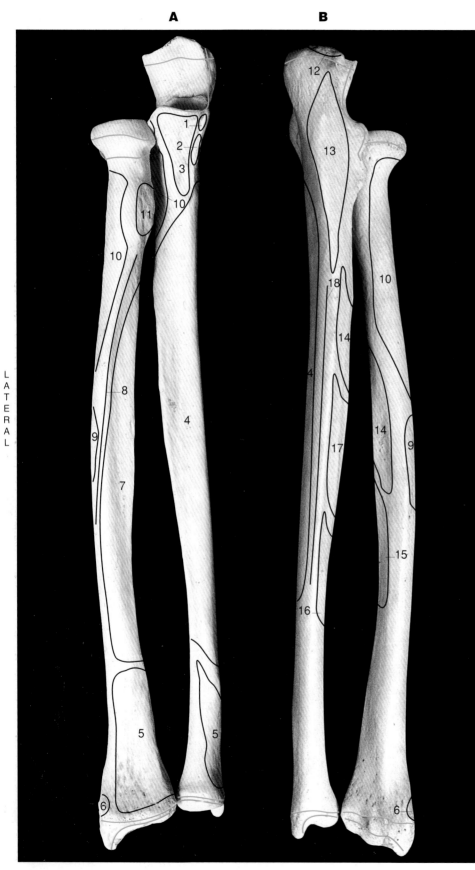

Right radius and ulna, **A** from the front, **B** from behind. Attachments

Blue lines = epiphysial lines; green lines = capsule attachments of elbow and wrist joints

1	Flexor digitorum superficialis, ulnar head
2	Pronator teres
3	Brachialis
4	Flexor digitorum profundus
5	Pronator quadratus
6	Brachioradialis
7	Flexor pollicis longus
8	Flexor digitorum superficialis, radial head
9	Pronator teres
10	Supinator
11	Biceps
12	Triceps
13	Anconeus
14	Abductor pollicis longus
15	Extensor pollicis brevis
16	Extensor indicis
17	Extensor pollicis longus
18	Aponeurotic attachment of flexor digitorum profundus, flexor carpi ulnaris and extensor carpi ulnaris

• Abductor pollicis longus (14) and extensor pollicis brevis (15) are the only two muscles to have an origin from the posterior surface of the radius (although both extend on to the interosseous membrane and the abductor also has an origin from the posterior surface of the ulna). These muscles remain companions as they wind round the lateral side of the radius (page 135, C4 and 5) and form the radial boundary of the anatomical snuffbox (page 146, A6 and 7).

• Flexor pollicis longus has an occasional small additional origin from the lateral (or rarely the medial) side of the coronoid process of the ulna (beside the lower part of the brachialis attachment).

• Note the positions of the epiphysial and capsular lines at the lower ends of the bones; the epiphyses are extracapsular.

• In the young subject the radius sometimes fractures across the lower epiphysis following an injury to the wrist, a 'slipped' epiphysis. In the adult the term 'Colles' fracture' refers to a transverse break across the lower radius within about 2.5 cm of the lower end of the bone. The ulnar styloid process is also often fractured.

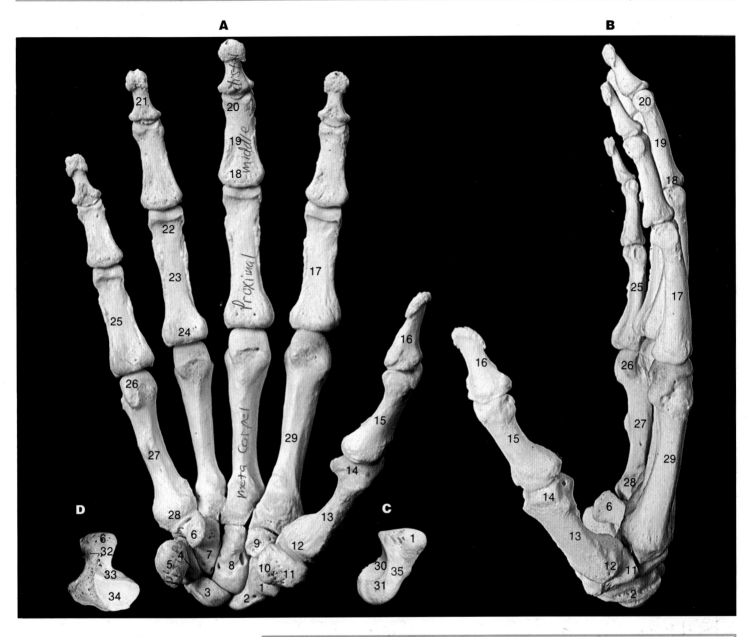

Bones of the right hand, A palmar surface, B from the lateral side, C scaphoid, palmar surface, D hamate from the medial side

• The scaphoid, lunate, triquetral and pisiform bones form the proximal row of carpal bones.
• The trapezium, trapezoid, capitate and hamate bones form the distal row of carpal bones.
• The tubercle (1) and waist (35) are the non-articular parts of the scaphoid and therefore contain nutrient foramina. A fracture across the waist may therefore interfere with the blood supply of the proximal pole of the bone and lead to avascular necrosis. The waist of the scaphoid lies in the anatomical snuffbox; the tubercle may be palpated in front of the radial boundary of the snuffbox.

1 Tubercle of scaphoid	18 Base ⎫
2 Scaphoid	19 Shaft ⎬ of middle phalanx of middle finger
3 Lunate	20 Head ⎭
4 Triquetral	21 Distal phalanx of ring finger
5 Pisiform	22 Head ⎫
6 Hook of hamate	23 Shaft ⎬ of proximal phalanx of ring finger
7 Hamate	24 Base ⎭
8 Capitate	25 Proximal phalanx of little finger
9 Trapezoid	26 Head ⎫
10 Tubercle of trapezium	27 Shaft ⎬ of fifth metacarpal
11 Trapezium	28 Base ⎭
12 Base ⎫	29 Second metacarpal
13 Shaft ⎬ of first metacarpal	30 Surface for capitate
14 Head ⎭	31 Surface for lunate
15 Proximal ⎫ phalanx of thumb	32 Groove for deep branch of ulnar nerve
16 Distal ⎭	33 Palmar surface
17 Proximal phalanx of index finger	34 Surface for triquetral
	35 Waist of scaphoid

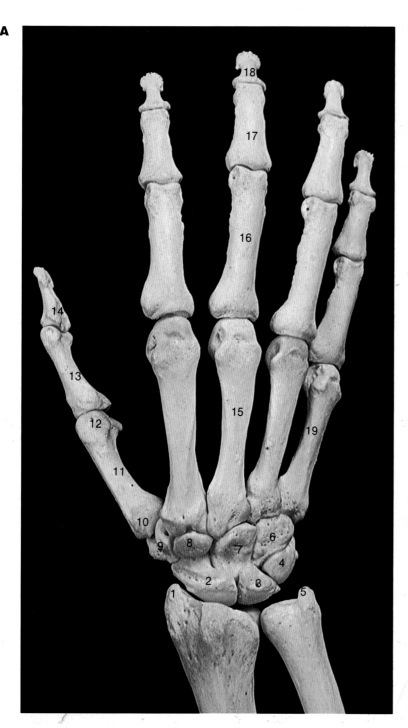

Bones of the right hand, A dorsal surface

1	Styloid process of radius	13	Proximal	phalanx of
2	Scaphoid	14	Distal	thumb
3	Lunate	15	Third metacarpal	
4	Triquetral	16	Proximal	phalanx
5	Styloid process of ulna	17	Middle	of middle
6	Hamate	18	Distal	finger
7	Capitate	19	Fifth metacarpal	
8	Trapezoid			
9	Trapezium			
10	Base — of first			
11	Shaft — meta-			
12	Head — carpal			

**Bones of the right hand, B palmar surface, C dorsal surface.
Attachments**
Pale green lines = ligament attachments

1 Flexor carpi ulnaris
2 Abductor digiti minimi
3 Pisohamate ligament
4 Pisometacarpal ligament
5 Flexor digiti minimi brevis
6 Opponens digiti minimi
7 Fourth ⎫
8 Third ⎪
9 Second ⎬ palmar interosseous
10 First ⎭
11 First ⎫
12 Second ⎪
13 Third ⎬ dorsal interosseous
14 Fourth ⎭
15 Transverse ⎫
16 Oblique ⎬ head of adductor pollicis
17 Flexor carpi radialis
18 Flexor pollicis brevis
19 Opponens pollicis
20 Abductor pollicis brevis
21 Abductor pollicis longus
22 Extensor pollicis brevis
23 Extensor pollicis longus
24 Flexor digitorum superficialis
25 Flexor digitorum profundus
26 Flexor pollicis longus
27 Extensor expansion
28 Extensor carpi ulnaris
29 Extensor carpi radialis brevis
30 Extensor carpi radialis longus

• The wrist joint (properly called the radiocarpal joint) is the joint between (proximally) the lower end of the radius and the interarticular disc which holds the lower ends of the radius and the ulna together, and (distally) the scaphoid, lunate and triquetral bones.
• The midcarpal joint is the joint between the proximal and distal rows of carpal bones (see the note on page 111).
• The carpometacarpal joint of the thumb is the joint between the trapezium and the base of the first metacarpal.

c

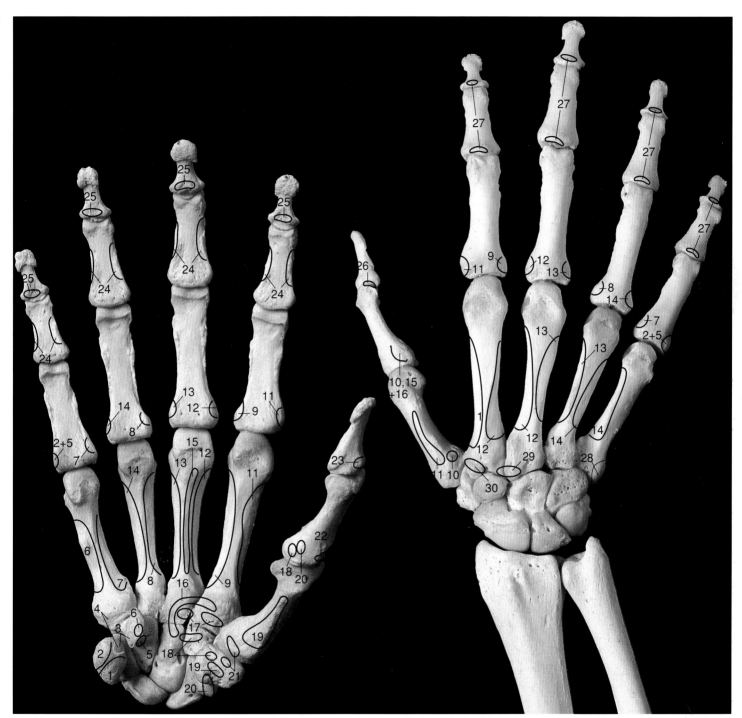

• The metacarpophalangeal joints are the joints between the heads of the metacarpals and the bases of the proximal phalanges.

• The interphalangeal joints are the joints between the head of one phalanx and the base of the adjoining phalanx.

• The pisiform is a sesamoid bone in the tendon of flexor carpi ulnaris and is anchored by the pisohamate and pisometacarpal ligaments.

• In official anatomical terminology, the origin of flexor pollicis brevis from the trapezium (and flexor retinaculum) is referred to as the superficial head, and that from the trapezoid and

capitate as the deep head (often small or even absent, and to be distinguished from the first palmar interosseous which is sometimes considered to be synonymous with the deep head).

• Dorsal interossei arise from the sides of two adjacent metacarpal bones (as at C12, from the sides of the second and third metacarpals); palmar interossei arise only from the metacarpal of their own finger (as at B9, from the second metacarpal). Compare with dissection B on page 144 and note that when looking at the palm, parts of the dorsal interossei can be seen as well as the palmar interossei, but when looking at the dorsum of the hand (as on page 151, C) only dorsal interossei are seen.

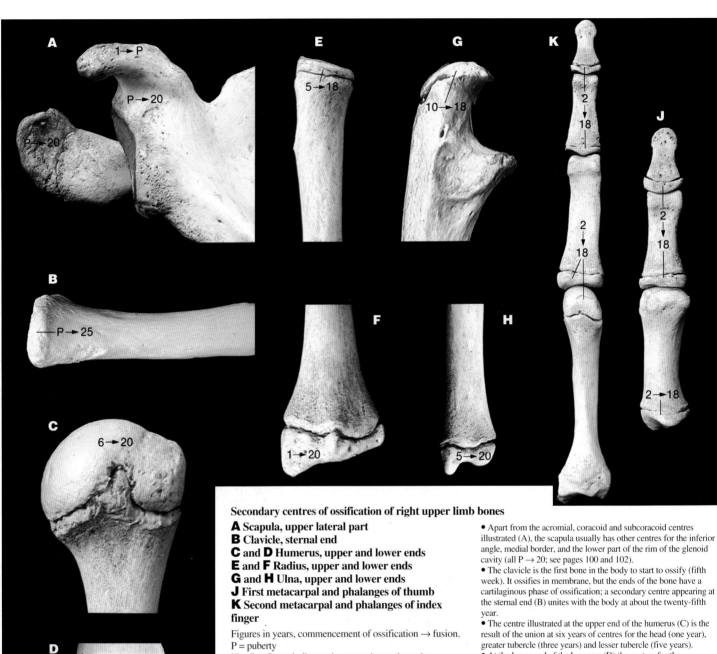

Secondary centres of ossification of right upper limb bones

A Scapula, upper lateral part
B Clavicle, sternal end
C and **D** Humerus, upper and lower ends
E and **F** Radius, upper and lower ends
G and **H** Ulna, upper and lower ends
J First metacarpal and phalanges of thumb
K Second metacarpal and phalanges of index finger

Figures in years, commencement of ossification → fusion. P = puberty
The first figure indicates the approximate date when ossification begins in the secondary centre, and the second figure (beyond the arrowhead) when the centre finally becomes fused with the rest of the bone. Single average dates have been given (both here and for the lower limb bone centres on pages 286 and 287) and although there may be considerable individual variations, the 'growing end' of the bone (when fusion occurs last) is constant. The dates in females are often a year or more earlier than in males

• Apart from the acromial, coracoid and subcoracoid centres illustrated (A), the scapula usually has other centres for the inferior angle, medial border, and the lower part of the rim of the glenoid cavity (all P → 20; see pages 100 and 102).
• The clavicle is the first bone in the body to start to ossify (fifth week). It ossifies in membrane, but the ends of the bone have a cartilaginous phase of ossification; a secondary centre appearing at the sternal end (B) unites with the body at about the twenty-fifth year.
• The centre illustrated at the upper end of the humerus (C) is the result of the union at six years of centres for the head (one year), greater tubercle (three years) and lesser tubercle (five years).
• At the lower end of the humerus (D) the centres for the capitulum, trochlea and lateral epicondyle fuse together before uniting with the shaft.
• All the phalanges (as in K), and the first metacarpal (J) have a secondary centre at their proximal ends; the other metacarpals (as in K) have one at their distal ends.
• All the carpal bones are cartilaginous at birth and none has a secondary centre. The largest, the capitate, is the first to begin to ossify (in the second month after birth), followed in a month or so by the hamate, with the triquetral at three years, lunate at four years, scaphoid, trapezoid and trapezium at five years and the pisiform last at nine years or later. There are often variations in the above common pattern.
• Primary centres for the body or shafts of bones usually begin to ossify about the eighth week of fetal life, but the clavicle is the first bone to commence ossification (see the second note above).

Right shoulder, from the front. Surface markings

The clavicle is subcutaneous throughout its length. Its acromial end (4) at the acromioclavicular joint (3) lies at a slightly higher level than the acromion of the scapula (2). At the most lateral part of the shoulder, deltoid overlies the humerus; the acromion of the scapula does not extend so far laterally. Compare the positions of the features noted here with the dissection on the next page

• The nipple in the male (15) normally lies at the level of the fourth intercostal space.
• The deltopectoral groove containing the cephalic vein (10) is formed by the adjacent borders of deltoid (9) and pectoralis major (8).
• The lower border of pectoralis major (11) forms the anterior axillary fold.
• Note that the most lateral bony point in the shoulder is the greater tubercle (1).

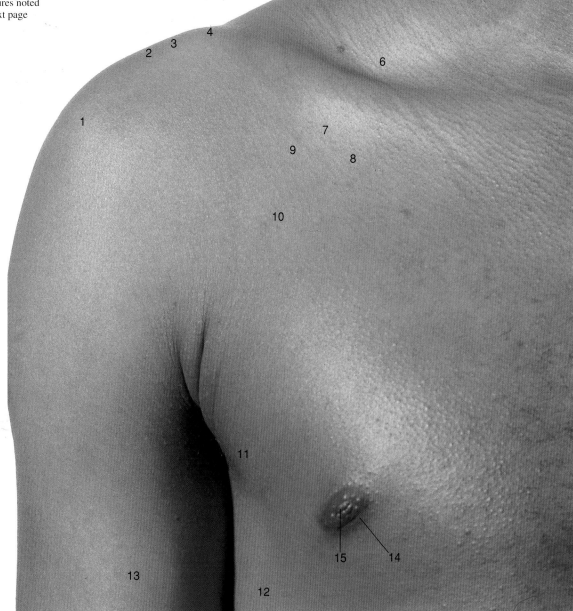

1 Deltoid overlying greater tubercle of humerus	6 Supraclavicular fossa	11 Lower margin of pectoralis major
2 Acromion	7 Infraclavicular fossa	12 Serratus anterior
3 Acromioclavicular joint	8 Upper margin of pectoralis major	13 Biceps
4 Acromial end of clavicle	9 Anterior margin of deltoid	14 Areola
5 Trapezius	10 Deltopectoral groove and cephalic vein	15 Nipple

A Right shoulder, from the front. Superficial dissection

Removal of skin and fascia displays branches of the supraclavicular nerve (9) crossing the clavicle (10), and the cephalic vein (17) lying in the deltopectoral groove between deltoid (2) and pectoralis major (15)

1 Tip of shoulder
2 Deltoid
3 Acromion of scapula
4 Acromioclavicular joint
5 Acromial end of clavicle
6 Trapezius
7 Accessory nerve
8 Cervical nerve to trapezius
9 Branches of supraclavicular nerve
10 Clavicle
11 A superficial venous plexus
12 Clavicular head ⎫ of sterno-
13 Sternal head ⎭ cleidomastoid
14 Sternocostal part ⎫ of pectoralis
15 Clavicular part ⎭ major
16 Clavipectoral fascia
17 Cephalic vein

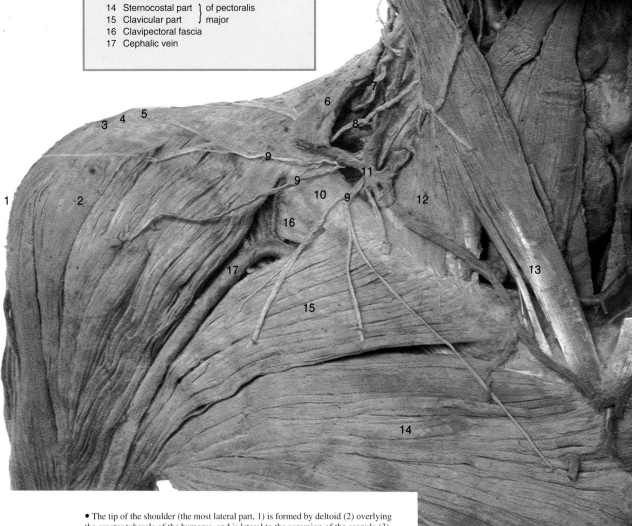

- The tip of the shoulder (the most lateral part, 1) is formed by deltoid (2) overlying the greater tubercle of the humerus, and is lateral to the acromion of the scapula (3).
- The position of the acromioclavicular joint (4) is indicated by the small 'step down' between the acromial end of the clavicle (5) and the acromion (3); compare with the surface feature 3 on page 115. This is the normal appearance; when the joint is dislocated, with the acromion being forced below the end of the clavicle, the 'step' is much exaggerated.
- The cephalic vein (17) runs in the deltopectoral groove between deltoid (2) and pectoralis major (15) and pierces the clavipectoral fascia (16) to drain into the axillary vein.

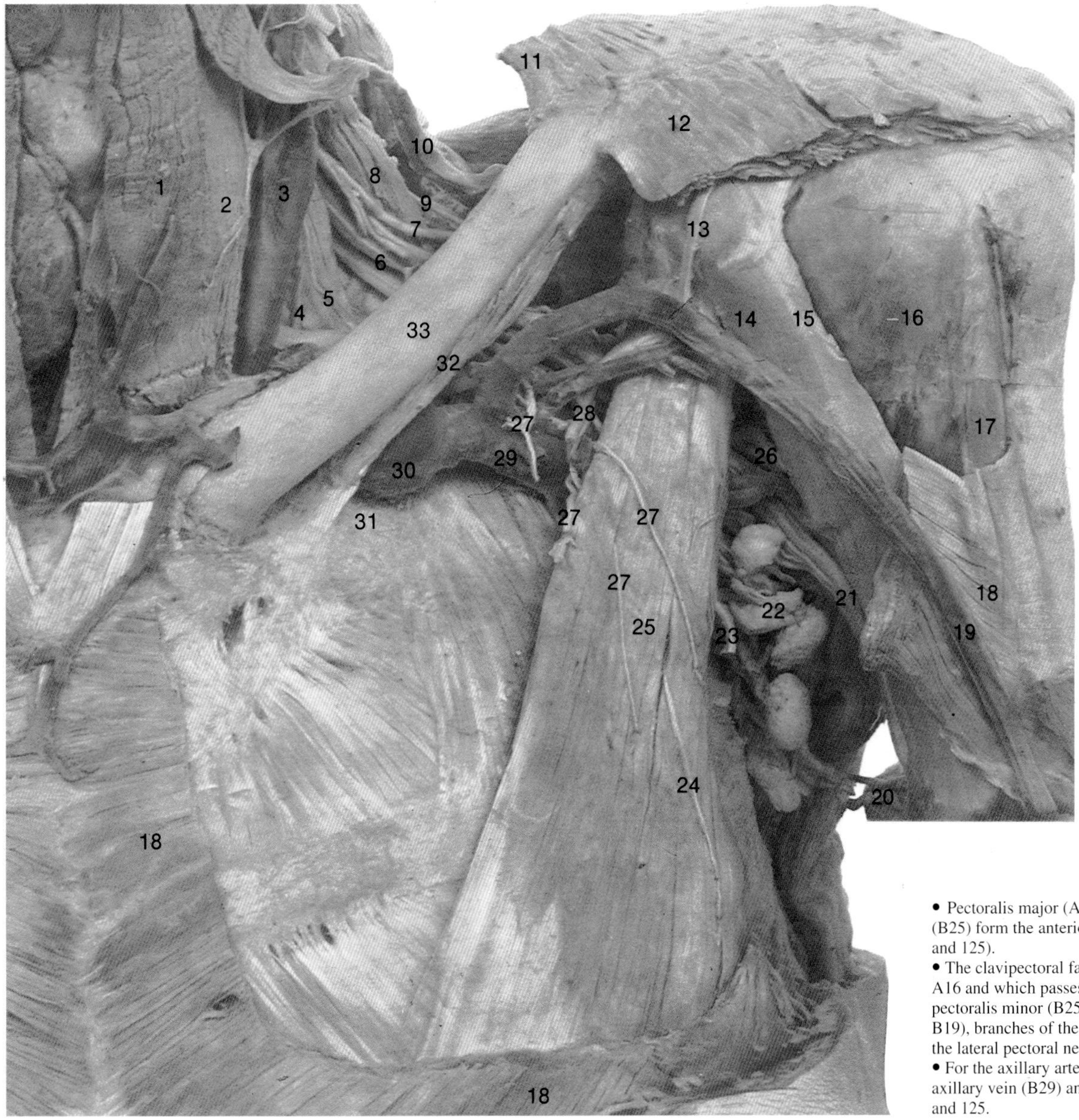

B Left shoulder, from the front. Deeper dissection

Most of deltoid (12) and pectoralis major (18) have been removed to show the underlying pectoralis minor (25) and its associated vessels and nerves. The clavipectoral fascia which passed between the clavicle (33) and the upper (medial) border of the pectoralis minor (25) has also been removed to show the axillary vein (29) receiving the cephalic vein (19) and continuing as the subclavian vein (30) as it crosses the first rib (31). Above the clavicle, the inferior belly of omohyoid (10) has been displaced upwards to give a clear view of the phrenic nerve (4) and some brachial plexus branches (5 to 7, and 9)

• Pectoralis major (A14 and A15) and pectoralis minor (B25) form the anterior wall of the axilla (see also pages 124 and 125).
• The clavipectoral fascia, a small part of which is seen at A16 and which passes between the clavicle (B33) and pectoralis minor (B25), is pierced by the cephalic vein (A17, B19), branches of the thoraco-acromial vessels (as at B28), the lateral pectoral nerve (B27) and lymph vessels.
• For the axillary artery, which in B is obscured by the axillary vein (B29) and adjacent structures, see pages 124 and 125.

1 Sternohyoid	18 Pectoralis major
2 Sternothyroid	19 Cephalic vein
3 Internal jugular vein	20 Intercostobrachial nerve
4 Phrenic nerve overlying scalenus anterior	21 Median nerve
5 Nerve to subclavius	22 Axillary lymph nodes
6 Trunks of brachial plexus	23 Lateral thoracic artery
7 Suprascapular nerve	24 Branch of medial pectoral nerve
8 Scalenus medius	25 Pectoralis minor
9 Long thoracic nerve (to serratus anterior)	26 Anterior circumflex humeral artery and musculocutaneous
10 Inferior belly of omohyoid (displaced upwards)	nerve
11 Trapezius	27 Branches of lateral pectoral nerve
12 Deltoid	28 Pectoral branch of thoraco-acromial artery
13 Coracoid process and acromial branch of thoraco-acromial	29 Axillary vein
artery	30 Subclavian vein
14 Coracobrachialis	31 First rib
15 Short head of biceps	32 Subclavius
16 Subscapularis	33 Clavicle
17 Tendon of long head of biceps	

A

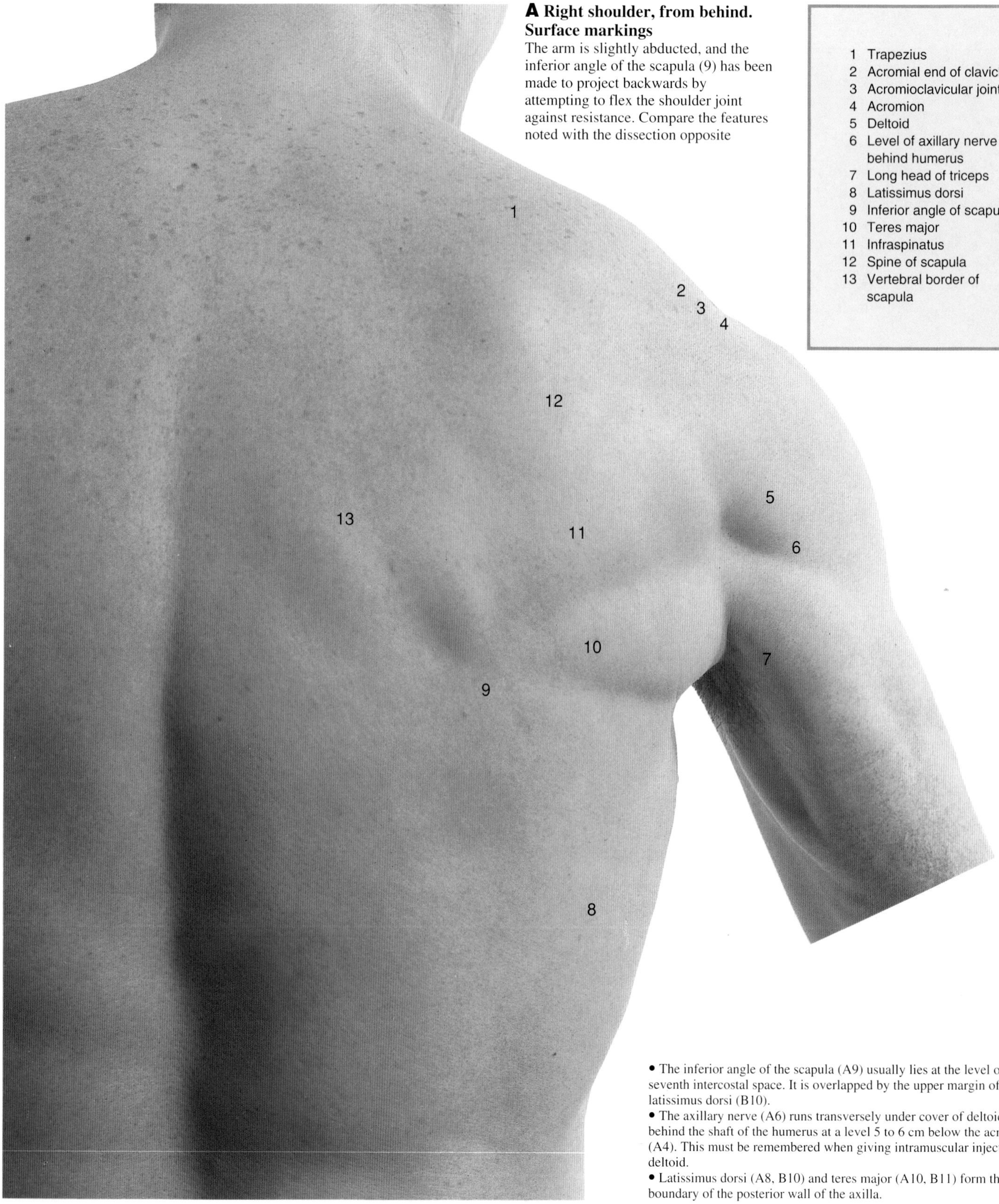

**A Right shoulder, from behind.
Surface markings**
The arm is slightly abducted, and the
inferior angle of the scapula (9) has been
made to project backwards by
attempting to flex the shoulder joint
against resistance. Compare the features
noted with the dissection opposite

1 Trapezius
2 Acromial end of clavicle
3 Acromioclavicular joint
4 Acromion
5 Deltoid
6 Level of axillary nerve
   behind humerus
7 Long head of triceps
8 Latissimus dorsi
9 Inferior angle of scapula
10 Teres major
11 Infraspinatus
12 Spine of scapula
13 Vertebral border of
   scapula

• The inferior angle of the scapula (A9) usually lies at the level of the
seventh intercostal space. It is overlapped by the upper margin of
latissimus dorsi (B10).
• The axillary nerve (A6) runs transversely under cover of deltoid (A5)
behind the shaft of the humerus at a level 5 to 6 cm below the acromion
(A4). This must be remembered when giving intramuscular injections into
deltoid.
• Latissimus dorsi (A8, B10) and teres major (A10, B11) form the lower
boundary of the posterior wall of the axilla.

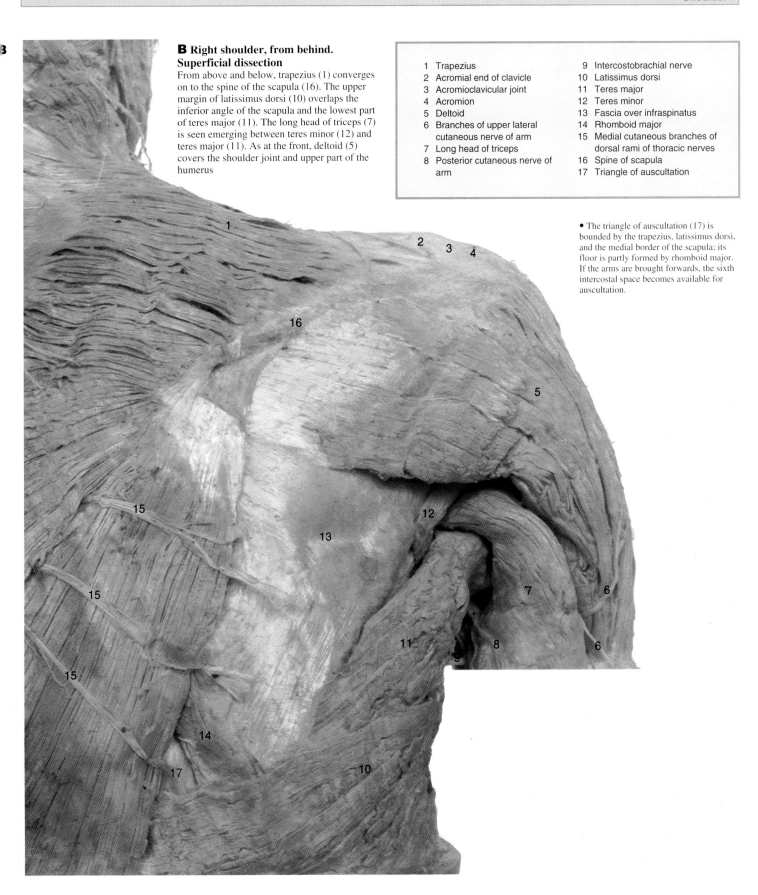

**B Right shoulder, from behind.
Superficial dissection**

From above and below, trapezius (1) converges
on to the spine of the scapula (16). The upper
margin of latissimus dorsi (10) overlaps the
inferior angle of the scapula and the lowest part
of teres major (11). The long head of triceps (7)
is seen emerging between teres minor (12) and
teres major (11). As at the front, deltoid (5)
covers the shoulder joint and upper part of the
humerus

1 Trapezius	9 Intercostobrachial nerve
2 Acromial end of clavicle	10 Latissimus dorsi
3 Acromioclavicular joint	11 Teres major
4 Acromion	12 Teres minor
5 Deltoid	13 Fascia over infraspinatus
6 Branches of upper lateral cutaneous nerve of arm	14 Rhomboid major
7 Long head of triceps	15 Medial cutaneous branches of dorsal rami of thoracic nerves
8 Posterior cutaneous nerve of arm	16 Spine of scapula
	17 Triangle of auscultation

• The triangle of auscultation (17) is
bounded by the trapezius, latissimus dorsi,
and the medial border of the scapula; its
floor is partly formed by rhomboid major.
If the arms are brought forwards, the sixth
intercostal space becomes available for
auscultation.

A Left shoulder, from behind

Interrupted line = outline of scapula

Most of trapezius (5) and deltoid (1) have been removed to show the underlying muscles. The medial cut edge of trapezius remains near the line of the thoracic spines (11). Levator scapulae (7), rhomboid minor (8) and rhomboid major (9) are seen converging on to the vertebral border of the scapula, and supraspinatus (6) lies above the spine of the scapula (20)

●Muscles producing movements at the shoulder joint:

Abduction: supraspinatus and deltoid (middle fibres) for about 120°; further abduction requires scapular rotation produced by serratus anterior and trapezius.
Adduction: pectoralis major, latissimus dorsi, teres major, teres minor.
Flexion: deltoid (anterior fibres), pectoralis major, biceps, coracobrachialis.
Extension: deltoid (posterior fibres), latissimus dorsi, teres major.
Lateral rotation: infraspinatus, teres minor.
Medial rotation: pectoralis major, subscapularis, latissimus dorsi, teres major.

1	Deltoid	11	Third thoracic spinous process
2	Acromion	12	Erector spinae
3	Acromioclavicular joint	13	Thoracic part of thoracolumbar fascia
4	Acromial end of clavicle	14	Latissimus dorsi
5	Trapezius	15	Teres major
6	Supraspinatus	16	Long head of triceps
7	Levator scapulae	17	Posterior circumflex humeral vessels and
8	Rhomboid minor		axillary nerve
9	Rhomboid major	18	Teres minor
10	Branch of dorsal ramus of a thoracic	19	Infraspinatus
	nerve	20	Spine of scapula

A

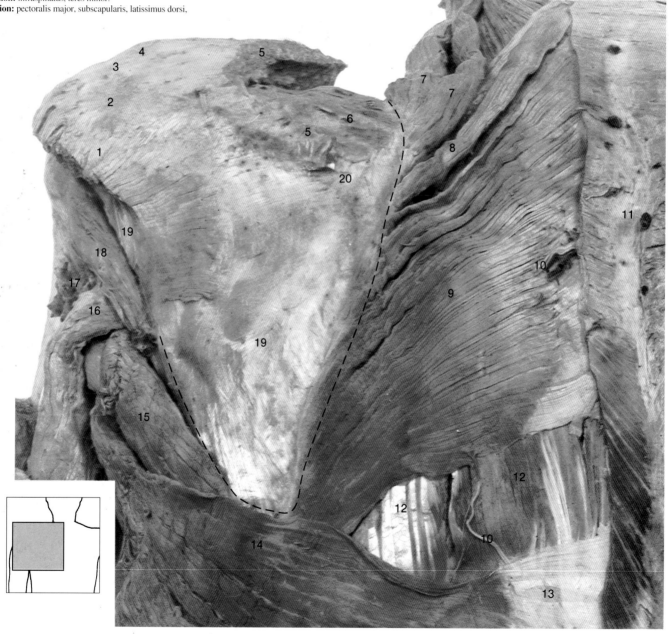

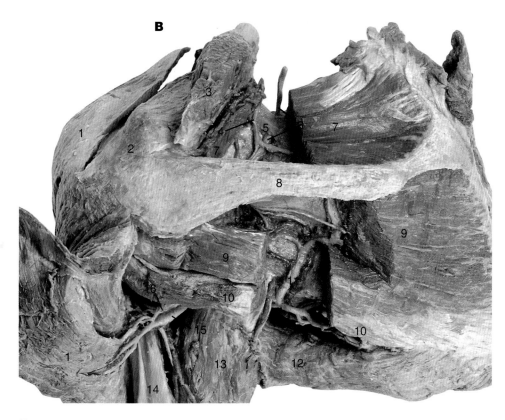

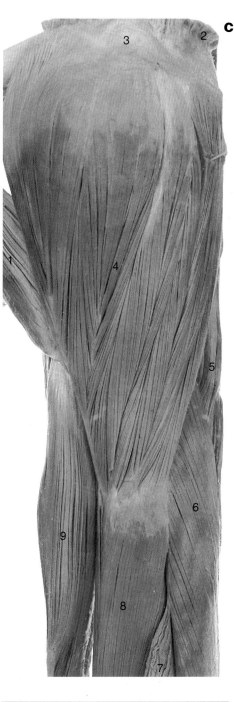

B Left shoulder, from the left and behind

The central parts of supraspinatus (7) and infraspinatus (9) have been removed to show the suprascapular nerve (6) which supplies both muscles. The removal of parts of infraspinatus and teres minor displays the anastomosis between the circumflex scapular branch of the subscapular artery and the suprascapular artery.Deltoid (1) has been reflected laterally to show the axillary nerve (16) and the posterior circumflex humeral vessels passing backwards through the quadrilateral space (see note below)

1	Deltoid	9	Infraspinatus
2	Acromioclavicular joint	10	Teres minor
3	Trapezius	11	Circumflex scapular artery
4	Suprascapular artery	12	Teres major
5	Superior transverse scapular	13	Long head of triceps
	(suprascapular) ligament	14	Lateral head of triceps
6	Suprascapular nerve	15	Posterior circumflex humeral artery
7	Supraspinatus	16	Axillary nerve
8	Spine of scapula		

• As it lies just beneath the capsule of the shoulder joint, the axillary nerve may be injured by dislocation of the joint.
• The suprascapular artery (B4) passes into the supraspinous fossa superficial to the superior transverse scapular ligament (B5); the suprascapular nerve (B6) passes deep to the ligament.
• The axillary nerve (B16) and posterior circumflex humeral vessels (B15) pass backwards through the quadrilateral space which (viewed from behind) is bounded by teres minor (B10), below by teres major (B12), medially by the long head of triceps (B13), and laterally by the humerus. (Viewed from the front, the upper boundary of the space is subscapularis – see page 126, A17.)

C Left shoulder and upper arm, from the left

Deltoid (4) extends over the tip of the shoulder to its attachment half way down the lateral side of the shaft of the humerus. Biceps (9) is on the front of the arm below pectoralis major (1) and triceps (5 and 6) is at the back

1	Pectoralis major
2	Trapezius
3	Acromion
4	Deltoid
5	Long head } of triceps
6	Lateral head } of triceps
7	Brachioradialis
8	Brachialis
9	Biceps

A

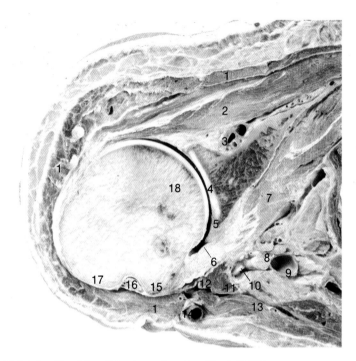

B

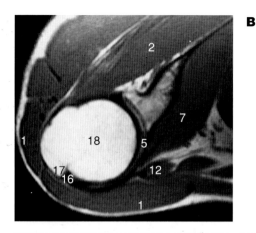

Right shoulder joint, A horizontal section, B axial MR image
Viewed from above, this section shows the articulation of the head of the humerus (18) with the glenoid cavity of the scapula (4). The tendon of the long head of biceps (16) lies in the groove between the greater and lesser tubercles of the humerus (17 and 15). Subscapularis (7) passes immediately in front of the joint, and infraspinatus (2) behind it. Compare the MR image in 3 with features in A

1	Deltoid	10	Musculocutaneous nerve
2	Infraspinatus	11	Coracobrachialis
3	Suprascapular nerve and vessels	12	Short head of biceps
4	Glenoid cavity	13	Pectoralis major
5	Glenoid labrum	14	Cephalic vein
6	Capsule	15	Lesser tubercle
7	Subscapularis	16	Tendon of long head of biceps in intertubercular groove
8	Cords of brachial plexus	17	Greater tubercle
9	Axillary artery	18	Head of humerus

C

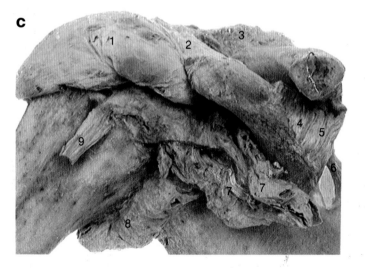

D

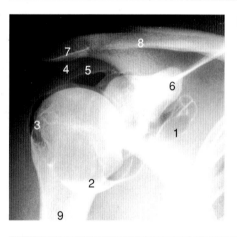

D Double contrast arthrogram of shoulder

1	Subscapularis bursa	6	Coracoid process
2	Axillary pouch	7	Acromion
3	Bicipital tendon sheath	8	Clavicle
4	Region of subacromial bursa	9	Humerus
5	Site of rotator cuff muscles		

C Right shoulder joint, from the front
The synovial joint cavity inside the capsule (8) and the subacromial bursa (1) have been injected separately with green resin

1	Subacromial bursa	6	Superior transverse scapular (suprascapular) ligament
2	Coraco-acromial ligament		
3	Acromioclavicular joint	7	Subscapularis bursa
4	Trapezoid ligament	8	Capsule of shoulder joint
5	Conoid ligament	9	Tendon of long head of biceps

• The subscapularis bursa (C7 and D1) normally communicates with the synovial cavity of the shoulder joint.
• The subacromial bursa (C1 and D4) does *not* normally communicate with the shoulder joint; it is separated from the joint by the supraspinatus tendon. Only if the tendon is ruptured can the two cavities become continuous with one another.

E

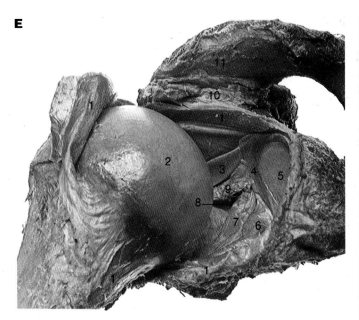

F

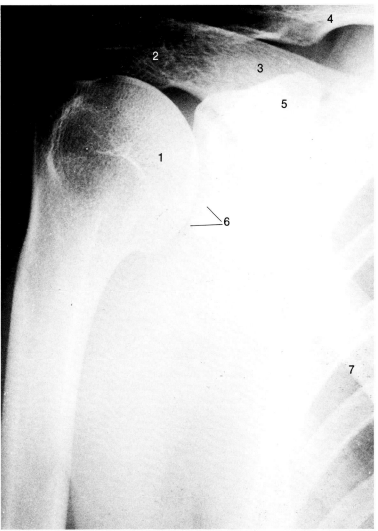

E Left shoulder joint, opened from behind

In this view, after removing all the posterior part of the capsule, the inner surface of the front of the capsule (1) is seen, with its reinforcing glenohumeral ligaments (6, 7 and 9)

1	Capsule	8	Opening into subscapularis bursa
2	Head of humerus		
3	Long head of biceps	9	Superior glenohumeral ligament
4	Glenoid labrum		
5	Glenoid cavity	10	Supraspinatus
6	Inferior glenohumeral ligament	11	Acromion
7	Middle glenohumeral ligament		

• The joint cavity communicates with the subscapularis bursa through an opening (8) between the superior (9) and middle (7) glenohumeral ligaments.
• The tendon of the long head of biceps (3) is continuous with the glenoid labrum (4).

G

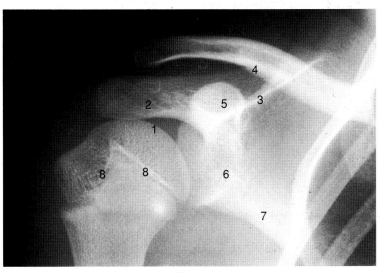

Shoulder radiographs, F anteroposterior projection, G of a nine-year-old child

In F the head of the humerus (1) lies against the glenoid cavity of the scapula (6), whose coracoid process (5) is seen end-on. In G note the epiphysial line (8) at the upper end of the humerus

1	Head of humerus
2	Acromion
3	Spine of scapula
4	Clavicle
5	Coracoid process
6	Rim of glenoid cavity
7	Lateral border of scapula
8	Epiphysial line

• The upper humeral epiphysis is a compound structure made up of epiphyses for the head, and greater and lesser tubercles. It rests on the spike-like upper humeral shaft, giving the appearance of an inverted 'V' to the epiphysial line on the radiograph (G8). Compare with page 114, C.

A

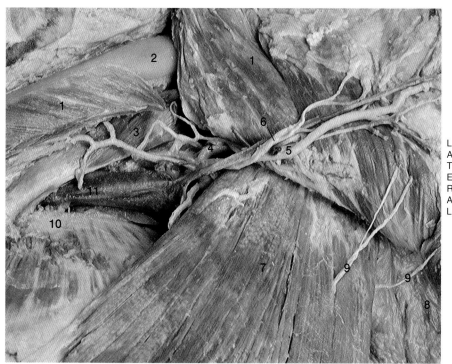
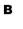
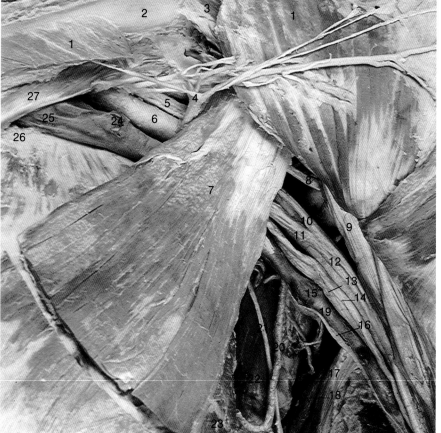

A Left axilla, anterior wall

Pectoralis major (1) has been reflected upwards and laterally, and the clavipectoral fascia which passes from subclavius (3) to pectoralis minor (7) has been removed

LATERAL

1 Pectoralis major
2 Clavicle
3 Subclavius
4 Cephalic vein
5 Thoraco-acromial vessels
6 Lateral pectoral nerve
7 Pectoralis minor
8 Axillary sheath surrounding axillary artery and brachial plexus
9 Branches of medial pectoral nerve
10 First rib
11 Subclavian vein

• The clavipectoral fascia (here removed, between subclavius, 3, and pectoralis minor, 7) is pierced by the cephalic vein (4), thoraco-acromial vessels (5), lateral pectoral nerve (6) and lymphatics.
• The axillary sheath (8) is the downward continuation of the prevertebral fascia of the neck and forms a dense covering for the axillary artery and the surrounding parts of the brachial plexus.
• The *lateral* pectoral nerve (6) is related to the *medial* (upper) border of pectoralis minor (7). The *medial* pectoral nerve (9) is related to the *lateral* (lower) border of pectoralis minor.

B

B Left axilla and brachial plexus, from the front

Pectoralis major (1) has been reflected and the clavipectoral fascia removed, together with the axillary sheath (A8) which surrounded the axillary artery and brachial plexus

LATERAL

1 Pectoralis major
2 Clavicle
3 Deltoid
4 Thoraco-acromial vessels and lateral pectoral nerve
5 Lateral cord of brachial plexus
6 Axillary artery
7 Pectoralis minor
8 Musculocutaneous nerve
9 Coracobrachialis
10 Lateral root ⎫ of median nerve
11 Medial root ⎭
12 Median nerve
13 Ulnar nerve
14 Medial cutaneous nerve of forearm
15 Axillary vein
16 Medial cutaneous nerve of arm
17 Latissimus dorsi
18 Teres major
19 Circumflex scapular artery
20 Thoracodorsal artery
21 Thoracodorsal nerve
22 Subscapularis
23 Serratus anterior
24 Entry of cephalic vein into axillary vein
25 Subclavian vein
26 First rib
27 Subclavius

C

C Left brachial plexus, from the front

Pectoralis major and minor (2 and 9) have been
reflected and the axillary sheath (A8) removed, together
with most of the axillary vein (36) and its tributaries

 1 Clavicle
 2 Pectoralis major
 3 Subclavius
 4 Lateral pectoral nerve
 5 Lateral cord
 6 Axillary artery
 7 Thoraco-acromial artery
 8 Loop between medial and lateral
    pectoral nerves
 9 Pectoralis minor
10 Musculocutaneous nerve
11 Lateral root } of median nerve
12 Medial root
13 Median nerve
14 Radial nerve
15 Axillary nerve
16 Anterior circumflex humeral artery
17 Coracobrachialis and short head of
    biceps
18 Long head of biceps
19 Deltoid
20 Ulnar nerve
21 Medial cutaneous nerve of forearm
22 Medial cutaneous nerve of arm
23 Latissimus dorsi
24 Teres major
25 Lower subscapular nerve
26 Circumflex scapular artery
27 Thoracodorsal artery
28 Thoracodorsal nerve
29 Subscapularis
30 Serratus anterior
31 Long thoracic nerve
32 Intercostobrachial nerve (cut end)
33 Communication between 22 and 32
34 Branch from first thoracic nerve to
    intercostobrachial nerve
35 Lateral thoracic artery
36 Axillary vein
37 Entry of cephalic vein
38 Subclavian vein
39 First rib

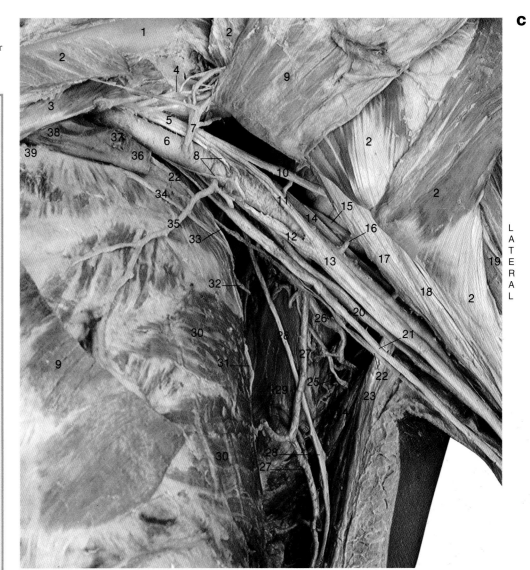

L
A
T
E
R
A
L

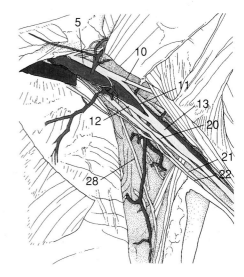

• The thoracodorsal artery (27) is the name given to the continuation of
the subscapular artery distal to the origin of the circumflex scapular
branch (26).
• To sort out the major branches of the medial and lateral cords, note
that the largest branches of the medial and lateral cords form the shape
of a capital M. Identify the median nerve (13, the middle stem of the M)
in front of the axillary artery. Follow its lateral root (11) upwards to the
lateral cord (5), from which the musculocutaneous nerve arises (10, as
the lateral stem of the M) to run into the coracobrachialis muscle (17).
Follow the medial root of the median nerve (12) upwards to the medial
cord (obscured by the axillary artery below the label 6), whose largest
branch is the ulnar nerve (20, the medial stem of the M).
• The radial nerve (14, one of the two terminal branches of the posterior
cord and the largest of all the branches of the plexus) is most easily
identified as it lies behind the axillary artery and in front of the
latissimus dorsi tendon. Follow the nerve upwards to find the axillary
nerve (15, the other terminal branch of the posterior cord) passing
laterally and backwards through the quadrilateral space (see page 121).

• Boundaries of the axilla:
Anterior wall: pectoralis major and minor (B1 and 7) and
the clavipectoral fascia with subclavius.
Posterior wall: subscapularis (C29), teres major (C24) and
latissimus dorsi (C23)**.**
Medial wall: serratus anterior (C30) overlying the first four
ribs and intercostal muscles.
Lateral wall: the intertubercular groove of the humerus,
coracobrachialis and biceps (C17).
Apex: the space between the clavicle (C1), first rib (C39)
and upper border of the scapula.
Base: the concavity of skin and axillary fascia between the
lower borders of pectoralis major and latissimus dorsi.

A Right brachial plexus and branches

In this front view of the plexus, all the blood vessels have been removed to show the cords of the plexus and their branches more clearly. Note the 'capital M' pattern (referred to in the notes on page 125) formed by the musculocutaneous nerve (5), the lateral root of the median nerve (7), the median nerve itself (24), the medial root of the median nerve (9) and the ulnar nerve (14). In this specimen the tendon of latissimus dorsi (19) is unusually broad and has become blended with the long head of triceps (20)

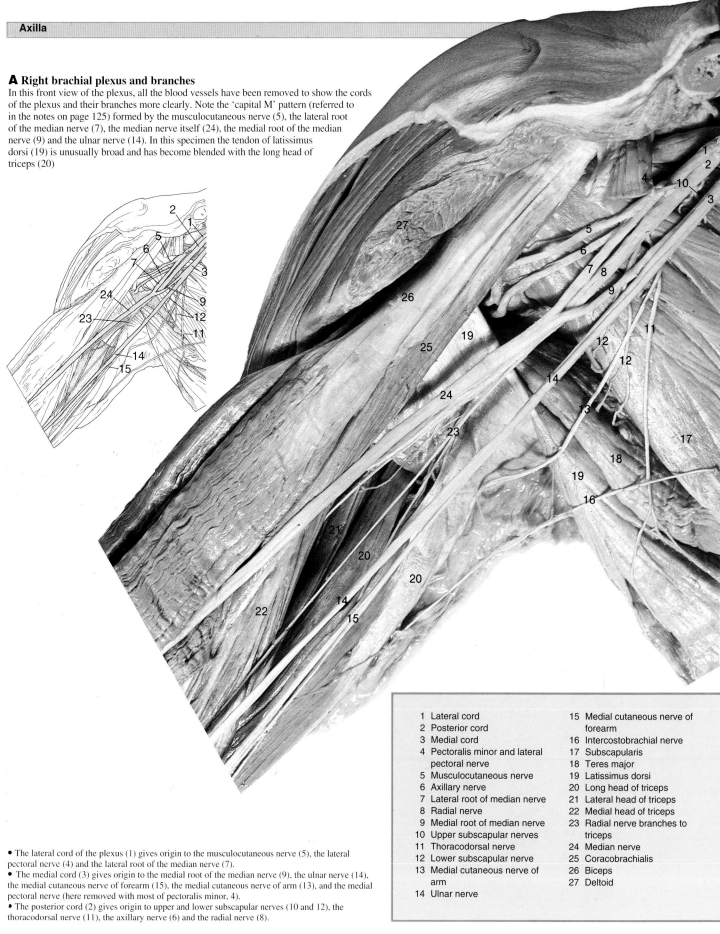

1 Lateral cord	15 Medial cutaneous nerve of
2 Posterior cord	forearm
3 Medial cord	16 Intercostobrachial nerve
4 Pectoralis minor and lateral	17 Subscapularis
pectoral nerve	18 Teres major
5 Musculocutaneous nerve	19 Latissimus dorsi
6 Axillary nerve	20 Long head of triceps
7 Lateral root of median nerve	21 Lateral head of triceps
8 Radial nerve	22 Medial head of triceps
9 Medial root of median nerve	23 Radial nerve branches to
10 Upper subscapular nerves	triceps
11 Thoracodorsal nerve	24 Median nerve
12 Lower subscapular nerve	25 Coracobrachialis
13 Medial cutaneous nerve of	26 Biceps
arm	27 Deltoid
14 Ulnar nerve	

- The lateral cord of the plexus (1) gives origin to the musculocutaneous nerve (5), the lateral pectoral nerve (4) and the lateral root of the median nerve (7).
- The medial cord (3) gives origin to the medial root of the median nerve (9), the ulnar nerve (14), the medial cutaneous nerve of forearm (15), the medial cutaneous nerve of arm (13), and the medial pectoral nerve (here removed with most of pectoralis minor, 4).
- The posterior cord (2) gives origin to upper and lower subscapular nerves (10 and 12), the thoracodorsal nerve (11), the axillary nerve (6) and the radial nerve (8).

B Left arm. Vessels and nerves, from the front

Biceps (6 and 8) has been turned laterally to show the musculocutaneous nerve (5) emerging from coracobrachialis (4), giving branches to biceps and brachialis (7 and 10) and becoming the lateral cutaneous nerve of the forearm (12) on the lateral side of the biceps tendon (11). The median nerve (3) gradually crosses over in front of the brachial artery (2) from the lateral to the medial side. The ulnar nerve (16) passes behind the medial intermuscular septum (15), and the end of the basilic vein (18) is seen joining a vena comitans (17) of the brachial artery to form the brachial vein (1)

1	Brachial vein	12	Lateral cutaneous nerve of forearm
2	Brachial artery	13	Brachioradialis
3	Median nerve	14	Pronator teres
4	Coracobrachialis	15	Medial intermuscular septum
5	Musculocutaneous nerve		
6	Short head of biceps	16	Ulnar nerve
7	Nerve to short head of biceps	17	Vena comitans of brachial artery
8	Long head of biceps	18	Basilic vein (cut end)
9	Brachialis	19	Long head of triceps
10	Nerve to brachialis		
11	Tendon of biceps		

- The musculocutaneous nerve (B5) supplies coracobrachialis (B4), biceps (B6 and 8) and brachialis (B9), and at the level where the muscle fibres of biceps become tendinous (B11) it pierces the deep fascia to become the lateral cutaneous nerve of the forearm (B12).
- The median nerve does not give off any muscular branches in the arm (unless the nerve to pronator teres has a high origin — page 132, C).
- The ulnar nerve (B16) leaves the anterior compartment of the arm by piercing the medial intermuscular septum (B15), and does not give off any muscular branches in the arm.

C Cross section of the left arm, from below

Looking from the elbow towards the shoulder, the section is taken through the middle of the arm. The musculocutaneous nerve (13) lies between brachialis (3) and biceps (2), and the median nerve (11) is on the medial side of the brachial artery (12) which has several venae comitantes adjacent (unlabelled). The ulnar nerve (7), with the superior ulnar collateral artery (8) beside it, is behind the median nerve (11) and the basilic vein (9). The radial nerve and the profunda brachii vessels (4) are in the posterior compartment at the lateral side of the humerus (5)

1	Cephalic vein
2	Biceps
3	Brachialis
4	Radial nerve and profunda brachii vessels
5	Humerus
6	Triceps
7	Ulnar nerve
8	Superior ulnar collateral artery
9	Basilic vein
10	Medial cutaneous nerve of forearm
11	Median nerve
12	Brachial artery
13	Musculocutaneous nerve

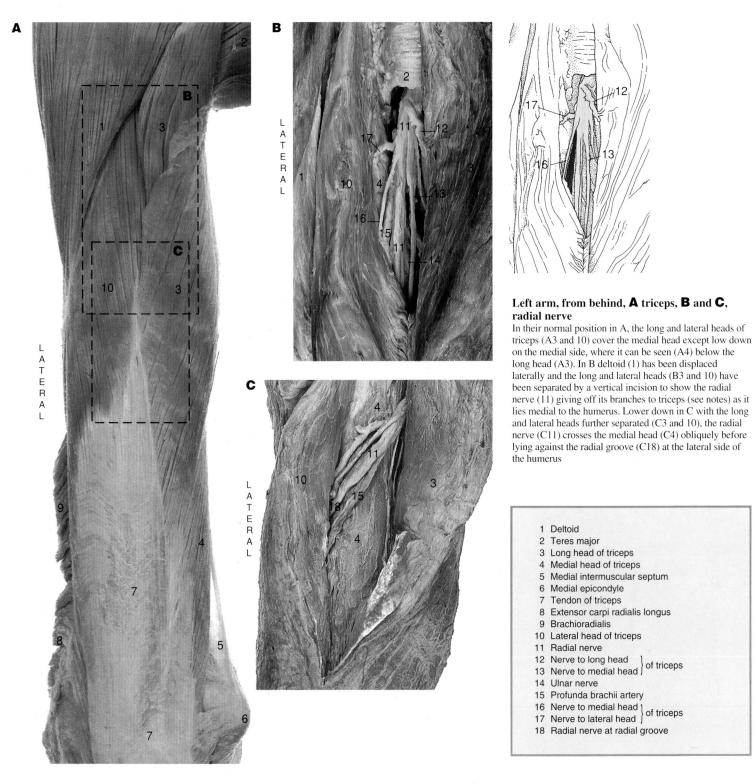

Left arm, from behind, A triceps, B and C, radial nerve

In their normal position in A, the long and lateral heads of triceps (A3 and 10) cover the medial head except low down on the medial side, where it can be seen (A4) below the long head (A3). In B deltoid (1) has been displaced laterally and the long and lateral heads (B3 and 10) have been separated by a vertical incision to show the radial nerve (11) giving off its branches to triceps (see notes) as it lies medial to the humerus. Lower down in C with the long and lateral heads further separated (C3 and 10), the radial nerve (C11) crosses the medial head (C4) obliquely before lying against the radial groove (C18) at the lateral side of the humerus

1	Deltoid
2	Teres major
3	Long head of triceps
4	Medial head of triceps
5	Medial intermuscular septum
6	Medial epicondyle
7	Tendon of triceps
8	Extensor carpi radialis longus
9	Brachioradialis
10	Lateral head of triceps
11	Radial nerve
12	Nerve to long head
13	Nerve to medial head } of triceps
14	Ulnar nerve
15	Profunda brachii artery
16	Nerve to medial head
17	Nerve to lateral head } of triceps
18	Radial nerve at radial groove

• Triceps has three heads but four nerves—the medial head receives two branches. All the muscular branches (B12, 13, 16 and 17) arise from the radial nerve (B11) high up, well before the nerve has reached the radial groove (C18) at the lateral side of the humerus (page 103, B8). The usual order of origin of the branches from above downwards is: nerve to the long head (B12), medial head (B13), lateral head (B17), and medial head (B16). The first branch to the medial head (B13) runs for part of its course close to the ulnar nerve (B14), and is therefore sometimes called the ulnar collateral nerve.

• The medial head (4) of triceps would be better known as the deep head, since most of it is under cover of the long and lateral heads (3 and 10 in A and B), but on the lower medial side of the arm part of the medial head (A4) does project below the long head (A3).

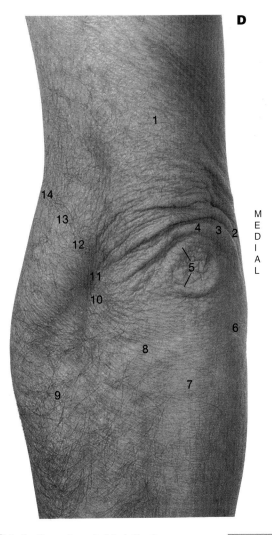

D

M
E
D
I
A
L

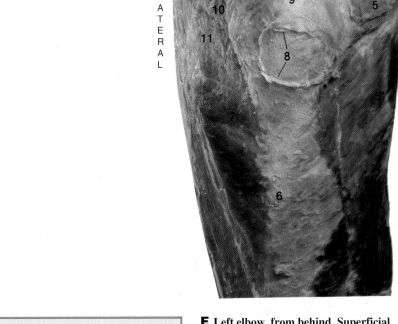

E

L
A
T
E
R
A
L

D Left elbow, from behind. Surface markings

With the elbow fully extended, the extensor muscles (9, 13) form a bulge on the lateral side. In the adjacent hollow can be felt the head of the radius (10) and the capitulum of the humerus (11) which indicate the line of the humeroradial part of the elbow joint. The lateral and medial epicondyles of the humerus (12 and 2) are palpable on each side. Wrinkled skin lies at the back of the prominent olecranon of the ulna (4), and in this arm the margin of the olecranon bursa (5) is outlined. The most important structure in this region is the ulnar nerve (3) which is palpable as it lies in contact with the humerus behind the medial epicondyle (2). The posterior border of the ulna (7) is subcutaneous throughout its whole length

1	Triceps
2	Medial epicondyle of humerus
3	Ulnar nerve
4	Olecranon of ulna
5	Margin of olecranon bursa
6	Flexor carpi ulnaris
7	Posterior border of ulna
8	Anconeus
9	Extensor muscles
10	Head of radius
11	Capitulum of humerus
12	Lateral epicondyle of humerus
13	Extensor carpi radialis longus
14	Brachioradialis

E Left elbow, from behind. Superficial dissection

Skin and subcutaneous tissue and some deep fascia have been removed, but the margin of the olecranon bursa (8) has been preserved. The ulnar nerve (3) is behind the medial epicondyle (4) and passes downwards under cover of flexor carpi ulnaris (5)

1	Triceps tendon
2	Medial head of triceps
3	Ulnar nerve
4	Medial epicondyle of humerus
5	Flexor carpi ulnaris
6	Posterior border of ulna
7	Anconeus
8	Margin of olecranon bursa
9	Olecranon of ulna
10	Lateral epicondyle of humerus
11	Common extensor origin

• With the elbow extended (straight) the medial and lateral epicondyles of the humerus (D2 and 12; E4 and 10) and the olecranon of the ulna (D4 and E9) are on the same level, but with flexion of the elbow the olecranon moves to a lower level.
• The subcutaneous position of the ulnar nerve (D3, E3) behind the medial epicondyle of the humerus (D2, E4) makes it easily palpable; here it can be rolled against the bone or injured, with paraesthesia (tingling sensation) in the distribution of the nerve on the ulnar side of the hand.
• The region of the medial epicondyle of the humerus is colloquially called the 'funny bone'.

A

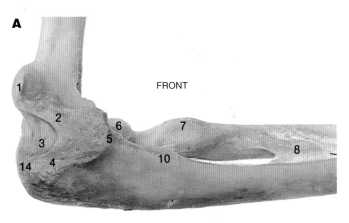

FRONT

D

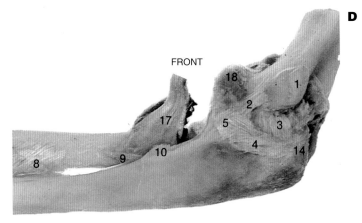

FRONT

B

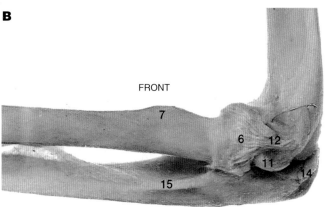

FRONT

E

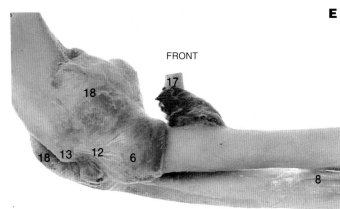

FRONT

C

L
A
T
E
R
A
L

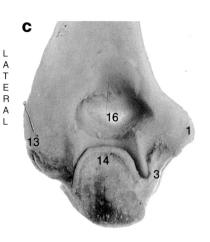

Left elbow joint and proximal radio-ulnar joint, A from the medial side, B from the lateral side, C from behind
Right elbow joint and proximal radio-ulnar joint, D from the medial side, E from the lateral side, F from behind
In A, B and C the forearm is flexed to a right angle. In D, E and F the forearm is partially flexed, and the synovial cavity within the capsule (18) and the bursa beneath the biceps tendon (17) have been injected with green resin

F

L
A
T
E
R
A
L

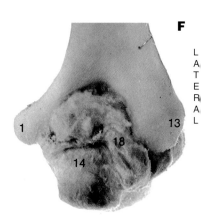

• The synovial cavity of the proximal radio-ulnar joint is continuous with that of the elbow joint (the synovial cavity of the distal radio-ulnar joint is *not* continuous with that of the wrist joint).
• Posteriorly and above, the capsule of the elbow joint is attached to the upper part of the *floor* of the olecranon fossa, not to the upper margin of the fossa (page 106, B).
• The main ligaments of the elbow and proximal radio-ulnar joints are the capsule (18), the ulnar and radial collateral ligaments (2 to 4 and 12) and the annular ligament (6).

1	Medial epicondyle
2	Upper band
3	Posterior band } of ulnar collateral ligament
4	Oblique band
5	Coronoid process of ulna
6	Head and neck of radius covered by annular ligament
7	Tuberosity of radius
8	Interosseous membrane
9	Oblique cord
10	Tuberosity of ulna
11	Capitulum
12	Radial collateral ligament
13	Lateral epicondyle
14	Olecranon of ulna
15	Supinator crest of ulna
16	Olecranon fossa
17	Biceps tendon and underlying bursa
18	Capsule (distended)

• Muscles producing movements at the elbow joint:
Flexion: brachialis, biceps, brachioradialis.
Extension: triceps, anconeus.

• Muscles producing movements at the proximal and distal radio-ulnar joints:
Pronation: pronator quadratus, pronator teres.
Supination: supinator, biceps.

A

L A T E R A L

A Left elbow joint, opened from behind

The joint has been 'forced open' from behind: the capitulum (1) and trochlea (2) of the lower end of the humerus are seen from below with the forearm in forced flexion to show the upper ends of the radius and ulna (7 and 5) from above

1 Capitulum	
2 Trochlea	of humerus
3 Medial epicondyle	
4 Olecranon	
5 Trochlear notch	of ulna
6 Coronoid process	
7 Head of radius	
8 Annular ligament	
9 Anterior part of capsule	

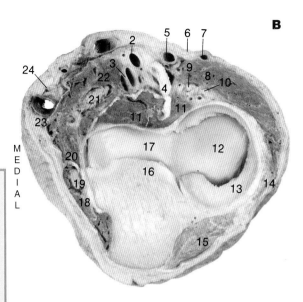

B

M E D I A L

B Cross section of the left elbow

The section is viewed from below, looking towards the shoulder, and is just below the point where the brachial artery has divided into radial and ulnar arteries (2 and 3). The cut has passed immediately below the trochlea (17) and capitulum (12) of the humerus, and has gone through the coronoid process of the ulna (16). The radial nerve (9) and its posterior interosseous branch (10) lie between brachioradialis (8) and brachialis (11). The median nerve (21) is under the main part of pronator teres (22), and the ulnar nerve (19) is passing under flexor carpi ulnaris (18)

1 Median basilic vein
2 Radial artery
3 Ulnar artery
4 Tendon of biceps
5 Median cephalic vein
6 Lateral cutaneous nerve of forearm
7 Cephalic vein
8 Brachioradialis
9 Radial nerve
10 Posterior interosseous nerve
11 Brachialis
12 Capitulum of humerus
13 Fringe of synovial membrane
14 Extensor carpi radialis longus and brevis
15 Anconeus
16 Coronoid process of ulna
17 Trochlea of humerus
18 Flexor carpi ulnaris
19 Ulnar nerve
20 Common flexor origin
21 Median nerve
22 Pronator teres
23 Basilic vein
24 Medial cutaneous nerve of forearm

C

D

Radiograph of the elbow, C in extension, D from the side in semiflexion

1 Lateral epicondyle of humerus	7 Coronoid process of ulna
2 Capitulum	8 Head of radius (in D superimposed on coronoid process of ulna)
3 Olecranon fossa	
4 Olecranon of ulna	9 Tuberosity of radius
5 Medial epicondyle	10 Medial supracondylar ridge
6 Medial margin of trochlea	

131

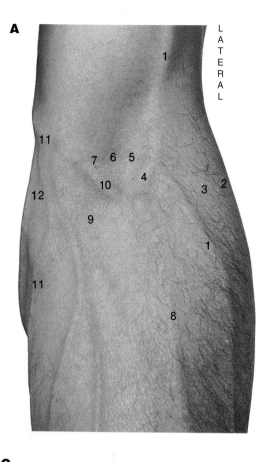

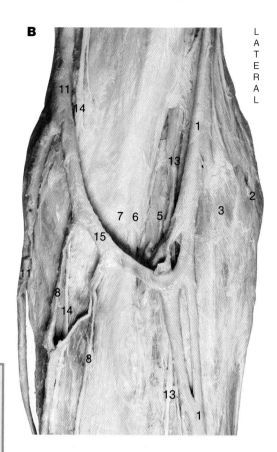

Left cubital fossa, **A** surface markings, **B** superficial veins, **C** after removal of the deep fascia, **D** brachial arteriogram

In A there is an M-shaped pattern of superficial veins (see notes). In B the cephalic (1) and basilic (11) veins are joined by a median cubital vein (15) into which drain two small median forearm veins (8). In C the deep fascia has been removed but the bicipital aponeurosis (18) is preserved; it runs downwards and medially from the biceps tendon (5), crossing the brachial artery (6) and the median nerve (7). The musculocutaneous nerve becomes the lateral cutaneous nerve of the forearm (13) at the lateral border of biceps where the muscle becomes tendinous. Brachioradialis (3) forms the lateral boundary and pronator teres (9) the medial boundary of the cubital fossa. The arteriogram in D outlines the main arteries (6, 17, 23)

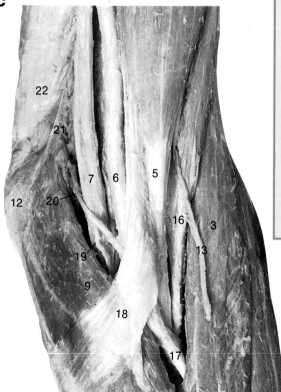

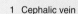

1	Cephalic vein
2	Lateral epicondyle
3	Brachioradialis
4	Median cephalic vein
5	Biceps tendon
6	Brachial artery
7	Median nerve
8	Median forearm vein
9	Pronator teres
10	Median basilic vein
11	Basilic vein
12	Medial epicondyle
13	Lateral cutaneous nerve of forearm
14	Medial cutaneous nerve of forearm
15	Median cubital vein
16	Brachialis
17	Radial artery
18	Bicipital aponeurosis
19	Nerve to pronator teres
20	A muscular artery
21	Medial intermuscular septum
22	Medial head of triceps
23	Ulnar artery

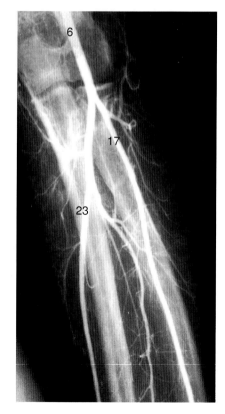

• The superficial veins on the front of the elbow such as the cephalic (1) and basilic (11) and their intercommunicating tributaries are those most commonly used for intravenous injections and obtaining specimens of venous blood. The pattern of veins is typically M-shaped (as in A) or H-shaped (as in B), but there is much variation and it is not always possible or necessary to name every vessel.
• The order of the structures in the cubital fossa from lateral to medial is: biceps tendon (5), brachial artery (6) and median nerve (7).

E Left forearm, from the front. Superficial muscles

Skin and fascia have been removed, but the larger superficial veins (2, 8 and 9) have been preserved. On the lateral side the radial artery (11) is largely covered by brachioradialis (10). At the wrist the tendon of flexor carpi radialis (15) has the radial artery (11) on its lateral side; on its medial side is the median nerve (5), slightly overlapped from the medial side by the tendon of palmaris longus (16) (if present; it is absent in 13% of arms)

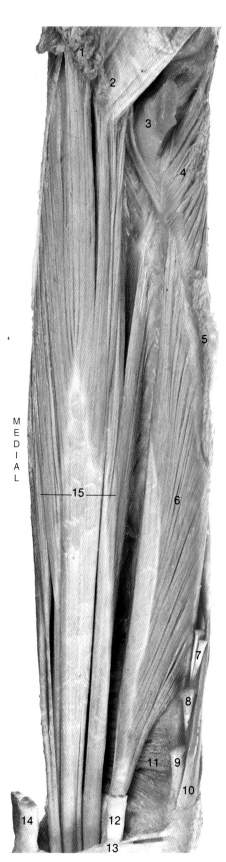

1	Medial epicondyle
2	Basilic vein
3	Common flexor origin
4	Pronator teres
5	Median nerve
6	Brachial artery
7	Biceps tendon
8	Cephalic vein
9	Median cubital vein
10	Brachioradialis
11	Radial artery
12	Ulnar artery
13	Bicipital aponeurosis
14	Median forearm vein
15	Flexor carpi radialis
16	Palmaris longus
17	Flexor carpi ulnaris
18	Flexor digitorum superficialis
19	Flexor pollicis longus
20	Pronator quadratus
21	Palmar branch of median nerve
22	Palmar branch of ulnar nerve
23	Ulnar nerve

F Left forearm, from the front, deep muscles

All vessels and nerves have been removed, together with the superficial muscles, to show the deep flexor group—flexor digitorum profundus (15), flexor pollicis longus (6) and pronator quadratus (11)

1	Common flexor origin
2	Brachialis
3	Biceps
4	Supinator
5	Pronator teres
6	Flexor pollicis longus
7	Extensor carpi radialis brevis
8	Extensor carpi radialis longus
9	Brachioradialis
10	Abductor pollicis longus
11	Pronator quadratus
12	Flexor carpi radialis
13	Flexor retinaculum
14	Flexor carpi ulnaris
15	Flexor digitorum profundus

133

A Right cubital fossa and forearm. Arteries

The arteries have been injected, and after removal of most of the superficial muscles the brachial artery (6) is seen dividing into the radial artery (18) and the ulnar artery (9). The radial artery gives off the radial recurrent (3) which runs upwards in front of supinator, giving branches to the carpal extensor muscles (2 and 20). The ulnar artery gives off the anterior and posterior ulnar recurrent vessels (11 and 10), and its common interosseous branch (12) is seen giving off the anterior interosseous (15) which passes down in front of the interosseous membrane between flexor pollicis longus (17) and flexor digitorum profundus (14)

1	Brachioradialis	12	Common interosseous artery
2	Extensor carpi radialis longus	13	Flexor carpi ulnaris
3	Radial recurrent artery overlying supinator	14	Flexor digitorum profundus
4	Biceps tendon	15	Anterior interosseous artery overlying interosseous membrane
5	Brachialis	16	Pronator quadratus
6	Brachial artery	17	Flexor pollicis longus
7	Medial epicondyle of humerus	18	Radial artery
8	Common flexor origin	19	Pronator teres
9	Ulnar artery	20	Extensor carpi radialis brevis
10	Posterior ulnar recurrent artery		
11	Anterior ulnar recurrent artery		

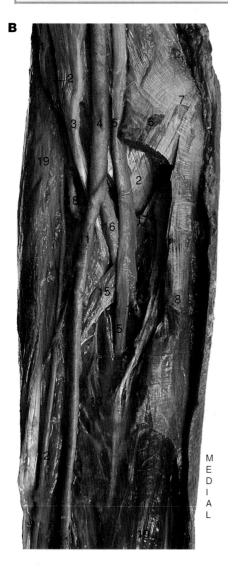

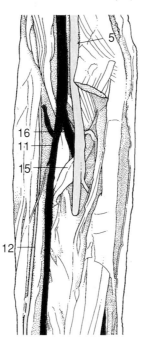

B Right cubital fossa and forearm. Arteries and nerves

Most of the humeral origins of pronator teres and flexor carpi radialis (from the common flexor origin, 6 and 7) and palmaris longus have been removed to show the median nerve (5) passing superficial to the deep head of pronator teres (15) and then deep to the upper border of the radial head of flexor digitorum superficialis (13)

- The radial artery (A18 and B11) usually appears to be the direct continuation of the brachial (A6 and B4), and the ulnar artery (A9 and B16) branches off from the parent trunk almost at a right angle.
- The unnamed vessels are muscular branches.
- The median nerve (B5) passes between the humeral (superficial) and ulnar (deep) heads of pronator teres; the ulnar artery (B16) passes deep to the ulnar head. In B most of the humeral head (B6) has been removed to show the ulnar head (B15) lying between the median nerve (B5) and the ulnar artery (B16).

- In the lower part of B flexor carpi ulnaris (B9) has been displaced medially to show the underlying ulnar nerve and artery (B10).

1	Lateral cutaneous nerve of forearm	12	Superficial terminal branch of radial nerve overlying extensor carpi radialis longus
2	Brachialis		
3	Biceps	13	Radial head of flexor digitorum superficialis
4	Brachial artery		
5	Median nerve	14	Anterior interosseous nerve
6	Humeral head of pronator teres	15	Ulnar head of pronator teres
7	Common flexor origin	16	Ulnar artery
8	Humero-ulnar head of flexor digitorum superficialis	17	A muscular branch of median nerve
9	Flexor carpi ulnaris (displaced medially)	18	Radial recurrent artery
10	Ulnar nerve and artery	19	Brachioradialis (displaced laterally)
11	Radial artery		

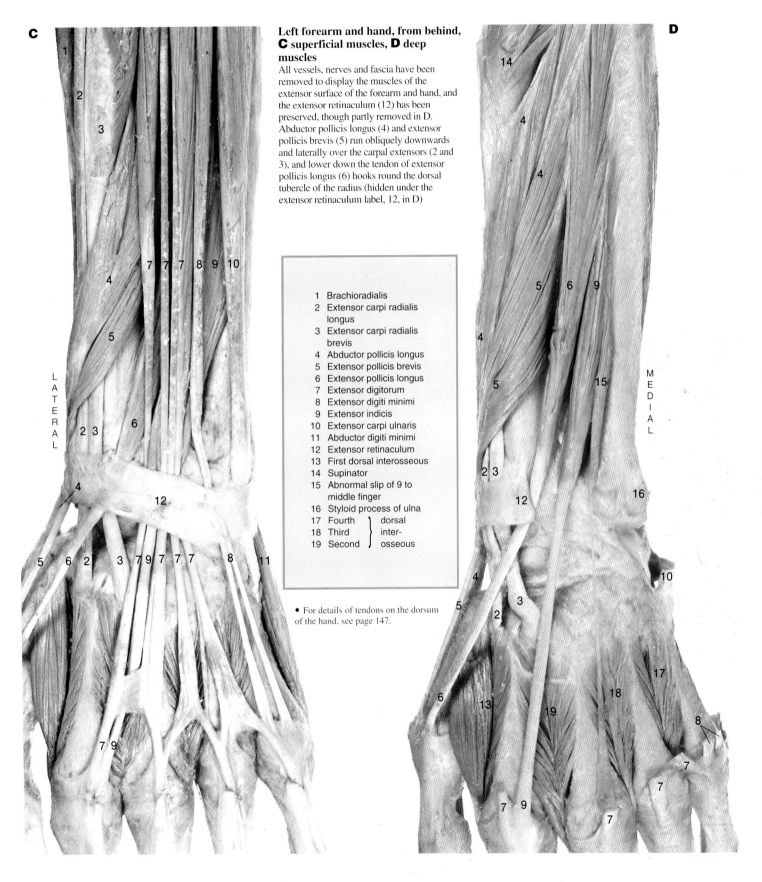

C

**Left forearm and hand, from behind,
C superficial muscles, D deep
muscles**

All vessels, nerves and fascia have been
removed to display the muscles of the
extensor surface of the forearm and hand, and
the extensor retinaculum (12) has been
preserved, though partly removed in D.
Abductor pollicis longus (4) and extensor
pollicis brevis (5) run obliquely downwards
and laterally over the carpal extensors (2 and
3), and lower down the tendon of extensor
pollicis longus (6) hooks round the dorsal
tubercle of the radius (hidden under the
extensor retinaculum label, 12, in D)

D

1   Brachioradialis
2   Extensor carpi radialis
    longus
3   Extensor carpi radialis
    brevis
4   Abductor pollicis longus
5   Extensor pollicis brevis
6   Extensor pollicis longus
7   Extensor digitorum
8   Extensor digiti minimi
9   Extensor indicis
10 Extensor carpi ulnaris
11 Abductor digiti minimi
12 Extensor retinaculum
13 First dorsal interosseous
14 Supinator
15 Abnormal slip of 9 to
    middle finger
16 Styloid process of ulna
17 Fourth ⎫ dorsal
18 Third   ⎬ inter-
19 Second ⎭ osseous

• For details of tendons on the dorsum
of the hand, see page 147.

A

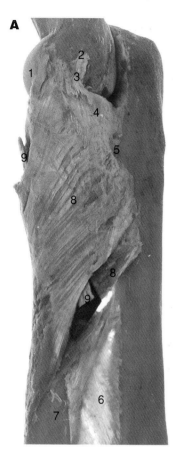

A Left elbow from the lateral side

With the forearm in midpronation and seen from the lateral side so that the radius (7) lies in front of the ulna, all muscles have been removed except supinator (8) to show its humeral and ulnar origins (see notes)

1	Capitulum of humerus
2	Lateral epicondyle
3	Radial collateral ligament
4	Annular ligament
5	Supinator crest of ulna
6	Interosseous membrane
7	Radius
8	Supinator
9	Posterior interosseous nerve

• The fibres of the interosseous membrane (6) pass obliquely downwards from the radius (7) to the ulna, so transmitting weight from the hand and radius to the ulna.

• The supinator muscle (8) arises from the lateral epicondyle of the humerus (2), radial collateral ligament (3), annular ligament (4), supinator crest of the ulna (5) and bone in front of the crest (page 108, D6), and an aponeurosis overlying the muscle. From these origins the fibres wrap themselves round the upper end of the radius above the pronator teres attachment, to be attached to the lateral surface of the radius and extending anteriorly and posteriorly as far as the tuberosity of the radius.

• The posterior interosseous nerve (9) passes through the muscle, dividing it into superficial and deep layers. In A there is a black marker behind the nerve as it emerges from between the two layers.

B Left forearm, from the lateral side. Deep muscles

All vessels, nerves and fascia and the superficial group of flexor muscles have been removed, but the attachment of pronator teres (3) halfway down the lateral side of the radius remains. Above it the radius is covered by supinator (2), and below it abductor pollicis longus (4) and extensor pollicis brevis (5) curl obliquely round the lower part of the radius. The three most radial compartments of the extensor retinaculum (8) have been preserved, containing the tendons of abductor pollicis longus and extensor pollicis brevis (4 and 5), extensor carpi radialis longus and brevis (10 and 9) and extensor pollicis longus (6)

1	Biceps
2	Supinator
3	Pronator teres
4	Abductor pollicis longus
5	Extensor pollicis brevis
6	Extensor pollicis longus
7	Extensor indicis
8	Extensor retinaculum
9	Extensor carpi radialis brevis
10	Extensor carpi radialis longus (double)
11	Flexor pollicis longus

B   **C**

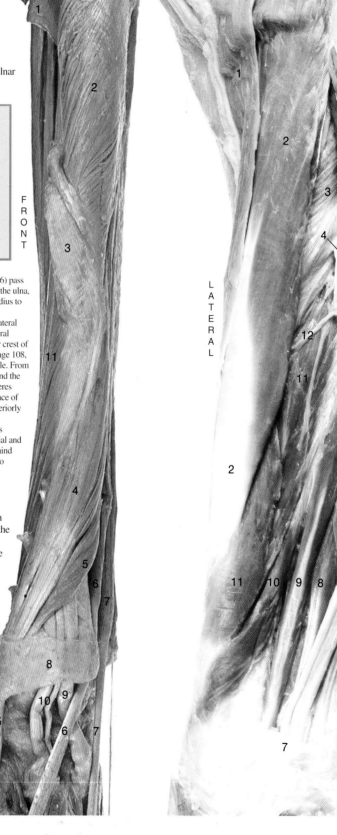

FRONT

LATERAL

• Distal to the extensor retinaculum (8) the tendons of extensor carpi radialis longus and brevis (10 and 9) pass deep to the tendon of extensor pollicis longus (6).

◁ **C Left forearm, from behind. Posterior interosseous nerve**

The forearm is in the midprone position. Most of the deep fascia has been removed and the extensor group of muscles has been split between extensor digitorum (5, which has been displaced medially) and extensor carpi radialis brevis (2). The posterior interosseous nerve (4) emerges from supinator (3) and gives off branches to the adjacent muscles

1 Extensor carpi radialis longus
2 Extensor carpi radialis brevis
3 Supinator
4 Posterior interosseous nerve
5 Extensor digitorum
6 Extensor carpi ulnaris
7 Extensor retinaculum
8 Extensor indicis
9 Extensor pollicis longus
10 Extensor pollicis brevis
11 Abductor pollicis longus
12 Branch of posterior interosseous artery

• Abductor pollicis longus (11) and extensor pollicis brevis (10) are the only muscles attached to the posterior surface of the radius. The abductor also has an attachment to the posterior surface of the ulna (as well as the intervening interosseous membrane), and below it on this bone extensor pollicis longus (9) and extensor indicis (8) have an origin (see page 110, B).

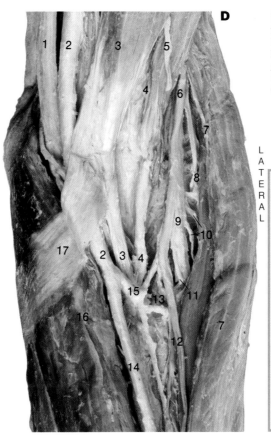

D Left elbow and upper forearm, from the front

Brachioradialis (7) and extensor carpi radialis longus (8) have been displaced laterally to show the radial nerve (6) giving off branches to those muscles and then dividing into the superficial (cutaneous) branch (12) and the deep (posterior interosseous) branch (9) which enters supinator

1 Median nerve
2 Brachial artery
3 Biceps
4 Brachialis
5 Lateral cutaneous nerve of forearm
6 Radial nerve
7 Brachioradialis and nerve
8 Extensor carpi radialis longus and nerve
9 Posterior interosseous nerve
10 Branches to extensor carpi radialis brevis
11 Nerve to supinator
12 Superficial branch of radial nerve
13 Supinator
14 Radial artery
15 Radial recurrent artery
16 Pronator teres
17 Bicipital aponeurosis

Left upper forearm, E cross section, from below, F axial MR image

The section, seen from below looking towards the elbow, shows the posterior interosseous nerve (15) within the supinator muscle (14) which curls round the radius (16). Compare the MR image in F with features in E

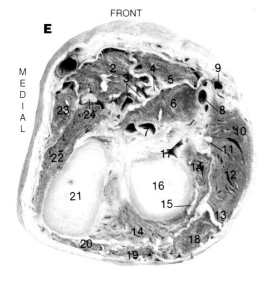

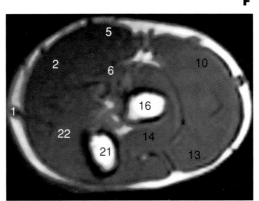

1 Basilic vein
2 Flexor digitorum superficialis
3 Anterior interosseous nerve and vessels
4 Median nerve
5 Flexor carpi radialis and palmaris longus
6 Pronator teres
7 Ulnar artery
8 Radial artery
9 Cephalic vein
10 Brachioradialis
11 Superficial branch of radial nerve
12 Extensor carpi radialis longus
13 Extensor carpi radialis brevis
14 Supinator
15 Posterior interosseous nerve
16 Radius
17 Tendon of biceps and bursa
18 Extensor digitorum
19 Extensor carpi ulnaris
20 Anconeus
21 Ulna
22 Flexor digitorum profundus
23 Flexor carpi ulnaris
24 Ulnar nerve

A Palm of the left hand

Interrupted lines = radial and ulnar arteries and palmar arches
The surface markings of various structures within the wrist and hand are indicated; not all of them are palpable, e.g. the superficial and deep palmar arches (5 and 6), but their relative positions are important

• The curved lines (1) proximal to the bases of the fingers indicate the ends of the heads of the metacarpals and the level of the metacarpophalangeal joints.
• The creases on the fingers indicate the level of the interphalangeal joints.
• The middle crease at the wrist indicates the level of the wrist joint.
• The radial artery at the wrist (20) is the commonest site for feeling the pulse. The vessel is on the radial side of the tendon of flexor carpi radialis (19) and can be compressed against the lower end of the radius.
• The median nerve at the wrist (18) lies on the ulnar side of the tendon of flexor carpi radialis (19) and is slightly overlapped from the ulnar side by the tendon of palmaris longus (17) (although this muscle is absent in 13 per cent of limbs).

1	Head of metacarpal	13	Distal
2	Longitudinal crease	14	Middle } wrist crease
3	Proximal } transverse	15	Proximal
4	Distal } crease	16	Flexor carpi ulnaris
5	Level of superficial palmar arch	17	Palmaris longus
6	Level of deep palmar arch	18	Median nerve
7	Abductor digiti minimi	19	Flexor carpi radialis
8	Flexor digiti minimi brevis	20	Radial artery
9	Palmaris brevis	21	Abductor pollicis brevis
10	Hook of hamate	22	Flexor pollicis brevis
11	Pisiform	23	Thenar eminence
12	Ulnar artery and nerve	24	Adductor pollicis

B Left wrist, from the front. Cutaneous nerves

The hand is in ulnar deviation at the wrist joint, so the radial border (with the base of the thumb and thenar muscles, 1) is in line with the radial border of the forearm. The palmar cutaneous branch of the median nerve (2) pierces the fascia between flexor carpi radialis (9) and palmaris longus (8). The palmar cutaneous branch of the ulnar nerve (6) in this specimen is on the ulnar side of flexor carpi ulnaris (5); it is usually on the radial side

1 Lateral part of palmar aponeurosis overlying thenar muscles
2 Palmar cutaneous branch of median nerve overlying palmaris longus attachment of flexor retinaculum
3 Medial part of palmar aponeurosis overlying hypothenar muscles
4 Branches of dorsal branch of ulnar nerve
5 Flexor carpi ulnaris
6 Palmar cutaneous branch of ulnar nerve
7 Medial cutaneous nerve of forearm and fascia overlying flexor digitorum superficialis
8 Palmaris longus
9 Flexor carpi radialis
10 Lateral cutaneous nerve of forearm
11 Superficial terminal branch of radial nerve

A

• The ulnar nerve and artery at the wrist (12) are on the radial side of the tendon of flexor carpi ulnaris (16) and the pisiform bone (11). The artery is on the radial side of the nerve and its pulsation can be felt, though less easily than that of the radial artery (20).
• Abductor pollicis brevis (21) and flexor pollicis brevis (22), together with the underlying opponens pollicis, are the muscles which form the thenar eminence, the 'bulge' at the base of the thumb. Abductor digiti minimi (7) and flexor digiti minimi brevis (8), together with the underlying opponens digiti minimi, form the muscles of the hypothenar eminence, the less prominent bulge on the ulnar side of the palm where palmaris brevis (9) lies subcutaneously.

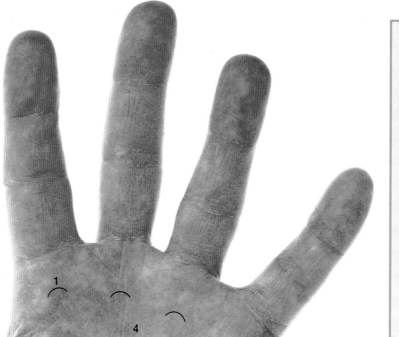

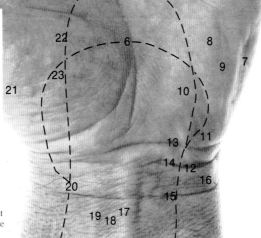

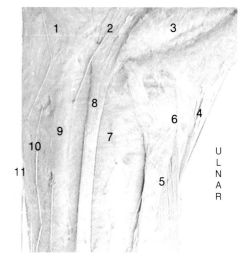

B

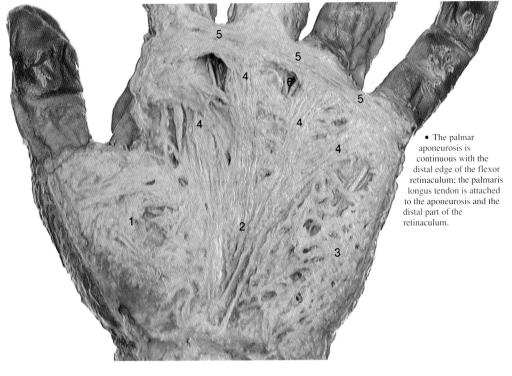

C Palm of the left hand. Palmar aponeurosis

Removal of skin reveals the palmar aponeurosis with its thick central part (2) and the thin lateral and medial parts (1 and 3) which overlie the thenar and hypothenar muscles, respectively. The central part divides into slips (4) for each finger; in the intervals between adjacent slips (as at 6) digital vessels and nerves are seen

• The palmar aponeurosis is continuous with the distal edge of the flexor retinaculum; the palmaris longus tendon is attached to the aponeurosis and the distal part of the retinaculum.

1 Lateral part of aponeurosis overlying thenar muscles
2 Central part of aponeurosis
3 Medial part of aponeurosis overlying hypothenar muscles
4 Digital slips of aponeurosis
5 Superficial transverse metacarpal ligaments
6 Palmar digital vessels and nerves in interval between slips

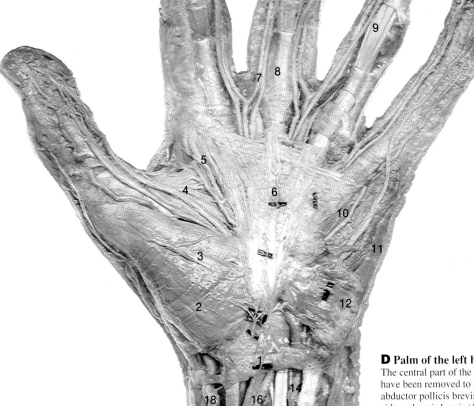

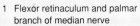

1 Flexor retinaculum and palmar branch of median nerve
2 Abductor pollicis brevis
3 Flexor pollicis brevis and muscular (recurrent) branch of median nerve
4 Adductor pollicis and digital branches of median nerve
5 First lumbrical
6 Central part of palmar aponeurosis and filaments of palmar branch of median nerve
7 Palmar digital vessels and nerves
8 Fibrous sheath (partly removed)
9 Flexor digitorum profundus tendon overlying superficialis tendon
10 Flexor digiti minimi brevis
11 Abductor digiti minimi
12 Palmaris brevis and filament of palmar branch of ulnar nerve
13 Flexor carpi ulnaris
14 Ulnar nerve and artery passing beneath superficial part of flexor retinaculum
15 Flexor digitorum superficialis
16 Median nerve and overlying palmar branch
17 Flexor carpi radialis
18 Radial artery

D Palm of the left hand. Superficial dissection

The central part of the aponeurosis remains (6) but the medial and lateral parts have been removed to show the underlying muscles. At the base of the thumb, abductor pollicis brevis (2) lies lateral to flexor pollicis brevis (3). On the ulnar side, palmaris brevis (12) overlies the proximal part of abductor digiti minimi (11) and flexor digiti minimi brevis (10). At the wrist the median nerve (16) is on the ulnar side of the tendon of flexor carpi radialis (17)

A

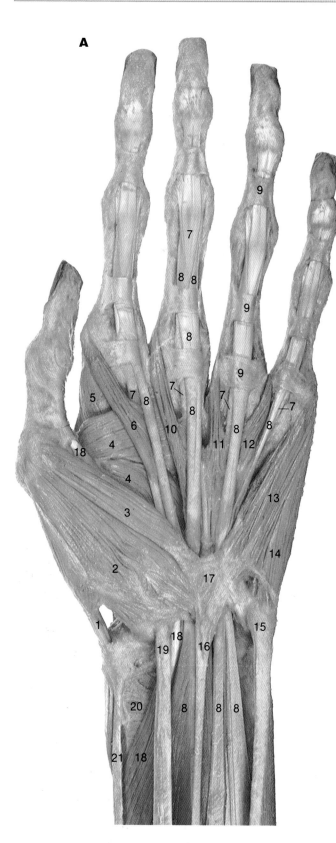

Left wrist and hand, A muscles and tendons of the palmar surface, B coronal MR image

All vessels, nerves and fascia have been removed, and parts of the fibrous flexor sheaths of the fingers (9) have also been excised to show the contained tendons of flexor digitorum superficialis (8) and flexor digitorum profundus (7). In the palm the lumbrical muscles (6, 10, 11 and 12) are seen arising from the profundus tendons. At the wrist, palmaris longus (16) becomes attached to the flexor retinaculum (17) and flexor carpi ulnaris to the pisiform bone (15). Compare features in the MR image with the dissection

1	Abductor pollicis longus overlying extensor pollicis brevis	11	Third lumbrical
2	Abductor pollicis brevis	12	Fourth lumbrical
3	Flexor pollicis brevis	13	Flexor digiti minimi brevis
4	Adductor pollicis	14	Abductor digiti minimi
5	First dorsal interosseous	15	Flexor carpi ulnaris and pisiform
6	First lumbrical	16	Palmaris longus
7	Flexor digitorum profundus	17	Flexor retinaculum
8	Flexor digitorum superficialis	18	Flexor pollicis longus
9	Remaining parts of fibrous flexor sheath	19	Flexor carpi radialis
		20	Pronator quadratus
10	Second lumbrical	21	Brachioradialis

• The lumbrical muscles have no bony attachments. They arise from the tendons of flexor digitorum profundus (A7)—the first and second (A6 and A10) from the tendons of the index and middle fingers respectively, and the third and fourth (A11 and A12) from adjacent sides of the middle and ring, and ring and little fingers respectively. Each is attached distally to the radial side of the dorsal digital expansion of each finger (page 146).

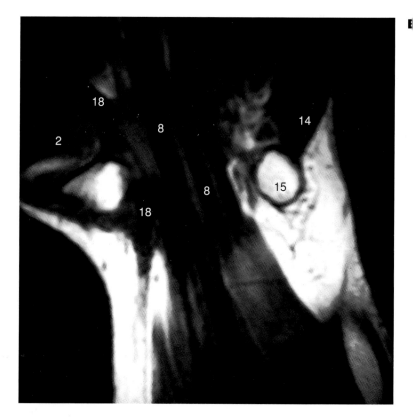

• Near the base of the proximal phalanges each flexor digitorum superficialis tendon divides (as at the two adjacent 8 labels on the middle finger) to allow the profundus tendon (as at 7 on the middle finger) to pass through to its attachment to the base of the distal phalanx. The divided superficialis slips reunite and partially decussate (cross over) before becoming attached to the sides of the shaft of the middle phalanx.

Superficial palmar arch, **A** incomplete in the left hand, **B** complete in the right hand

The superficial palmar (arterial) arch (6) and its branches (as at 7) in the palm are superficial to branches of the median and ulnar nerves (4 and 13). The arch, the continuation of the ulnar artery (21) in the palm, is usually incomplete as in A (see notes), but in B is completed by the superficial palmar branch (32) of the radial artery (26). In B the thenar muscles and long flexor tendons have been removed, and in both hands flexor digiti minimi brevis has been excised to show the deep branches of the ulnar nerve and artery (18 and 17) passing through opponens digiti minimi (14)

1 Abductor pollicis brevis
2 Flexor pollicis brevis
3 Muscular (recurrent) branch of median nerve
4 Median nerve dividing into common palmar digital branches
5 First lumbrical
6 Superficial palmar arch
7 A common palmar digital artery
8 A palmar digital nerve
9 A palmar digital artery
10 Flexor digitorum superficialis
11 Flexor digitorum profundus
12 Fourth lumbrical
13 Common palmar digital branch of ulnar nerve
14 Opponens digiti minimi
15 Abductor digiti minimi
16 Palmaris brevis
17 Deep branch of ulnar artery
18 Deep branch of ulnar nerve
19 Flexor carpi ulnaris and pisiform
20 Ulnar nerve
21 Ulnar artery
22 Flexor retinaculum
23 Median nerve
24 Flexor pollicis longus
25 Flexor carpi radialis
26 Radial artery
27 Abductor pollicis longus
28 Deep palmar arch
29 Common stem of 30 and 31
30 Radialis indicis artery
31 Princeps pollicis artery
32 Superficial palmar branch of radial artery

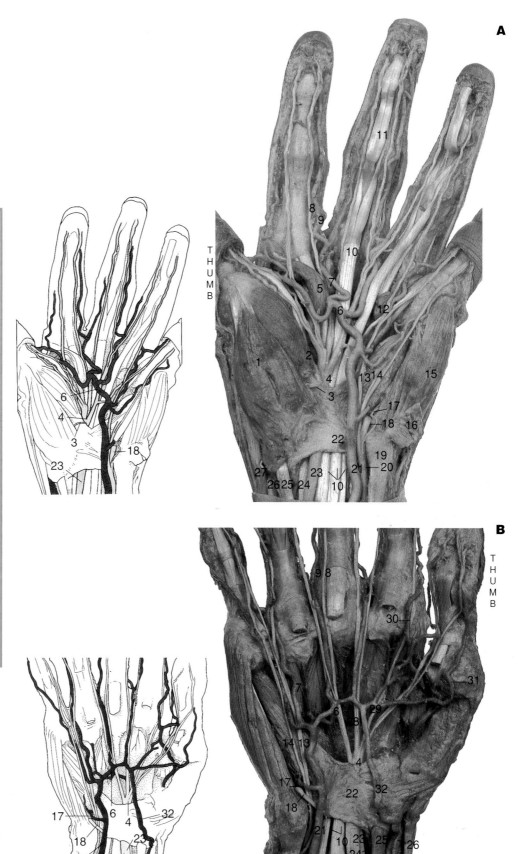

• In two-thirds of hands the superficial palmar arch is not complete (as in A6). In the other third it is usually completed by the superficial palmar branch of the radial artery (B32).
• In the palm the superficial arterial arch (6) and its branches (as at 7) lie superficial to the common palmar digital nerves (4 and 13), but on the fingers the palmar digital nerves (as at 8) lie superficial (anterior) to the palmar digital arteries (as at 9).
• The ulnar nerve (20) supplies the skin of the ulnar side of the palm and of the ulnar one-and-a-half or two fingers; the rest of the palm and the palmar surfaces of the remaining fingers and thumb are supplied by the median nerve (23).
• In B the radial side of the superficial arch gives off a common stem (B29), which divides into the radialis indicis and princeps pollicis arteries (B30 and 31); these vessels usually arise from the terminal part of the radial artery.

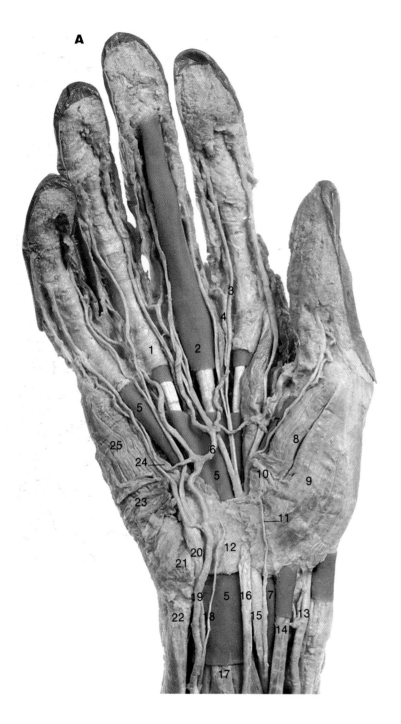

A

A Palm of the right hand, with synovial sheaths

The synovial sheaths of the wrist and fingers have been emphasized by blue tissue. On the middle finger the fibrous flexor sheath has been removed (but retained on the other fingers, as at 1) to show the whole length of the synovial sheath (2). On the index and ring fingers the synovial sheath projects slightly proximal to the fibrous sheath. The synovial sheath of the little finger is continuous with the sheath surrounding the finger flexor tendons under the flexor retinaculum (the ulnar bursa, 5), and the sheath of flexor pollicis longus is the radial bursa (7), which also continues under the retinaculum (12)

1	Fibrous flexor sheath	13	Radial artery
2	Synovial sheath	14	Flexor carpi radialis
3	Palmar digital nerve	15	Median nerve
4	Palmar digital artery	16	Palmaris longus
5	Ulnar bursa	17	Flexor digitorum
6	Superficial palmar arch		superficialis
7	Radial bursa and flexor	18	Palmar branch of ulnar
	pollicis longus		nerve
8	Flexor pollicis brevis	19	Ulnar artery
9	Abductor pollicis brevis	20	Ulnar nerve
10	Muscular (recurrent)	21	Pisiform bone
	branch of median nerve	22	Flexor carpi ulnaris
11	Palmar branch of median	23	Palmaris brevis
	nerve	24	Flexor digiti minimi brevis
12	Flexor retinaculum	25	Abductor digiti minimi

• In the carpal tunnel (beneath the flexor retinaculum), one synovial sheath envelops the eight tendons of flexor digitorum superficialis and profundus (A5), another envelops the flexor pollicis longus tendon (A7), and flexor carpi radialis (in its own compartment of the flexor retinaculum) has its own sheath also (A14). The synovial sheaths for flexor carpi radialis and flexor pollicis longus extend as far as the tendon insertions.
• The sheath of the long finger flexors is continuous with the digital synovial sheath of the little finger, but is *not* continuous with the digital synovial sheaths of the ring, middle or index fingers; these fingers have their own synovial sheaths whose proximal ends project slightly beyond the *fibrous* sheaths within which the digital *synovial* sheaths lie.
• The muscular (recurrent) branch (A10) of the median nerve usually supplies abductor pollicis brevis, flexor pollicis brevis and opponens pollicis, but of all the muscles in the body flexor pollicis brevis (A8) is the one most likely to have an anomalous supply: in about one-third of hands by the median nerve, in another third by the ulnar nerve, and in the rest by both the median and ulnar nerves.

B Long flexor tendons and vincula of the right middle finger, from the front and the right

The fibrous and synovial sheaths have been removed, and the flexor tendons (1 and 2) have been pulled anteriorly to show the vincula (3 to 6), which are small fibrous bands carrying blood vessels from the sheaths to the tendons

1	Flexor digitorum superficialis
2	Flexor digitorum profundus
3	Short vinculum of profundus tendon
4	Long vinculum of profundus tendon
5	Position of short vinculum of superficialis tendon
6	Long vincula of superficialis tendon

B

FRONT

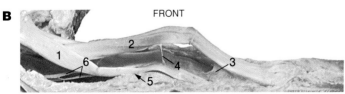

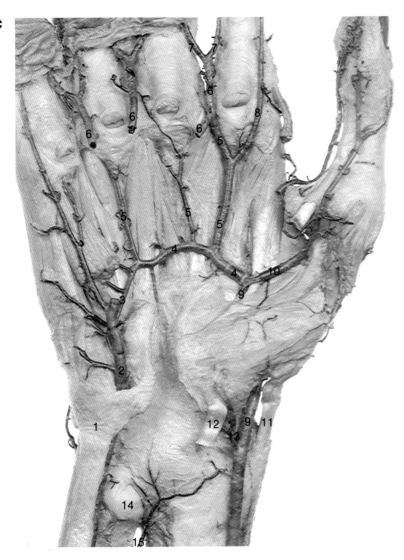

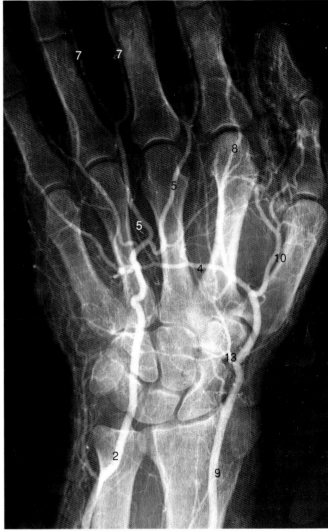

Palm of the right hand, C deep palmar arch, D arteriogram of palmar arteries
Most muscles and tendons have been removed and the arteries have been distended by injection.
The deep palmar arch (4) is seen giving off the palmar metacarpal arteries (5) which join the
common palmar digital arteries (6) from the superficial arch. Compare C with the vessels in the
arteriogram

1   Flexor carpi ulnaris and pisiform
2   Ulnar artery
3   Deep branch of ulnar artery
4   Deep palmar arch
5   Palmar metacarpal arteries
6   Common palmar digital arteries (from superficial arch)
7   Palmar digital arteries
8   Radialis indicis artery (anomalous origin)
9   Radial artery
10 Princeps pollicis artery
11 Abductor pollicis longus
12 Flexor carpi radialis
13 Superficial palmar branch of radial artery
14 Head of ulna
15 Branch of anterior interosseous artery to anterior carpal arch

• Unlike the superficial arch (page 141), the deep palmar arch (C4) is usually complete,
being formed by the terminal part of the radial artery (C9) anastomosing with the deep
branch of the ulnar artery (C3).
• The most distal part of the deep arch lies about 1 cm proximal to the superficial arch.
For the surface markings, see page 138.
• The radialis indicis artery (C8) is usually a branch of the deep arch (C4), but in C it
has arisen from the first palmar metacarpal artery (C5).
• For identification of the interossei see next page.

A

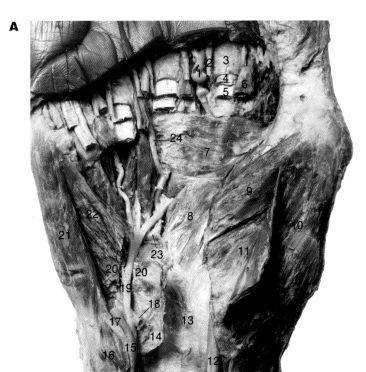

B

R
A
D
I
A
L

U
L
N
A
R

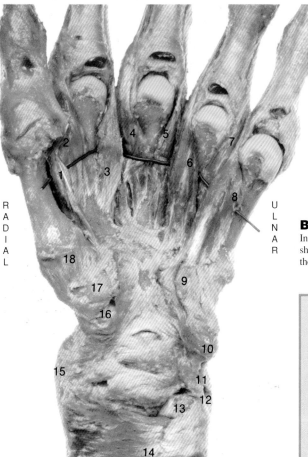

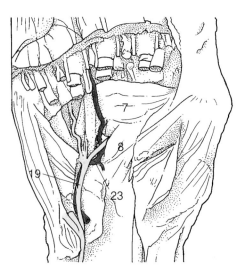

A Palm of the right hand. Deep branch of the ulnar nerve

The long flexor tendons (4 and 5) and lumbricals (6) have been cut off near the heads of the metacarpals, and parts of the hypothenar muscles removed to show the deep branches of the ulnar nerve and artery (19 and 18) running into the palm and curling laterally to pass between the transverse and oblique heads of adductor pollicis (7 and 8)

1	A common palmar digital artery	13	Carpal tunnel
2	A palmar digital nerve	14	Flexor retinaculum (cut edge)
3	Fibrous flexor sheath	15	Ulnar nerve
4	Flexor digitorum superficialis	16	Pisiform
5	Flexor digitorum profundus	17	Digital branches of ulnar nerve
6	First lumbrical	18	Deep branch of ulnar artery
7	Transverse head } of adductor	19	Deep branch of ulnar nerve
8	Oblique head } pollicis	20	Opponens digiti minimi
9	Flexor pollicis brevis	21	Abductor digiti minimi
10	Abductor pollicis brevis	22	Flexor digiti minimi brevis
11	Opponens pollicis	23	Deep palmar arch
12	Flexor pollicis longus	24	A palmar metacarpal artery

• The deep branch of the ulnar nerve (A19) normally supplies all the interossei, the hypothenar muscles (A20, A21 and A22), adductor pollicis (A7 and A8), and the two medial (third and fourth) lumbricals (not labelled in A but their cut ends are seen adjacent to the cut flexor tendons of the ring and little fingers). This branch may thus be said to supply all the small muscles of the hand except those supplied by the median nerve (the three thenar muscles—flexor and abductor pollicis brevis (A9 and A10) and opponens pollicis (A11)—and the two lateral lumbricals; but see the note on page 142 for the nerve supply of flexor pollicis brevis).

B Left wrist and palm. Interosseous muscles

In this deep dissection with most other muscles removed, the palmar interossei (1, 3, 6 and 8) are shown superficial to the blue marker and the dorsal interossei (2, 4, 5 and 7) deep to it. The capsule of the distal radio-ulnar joint has been opened up to show the head of the ulna (13)

1	First palmar	11	Ulnar collateral ligament
2	First dorsal	12	Styloid process of ulna
3	Second palmar	13	Head of ulna
4	Second dorsal	14	Pronator quadratus
5	Third dorsal } interosseous	15	Styloid process of radius
6	Third palmar	16	Scaphoid
7	Fourth dorsal	17	Trapezium
8	Fourth palmar	18	Capsule of carpometacarpal joint of
9	Hook of hamate		thumb
10	Pisiform		

C Palm of the right hand. Ligaments and joints

The capsule of the carpometacarpal joint of the thumb (between the base of the first metacarpal and the trapezium) has been removed, to show the saddle-shaped joint surfaces which allow the unique movement of opposition of the thumb to occur. The palmar and lateral ligaments (14 and 13) of the joint remain intact. The capsule of the distal radio-ulnar joint has also been removed to show the articular disc, but the wrist joint, the ulnar part of which lies distal to the disc, has not been opened

1 Ulnar collateral ligament of wrist joint
2 Pisiform
3 Pisometacarpal ligament
4 Pisohamate ligament
5 Hook of hamate
6 Interosseous metacarpal ligament
7 Deep transverse metacarpal ligament
8 Palmar ligament of metacarpophalangeal joint with groove for flexor tendon
9 Collateral ligament of interphalangeal joint
10 Sesamoid bones of flexor pollicis brevis tendons (with adductor pollicis on ulnar side)
11 Base of first metacarpal
12 Trapezium
13 Lateral ligament of carpometacarpal joint of thumb
14 Palmar ligament of carpometacarpal joint
15 Tubercle of trapezium
16 Marker in groove on trapezium for flexor carpi radialis tendon
17 Head of capitate
18 Tubercle of scaphoid
19 Lunate
20 Palmar radiocarpal ligament
21 Palmar ulnocarpal ligament
22 Articular disc of distal radio-ulnar joint
23 Sacciform recess of capsule of distal radio-ulnar joint

• The collateral ligaments of the metacarpophalangeal and interphalangeal joints (C9, D2) pass obliquely forwards from the posterior part of the side of the head of the proximal bone to the anterior part of the side of the base of the distal bone. They become tightest in flexion.
• Opposition of the thumb is a combination of flexion and abduction with medial rotation of the first metacarpal (page 149). The saddle-shape of the joint between the base of the first metacarpal and the trapezium, together with the way that the capsule and its reinforcing ligaments are attached to the bones, ensures that when flexor pollicis brevis and opponens pollicis contract they produce the necessary metacarpal rotation.
• The articular disc (22) holds the lower ends of the radius and ulna together, and separates the distal radio-ulnar joint from the wrist joint, so that the cavities of these joints are not continuous (unlike those of the elbow and proximal radio-ulnar joints, which have one continuous cavity—page 130).

DORSAL

D

D Metacarpophalangeal joint of the right index finger, from the radial side

Part of the capsule has been removed to define the collateral ligament (2)

1 Head of second metacarpal
2 Collateral ligament
3 Base of proximal phalanx
4 Fibrous flexor sheath

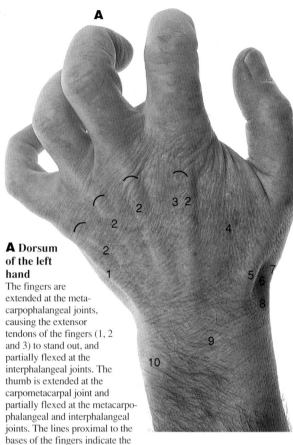

A Dorsum of the left hand

The fingers are extended at the meta-carpophalangeal joints, causing the extensor tendons of the fingers (1, 2 and 3) to stand out, and partially flexed at the interphalangeal joints. The thumb is extended at the carpometacarpal joint and partially flexed at the metacarpo-phalangeal and interphalangeal joints. The lines proximal to the bases of the fingers indicate the ends of the heads of the metacarpals and the level of the metacarpophalangeal joints. The anatomical snuffbox (6) is the hollow between the tendons of abductor pollicis longus and extensor pollicis brevis (7) laterally and extensor pollicis longus (5) medially

1 Extensor digiti minimi	7 Extensor pollicis brevis and abductor pollicis longus
2 Extensor digitorum	
3 Extensor indicis	
4 First dorsal interosseous	8 Styloid process of radius
5 Extensor pollicis longus	9 Extensor retinaculum
6 Anatomical snuffbox	10 Head of ulna

B Dorsum of the left wrist. Cutaneous nerves

Cutaneous nerves have been dissected out from the subcutaneous tissues. Branches of the radial nerve (5) overlie the region of the anatomical snuffbox (A6), while on the ulnar side are filaments from the dorsal branch of the ulnar nerve (1)

1 Branches of dorsal branch of ulnar nerve
2 Head of ulna
3 Extensor retinaculum
4 Lower end of radius
5 Superficial terminal branches of radial nerve
6 Branches of lateral cutaneous nerve of forearm

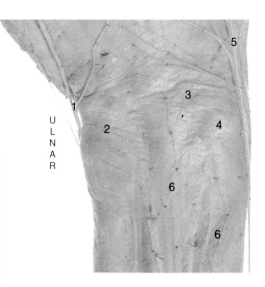

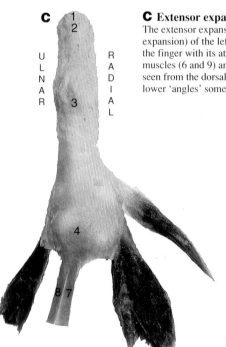

C Extensor expansion of the left index finger

The extensor expansion (often called the dorsal digital expansion) of the left index finger has been removed from the finger with its attached lumbrical (5) and interosseous muscles (6 and 9) and extensor tendons (7 and 8), and is seen from the dorsal surface (as in D opposite) but with the lower 'angles' somewhat spread out

1 End attached to distal phalanx
2 Part overlying distal interphalangeal joint
3 Part overlying proximal interphalangeal joint
4 Part overlying metacarpophalangeal joint
5 First lumbrical
6 First dorsal interosseous (two heads)
7 Extensor digitorum tendon
8 Extensor indicis tendon
9 Second palmar interosseous

• The expansions of the index, middle and ring fingers belong to the tendons of extensor digitorum, with extensor indicis joining that of the index finger (C7 and 8); that of the little finger belongs to the double tendon of extensor digiti minimi (as in D2).
• On all four fingers the lumbrical muscle (as at C5) is attached to the radial side of the expansion, distal to the interosseous muscle of that side (as at C6).
• The interossei are inserted partly into the sides of the proximal phalanges and partly into the extensor expansions. The lumbricals are not attached to the phalanges.
• Apart from their actions as flexors of the metacarpophalangeal joints and extensors of the interphalangeal joints (see page 148), the dorsal interossei abduct the fingers and the palmar interossei

adduct them (remembered by the mnemonics DAB and PAD; the baseline for these movements is the line of the middle finger). The movements occur at the metacarpophalangeal joints, and with the above facts in mind the attachments of the interossei to the fingers can be worked out as follows (omitting constant repetition of the word interosseous):
• The expansion of the index finger (shown in C) has the first dorsal on its radial side (C6), and the second palmar on its ulnar side (C9).
• The expansion of the middle finger has the second dorsal on its radial side and the third dorsal on its ulnar side (to abduct the finger to either side of its own baseline).
• The expansion of the ring finger has the third palmar on its radial side and the fourth dorsal on its ulnar side.

• The expansion of the little finger has the fourth palmar on its radial side and part of abductor digiti minimi on its ulnar side.
• The first palmar (page 144, B1) belongs to the thumb, not to a finger.
• The above attachments reflect the order of the interossei as seen in the palm dissection B on page 144.
• For the bony attachments of the interossei, see page 113. Note that the dorsal interossei have two heads of origin, from adjacent metacarpals, but the palmar interossei have only one, arising from the metacarpal of the digit into which they are inserted.
• When viewing a palmar dissection, as in B on page 144, all the interossei (palmar and dorsal) can be seen, but on the dorsum of the hand, as in D opposite, only the dorsal interossei are visible.

D Dorsum of the left hand. Muscles and tendons

All vessels, nerves and fascia have been removed to show the long tendons passing under the extensor retinaculum (15). See the notes below for the identification of finger tendons

1	Abductor digiti minimi
2	Extensor digiti minimi
3	Slip from extensor digitorum to little finger
4	Extensor digitorum
5	Extensor indicis
6	First
7	Second
8	Third
9	Fourth
10	Abductor pollicis longus
11	Extensor pollicis brevis
12	Extensor pollicis longus
13	Extensor carpi radialis longus
14	Extensor carpi radialis brevis
15	Extensor retinaculum
16	Extensor carpi ulnaris

(items 6–9: dorsal interosseous)

• On the dorsum of the hand the tendon of extensor indicis (D5) lies on the ulnar side of the extensor digitorum tendon (D4) to the index finger.
• It is normal for the tendon of extensor digiti minimi (D2) to be double. In this specimen the extensor digitorum tendon (D4) to the ring finger is also double, with a slip passing to the middle finger.
• The 'tendon' of extensor digitorum (D3) to the little finger normally consists, as here, of a slip from the digitorum tendon (D4) to the ring finger , joining the digiti minimi tendon (D2) just proximal to the metacarpophalangeal joint. Similar slips may join adjacent digitorum tendons on other fingers, as here between the ring and middle fingers.

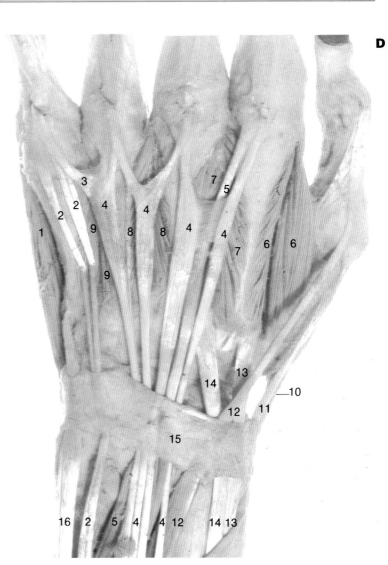

E Dorsum of the right wrist and hand. Synovial sheaths

Fascia and cutaneous branches of the ulnar nerve have been removed; the extensor retinaculum (10) and the radial nerve (2) have been preserved and the synovial sheaths have been emphasized by blue tissue. From the radial to the ulnar side, the six compartments of the extensor retinaculum contain the tendons of: a, abductor pollicis longus and extensor pollicis brevis (13 and 12); b, extensor carpi radialis longus and brevis (4 and 5); c, extensor pollicis longus (3); d, extensor digitorum and extensor indicis (7 and 8); e, extensor digiti minimi (9); f, extensor carpi ulnaris (11)

1	Cephalic vein
2	Branches of radial nerve
3	Extensor pollicis longus
4	Extensor carpi radialis longus
5	Extensor carpi radialis brevis
6	Common sheath for 4 and 5
7	Extensor digitorum
8	Extensor indicis
9	Extensor digiti minimi
10	Extensor retinaculum
11	Extensor carpi ulnaris
12	Extensor pollicis brevis
13	Abductor pollicis longus

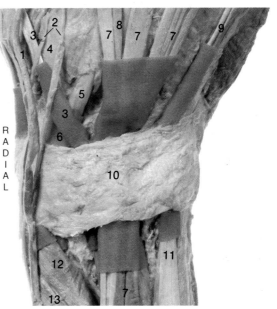

Movements of the fingers, A flexion of the metacarpophalangeal joints and flexion of the interphalangeal joints, **B** extension of the metacarpophalangeal joints and flexion of the interphalangeal joints, **C** extension of the metacarpophalangeal and interphalangeal joints

When 'making a fist' with all finger joints flexed (A), the heads of the metacarpals (2) form the knuckles. To extend the metacarpophalangeal joints (B3) requires the activity of the long extensor tendons of the fingers, but to extend the interphalangeal joints (C6 and 9) as well requires the activity of the interossei and lumbricals, pulling on the dorsal extensor expansions (page 146). Only if the metacarpophalangeal joints remain flexed can the long extensors extend the interphalangeal joints

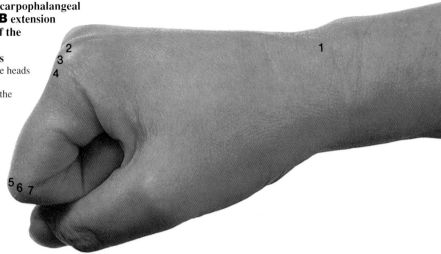

A

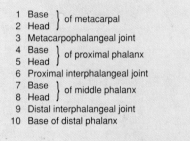

1 Base ⎫
           ⎬ of metacarpal
2 Head ⎭
3 Metacarpophalangeal joint
4 Base ⎫
           ⎬ of proximal phalanx
5 Head ⎭
6 Proximal interphalangeal joint
7 Base ⎫
           ⎬ of middle phalanx
8 Head ⎭
9 Distal interphalangeal joint
10 Base of distal phalanx

B

• Muscles producing movements at the metacarpophalangeal joints:
Flexion: flexor digitorum profundus, flexor digitorum superficialis, lumbricals, interossei, with flexor digiti minimi brevis for the little finger and flexor pollicis longus, flexor pollicis brevis and the first palmar interosseous for the thumb.
Extension: extensor digitorum, extensor indicis (index finger) and extensor digiti minimi (little finger), with extensor pollicis longus and extensor pollicis brevis for the thumb.
Adduction: palmar interossei; when flexed, the long flexors assist.
Abduction: dorsal interossei and the long extensors, with abductor digiti minimi for the little finger.
• Muscles producing movements at the interphalangeal joints:
Flexion: at the proximal joints, flexor digitorum superficialis and flexor digitorum profundus; at the distal joints, flexor digitorum profundus. For the thumb, flexor pollicis longus.
Extension: with the metacarpophalangeal joints flexed, extensor digitorum, extensor indicis and extensor digiti minimi; with the metacarpophalangeal joints extended, interossei and lumbricals. For the thumb, extensor pollicis longus.

C

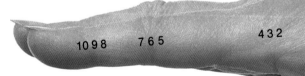

• Muscles producing movements at the wrist joint:
Flexion: flexor carpi radialis, flexor carpi ulnaris, palmaris longus, with assistance from flexor digitorum superficialis, flexor digitorum profundus, flexor pollicis longus and abductor pollicis longus.
Extension: extensor carpi radialis longus and brevis, extensor carpi ulnaris, assisted by extensor digitorum, extensor indicis, extensor digiti minimi and extensor pollicis longus.
Abduction: flexor carpi radialis, extensor carpi radialis longus and brevis, abductor pollicis longus and extensor pollicis brevis.
Adduction: flexor carpi ulnaris, extensor carpi ulnaris.

A **B** **C**

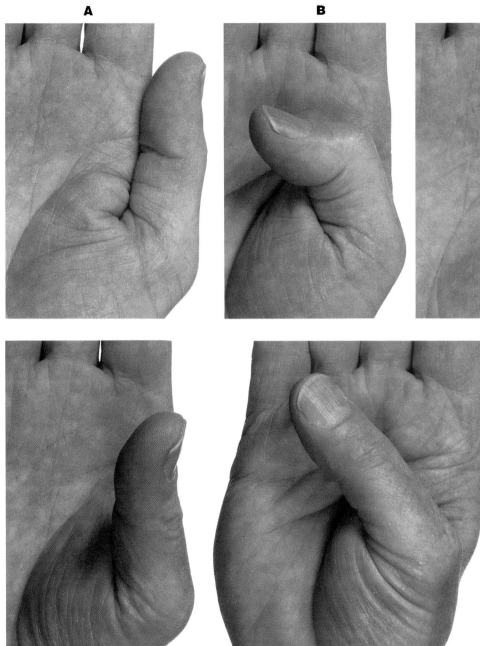

D **E**

Movements of the thumb, **A** in the anatomical position, **B** in flexion, **C** in extension, **D** in abduction, **E** in opposition

With the thumb in the anatomical position (A), the thumb nail is at right angles to the fingers because the first metacarpal is at right angles to the others (page 111). This is a rather artificial position; in the normal position of rest the thumb makes an angle of about 60° with the plane of the palm (i.e. it is partially abducted). Flexion (B) means bending the thumb across the palm, keeping the phalanges at right angles to the palm. Extension (C) is the opposite movement, away from the palm. In abduction (D) the thumb is lifted forwards from the plane of the palm, and continuation of this movement inevitably leads to opposition (E), with rotation of the first metacarpal, twisting the whole digit so that the pulp of the thumb can be brought towards the palm at the base of the little finger (or more commonly in everyday use, to contact or overlap any of the flexed fingers). Opposition is a combination of abduction with flexion and medial rotation at the carpometacarpal joint; it is not necessarily accompanied by flexion at the other thumb joints

• Muscles producing movements at the carpometacarpal joint of the thumb:

Flexion: flexor pollicis brevis, opponens pollicis, and (when the other thumb joints are flexed) flexor pollicis longus.
Extension: abductor pollicis longus, extensor pollicis longus, extensor pollicis brevis.
Abduction: abductor pollicis brevis, abductor pollicis longus.
Adduction: adductor pollicis.
Opposition: opponens pollicis, flexor pollicis brevis, reinforced by adductor pollicis and flexor pollicis longus.

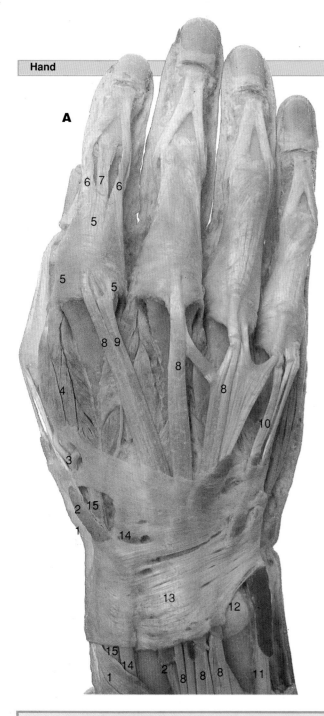

A

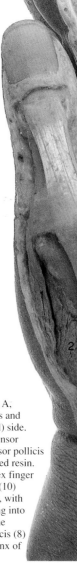

B

A Dorsum of the right hand. Muscles and tendons

All vessels and nerves (except the radial artery, 3) have been removed; the extensor retinaculum (13) is preserved, together with some fascia distal to it to give it some support to synovial sheaths which have been partially injected with green resin (compare with page 147, E). The margins of the distal parts of the extensor digital expansions (as at 5 and 6) have been emphasized by removal of the intervening connective tissue

B Right hand. Muscles and tendons, from the radial side

This is the specimen seen in A, now rotated to show muscles and tendons on the radial (lateral) side. The synovial sheaths of extensor pollicis brevis (4) and extensor pollicis longus (6) show some injected resin. Between the thumb and index finger the first dorsal interosseous (10) passes to the expansion (11), with the first lumbrical (9) running into the expansion just beyond the interosseous. Adductor pollicis (8) passes to the proximal phalanx of the thumb

1	Extensor pollicis brevis	8	Extensor digitorum
2	Extensor pollicis longus	9	Extensor indicis
3	Radial artery	10	Extensor digiti minimi
4	First dorsal interosseous	11	Extensor carpi ulnaris
5	Extensor expansion	12	Head of ulna
6	Collateral slip of expansion to distal phalanx	13	Extensor retinaculum
7	Intermediate part of expansion to middle phalanx	14	Extensor carpi radialis brevis
		15	Extensor carpi radialis longus

1	Abductor pollicis brevis	8	Adductor pollicis
2	Opponens pollicis	9	First lumbrical
3	Abductor pollicis longus	10	First dorsal interosseous
4	Extensor pollicis brevis	11	Extensor expansion
5	Radial artery	12	Extensor carpi radialis brevis
6	Extensor pollicis longus	13	Extensor carpi radialis longus
7	Princeps pollicis artery (unusual origin)	14	Extensor retinaculum

• In A the extensor digitorum tendon to the ring finger (8) is double, as well as giving a slip to the digiti minimi tendon (10), and to the extensor tendon of the middle finger. Some fascia distal to the extensor retinaculum (13) is preserved.

• At the lateral side of the wrist the radial artery (B5) lies in the 'anatomical snuffbox', which is bounded laterally by the tendons of abductor pollicis longus and extensor pollicis brevis (B3 and B4) and medially by the tendon of extensor pollicis longus (B6).

• The princeps pollicis artery (B7) has a more proximal origin than usual; it normally arises from the radial artery after that artery has passed through the first dorsal interosseous muscle (B10) to enter the palm.

• The radial artery (B5 and C15) enters the palm by passing through the first dorsal interosseous muscle (B10 and C2), in B just after giving off the princeps pollicis artery (B7), and in C after giving off the first dorsal metacarpal artery (C2).

• The anterior interosseous artery (C7) pierces the interosseous membrane above pronator quadratus (here removed) to anastomose with the posterior interosseous artery (C8) and join the dorsal carpal arch (C6).

C

C Dorsum of the right hand. Arteries
The arteries have been injected and the long finger tendons removed to display the dorsal carpal arch (6) and dorsal metacarpal arteries (as at 2 and 3). Above the wrist pronator quadratus has been removed to show the branch (9) of the anterior interosseous artery (7), which continues towards the palm; the anterior interosseous itself passes to the dorsal surface to join the posterior interosseous artery (8)

D

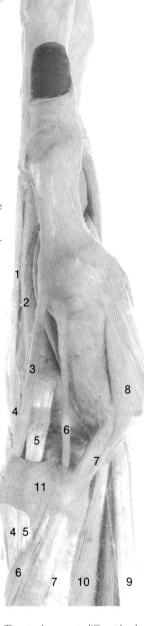

D Left wrist and hand, from the lateral side
This side view of the specimen seen on page 140 (A) shows the two most lateral compartments of the extensor retinaculum (11), one containing the tendons of abductor pollicis longus (7) and extensor pollicis brevis (6), and the other containing the two extensor carpi radialis tendons, longus (5) and brevis (4)

1 Extensor digitorum
2 First dorsal interosseous
3 Extensor pollicis longus
4 Extensor carpi radialis brevis
5 Extensor carpi radialis longus
6 Extensor pollicis brevis
7 Abductor pollicis longus (giving slip to brevis)
8 Abductor pollicis brevis
9 Flexor carpi radialis
10 Flexor pollicis longus
11 Extensor retinaculum

• Three tendons pass to different levels of the thumb: abductor pollicis longus (D7) to the base of the first metacarpal, extensor pollicis brevis (D6) to the base of the proximal phalanx, and extensor pollicis longus (D3) to the base of the distal phalanx.

1 Adductor pollicis and branch of princeps pollicis artery
2 First dorsal interosseous and first dorsal metacarpal artery
3 Second dorsal interosseous and second dorsal metacarpal artery
4 Abductor digiti minimi
5 Extensor carpi ulnaris
6 Dorsal carpal arch
7 Anterior interosseous artery
8 Posterior interosseous artery
9 Branch of anterior interosseous artery to anterior carpal arch
10 Extensor pollicis brevis
11 Abductor pollicis longus
12 Brachioradialis
13 Extensor carpi radialis brevis
14 Extensor carpi radialis longus
15 Radial artery
16 Extensor pollicis longus

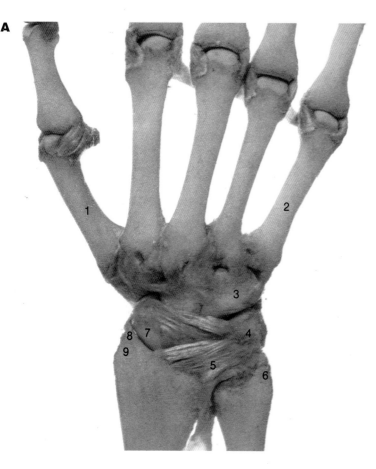

A Dorsum of the right hand. Ligaments and joints

Most joint capsules have been removed, including the radial part of the wrist joint capsule, so showing the articulation between the scaphoid (7) and the lower end of the radius (9)

1	First metacarpal	6	Styloid process of ulna
2	Fifth metacarpal	7	Scaphoid
3	Hamate	8	Radial collateral ligament of
4	Triquetral		wrist joint
5	Dorsal radiocarpal ligament	9	Styloid process of radius

• The wrist (radiocarpal) joint is the joint between the lower end of the radius and the articular disc of the distal radio-ulnar joint proximally, and the scaphoid, lunate and triquetral bones distally.
• The midcarpal joint is the joint between the scaphoid, lunate and triquetral proximally, and the trapezium, trapezoid, capitate and hamate distally.
• Extension of the wrist occurs at the wrist and midcarpal joints, but most of the movement takes place at the wrist joint.
• Flexion of the wrist occurs at the wrist and midcarpal joints, but most of the movement takes place at the midcarpal joint.

Coronal section of the right wrist, B dissection, C MR image

Viewed from the dorsal surface, the section has passed through the wrist near this surface, and the first and fifth metacarpals have not been included in the cut. The arrows between the two rows of carpal bones indicate the line of the midcarpal joint. Compare the MR image with the section

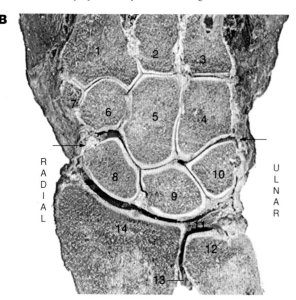

1	Base of second metacarpal
2	Base of third metacarpal
3	Base of fourth metacarpal
4	Hamate
5	Capitate
6	Trapezoid
7	Trapezium
8	Scaphoid
9	Lunate
10	Triquetral
11	Articular disc
12	Head of ulna
13	Sacciform recess of distal radio-ulnar joint
14	Lower end of radius

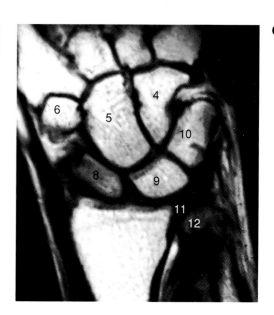

D

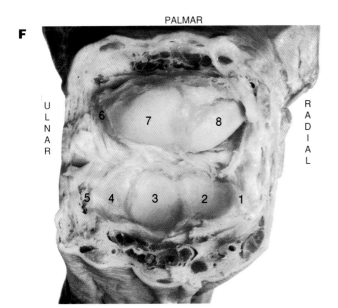

R A D I A L

U L N A R

Right wrist, D cross section of the wrist joint, from below, E MR image

The section, seen as when looking towards the elbow, is at the level of the scaphoid (14) and pisiform (9), and shows the flexor retinaculum (2) and the structures deep to it (in the carpal tunnel), in particular the median nerve (4). Compare features seen in the MR image with those in the section

E

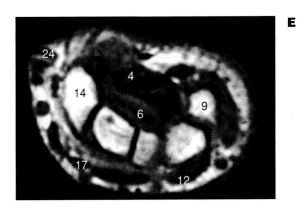

1 Flexor carpi radialis	7 Ulnar artery	13 Lunate with surface for capitate	19 Radial nerve
2 Flexor retinaculum	8 Ulnar nerve	14 Scaphoid with surface for capitate	20 Cephalic vein
3 Flexor pollicis longus	9 Pisiform	15 Extensor digitorum	21 Extensor carpi radialis longus
4 Median nerve	10 Triquetral	16 Extensor indicis	22 Radial artery
5 Flexor digitorum superficialis	11 Extensor carpi ulnaris	17 Extensor carpi radialis brevis	23 Extensor pollicis brevis
6 Flexor digitorum profundus	12 Extensor digiti minimi	18 Extensor pollicis longus	24 Abductor pollicis longus

F

PALMAR

ULNAR

RADIAL

DORSAL

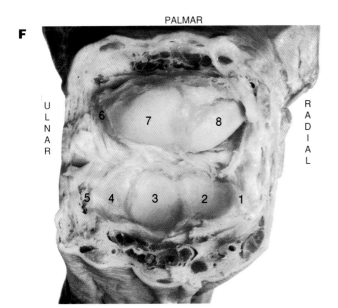

G

PALMAR

ULNAR

RADIAL

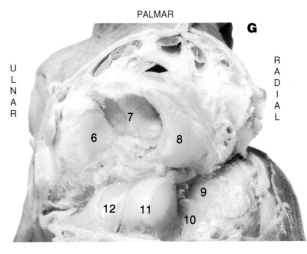

1 Styloid process of radius
2 Surface on radius for scaphoid
3 Surface on radius for lunate
4 Articular disc
5 Styloid process of ulna
6 Triquetral
7 Lunate
8 Scaphoid
9 Trapezium
10 Trapezoid
11 Capitate
12 Hamate

Right wrist and midcarpal joints, F wrist joint, opened up in forced extension, G midcarpal joint, opened up in forced flexion

Both joints have been opened up (far beyond the normal range of movement) in order to demonstrate the bones of the joint surfaces. The wrist joint in A has been forced open in extension, since extension takes place mostly at this joint, and the midcarpal joint in B has been forced open in flexion, since flexion takes place mostly at this joint. The proximal (wrist joint) surfaces of the scaphoid (8), lunate (7) and triquetral (6) are seen in F, and their distal (midcarpal joint) surfaces in G

A

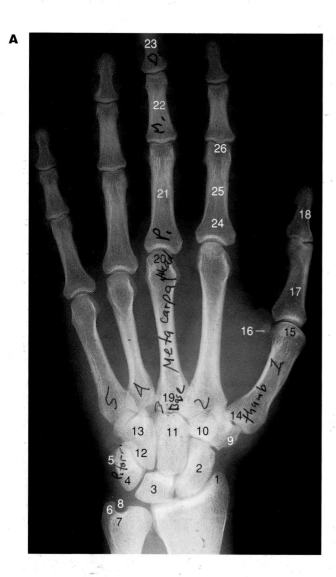

B

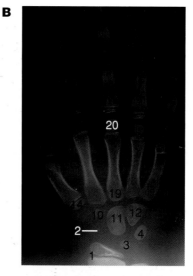

C

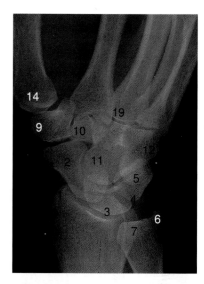

D

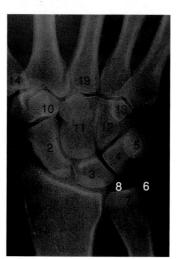

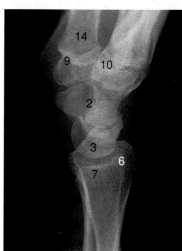

Wrist and hand radiographs, **A** dorsopalmar projection, **B** of a four-year-old child, **C** oblique projection, **D** postero-anterior projection, **E** lateral projection

Compare the epiphyses of the metacarpals and phalanges seen in B with the bony specimens in K and J on page 114

• The wrist (radiocarpal) joint is the joint between the lower end of the radius (1) and articular disc (8) of the distal radio-ulnar joint proximally, and the scaphoid (2), lunate (3) and triquetral (4) distally.

• In the normal position the lunate (A3) articulates with the radius and the articular disc, but in adduction it moves competely on to the radius. In extreme adduction part of the triquetral may also make contact with the radius.

• The epiphysis at the lower end of the radius appears on a radiograph at 2 years and in the ulna at 6 years. The first carpal bone to appear is the capitate at 1 year.

1	Styloid process at lower end of radius	14	Base	} of first metacarpal
2	Scaphoid	15	Head	
3	Lunate	16	Sesamoid bone in flexor pollicis brevis	
4	Triquetral	17	Proximal phalanx	} of thumb
5	Pisiform	18	Distal phalanx	
6	Styloid process of ulna	19	Base	} of third metacarpal
7	Head of ulna	20	Head	
8	Position of articular disc of distal radio-ulnar joint	21	Proximal	} phalanx of middle finger
9	Trapezium	22	Middle	
10	Trapezoid	23	Distal	
11	Capitate	24	Base	} of phalanx
12	Hamate	25	Shaft	
13	Hook of hamate	26	Head	

Typical ribs, from behind, **A** the left fifth rib (a typical upper rib), **B** the left seventh rib (a typical lower rib)

1	Articular facets of head
2	Crest of head
3	Neck
4	Articular facet of tubercle
5	Non-articular part of tubercle
6	Angle
7	Costal groove
8	Shaft

• The typical ribs are the third to the ninth.
• Typical ribs have a head with two facets (1), and a tubercle with articular and non-articular parts (4 and 5) at the junction of the neck (3) and shaft. The shaft has external and internal surfaces, an angle (6) and a costal groove (7).
• In typical upper ribs the articular facet of the tubercle is curved (A4) but becomes increasingly flattened in lower ribs (B4).

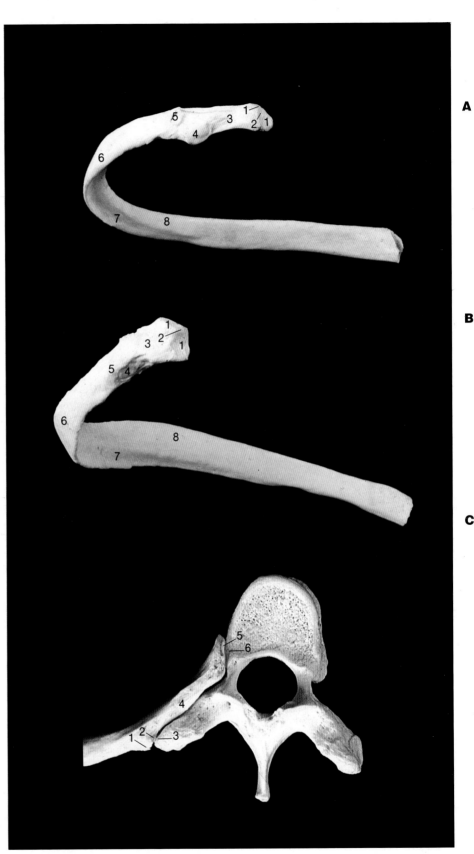

A

B

C

C Typical rib and vertebra articulated, from above

1	Non-articular ⎫ part of tubercle
2	Articular ⎭
3	Articular facet of transverse process
4	Neck of rib
5	Upper costal facet of head of rib
6	Upper costal facet of vertebral body

• The lower of the two facets on the head of a typical rib articulates with the upper costal facet (6) on the vertebral body having the same number as the rib. The upper facet on the head of the rib (5) articulates with the vertebral body above. These form the joints of the heads of ribs.
• The articular facet of the tubercle of a rib (C2) articulates with the costal facet of the transverse process of a vertebra. These are the costotransverse joints.
• The joints of the heads of the ribs and the costotransverse joints collectively form the costovertebral joints.

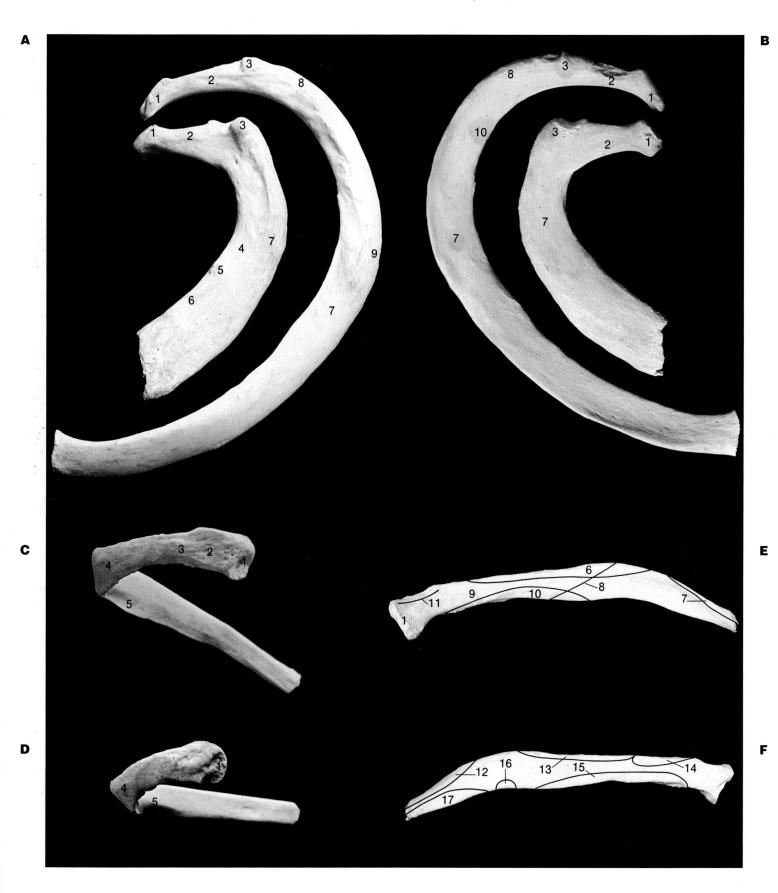

G   **H**

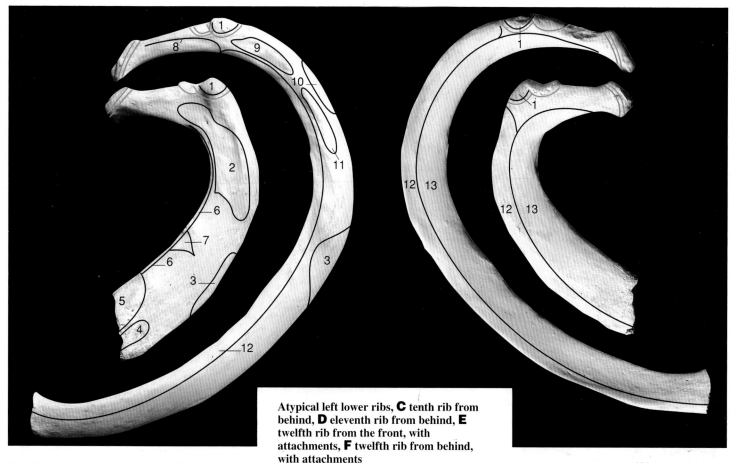

Atypical left lower ribs, **C** tenth rib from behind, **D** eleventh rib from behind, **E** twelfth rib from the front, with attachments, **F** twelfth rib from behind, with attachments

Left first rib (inner) and second rib (outer), A from above, B from below

Left first rib (inner) and second rib (outer), G from above, H from below. Attachments
Blue lines = epiphysial lines; green lines = capsule attachments of costovertebral joints

1	Head
2	Neck
3	Tubercle
4	Groove for subclavian artery and first thoracic nerve
5	Scalene tubercle
6	Groove for subclavian vein
7	Shaft
8	Angle
9	Serratus anterior tuberosity
10	Costal groove

1	Head
2	Neck
3	Tubercle
4	Angle
5	Costal groove
6	Internal intercostal
7	Diaphragm
8	Line of pleural reflexion
9	Area covered by pleura
10	Quadratus lumborum
11	Costotransverse ligament
12	Latissimus dorsi
13	External intercostal
14	Levator costae
15	Erector spinae
16	Serratus posterior inferior
17	External oblique

1	Lateral costotransverse ligament
2	Scalenus medius
3	Serratus anterior
4	Subclavius
5	Costoclavicular ligament
6	Suprapleural membrane
7	Scalenus anterior
8	Superior costotransverse ligament
9	Levator costae
10	Serratus posterior superior
11	Scalenus posterior
12	Intercostal muscles and membranes
13	Area covered by pleura

• The second rib gives origin to part of the first, and the whole of the second, digitation of serratus anterior.
• The atypical ribs are the first, second, tenth, eleventh and twelfth.
• The first rib has a head with one facet (A1), a prominent tubercle (A3), no angle and no costal groove. The shaft has superior and inferior surfaces.
• The second rib has a head with two facets (B1), an angle (B8) near the tubercle (B3), a broad costal groove (B10) posteriorly, and an external surface facing upwards and outwards with the inner surface facing correspondingly downwards and inwards.
• The tenth rib has a head with one or two facets (C1), a tubercle with or without an articular facet (C3), and a costal groove (C5).

• The eleventh rib has a head with one facet (D1), no tubercle but there is an angle (D4) and a slight costal groove (D5).
• The twelfth rib has a head with one facet (E1) but there is no tubercle, no angle and no costal groove. The shaft tapers at its end (the ends of all other ribs widen slightly).

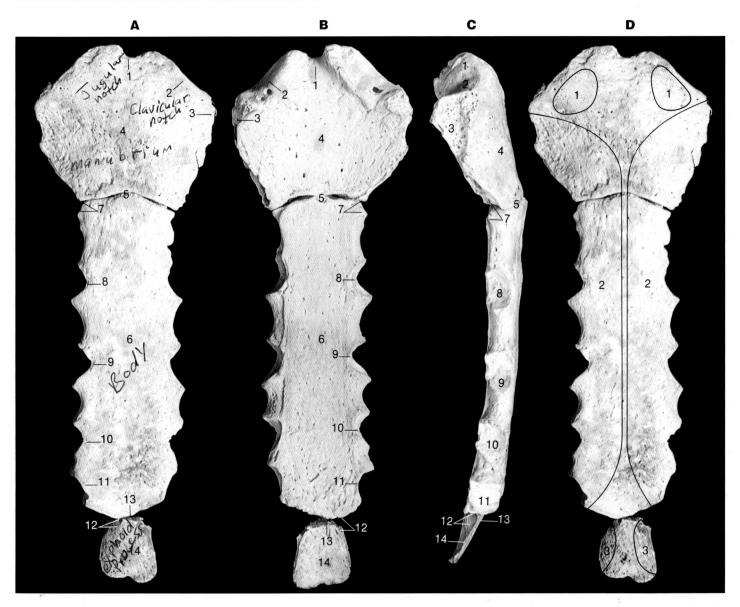

A   **B**   **C**   **D**

The sternum, A from the front, B from behind, C from the right

1	Jugular notch
2	Clavicular notch
3	Notch for first costal cartilage
4	Manubrium
5	Sternal angle and manubriosternal joint
6	Body
7	Notches for second
8	Notch for third
9	Notch for fourth
10	Notch for fifth
11	Notch for sixth
12	Notches for seventh
13	Xiphisternal joint
14	Xiphoid process

costal cartilage *(bracket spanning 7–12)*

• The sternum consists of the manubrium (4), body (6) and xiphoid process (14).

• The body of the sternum (6) is formed by the fusion of four sternebrae, the sites of the fusion sometimes being indicated by three slight transverse ridges.

• The manubrium (4) and body (6) are bony but the xiphoid process (14), which varies considerably in size and shape, is cartilaginous although it frequently shows some degree of ossification.

• The manubriosternal and xiphisternal joints (5 and 13) are both symphyses, the surfaces being covered by hyaline cartilage and united by a fibrocartilaginous disc.

The sternum, D from the front, E from behind. Attachments

1	Sternocleidomastoid
2	Pectoralis major
3	Rectus abdominis
4	Sternohyoid
5	Sternothyroid
6	Area covered by right pleura
7	Area covered by left pleura
8	Area in contact with pericardium
9	Transversus thoracis
10	Diaphragm

• The two pleural sacs are in contact from the levels of the second to fourth costal cartilages (E6 and 7).

E   **F**

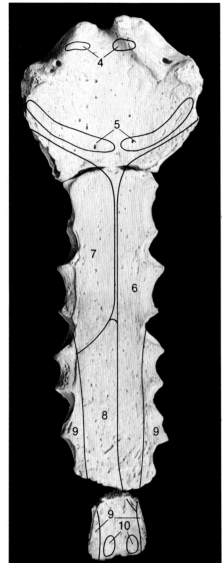

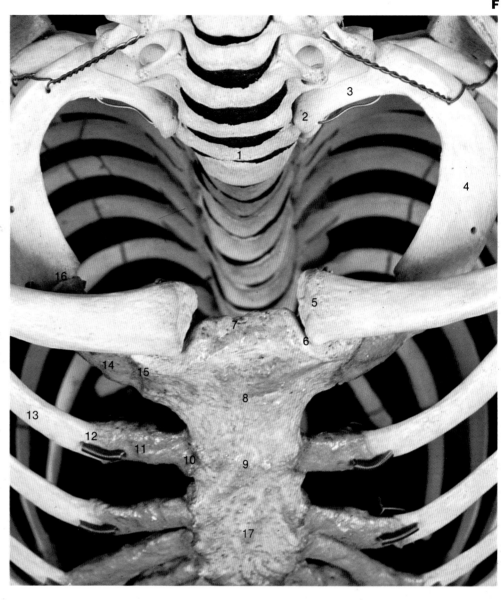

F Thoracic inlet, from above and in front, in an
articulated skeleton

• The thoracic inlet (upper aperture of the thorax) is
approximately the same size and shape as the outline of the
kidney, and is bounded by the first thoracic vertebra (1), first
ribs (4), and costal cartilages (14), and the upper border of the
manubrium of the sternum (jugular notch, 7). It does not lie in a
horizontal plane but slopes downwards and forwards.
• The second costal cartilage (11) joins the manubrium and
body of the sternum (8 and 17) at the level of the
manubriosternal joint (9). This is an important landmark, since
the joint line is palpable as a ridge at the slight angle between
the manubrium and body, and the second costal cartilage and rib
can be identified lateral to it. Other ribs can be identified by
counting down from the second; the first costal cartilage and the
end of the first rib are under cover of the clavicle and not easily
felt.
• The thoracic 'inlet' is sometimes known clinically as the
thoracic 'outlet'.

1	First thoracic vertebra
2	Head ⎫
3	Neck ⎬ of first rib
4	Shaft ⎭
5	Sternal end of clavicle
6	Sternoclavicular joint
7	Jugular notch
8	Manubrium of sternum
9	Manubriosternal joint (angle of Louis)
10	Second sternocostal joint
11	Second costal cartilage
12	Costochondral joint
13	Second rib
14	First costal cartilage
15	First sternocostal joint
16	First costochondral joint
17	Body of sternum

A

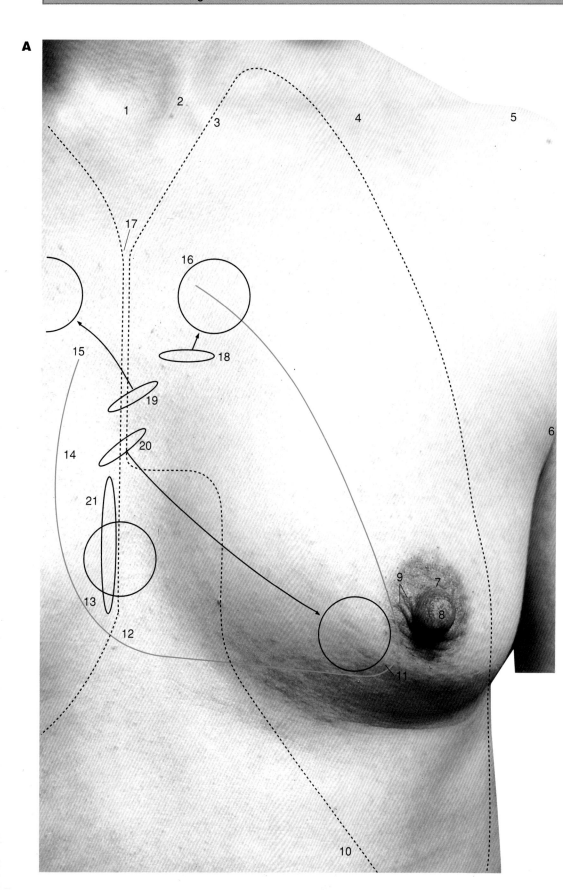

A Surface markings of the heart, left pleura and lung, in the female
Blue line = heart; dotted line = pleura
The positions of the four heart valves are indicated by ellipses, and the sites where the sounds of the corresponding valves are best heard with the stethoscope are indicated by the circles

1	Jugular notch
2	Sternocleidomastoid
3	Sternoclavicular joint
4	Midpoint of clavicle
5	Acromioclavicular joint
6	Axillary tail ⎫
7	Areola ⎬ of breast
8	Nipple ⎪
9	Areolar gland ⎭
10	Costal margin (at eighth costal cartilage)
11	Apex of heart
12	Xiphisternal joint
13	Sixth ⎫
14	Fourth ⎬ costal cartilage
15	Third ⎪
16	Second ⎭
17	Manubriosternal joint
18	Pulmonary ⎫
19	Aortic ⎬ valve
20	Mitral ⎪
21	Tricuspid ⎭

• The manubriosternal joint (17) is palpable and a guide to identifying the second costal cartilage (16) which joins the sternum at this level (see page 159, F9 to 11).
• The pleura and lung extend into the neck for 2.5 cm above the medial third of the clavicle.
• In the midclavicular line the lower limit of the *pleura* reaches the eighth costal cartilage, in the midaxillary line it reaches the tenth rib, and at the lateral border of the erector spinae muscle it crosses the twelfth rib. The lower border of the *lung* is about two ribs higher than the pleural reflexion.
• Behind the sternum the pleural sacs are adjacent to one another in the midline from the level of the second to fourth costal cartilages, but then diverge due to the mass of the heart on the left.
• The four heart valves are approximately in or just to the left of the midline—pulmonary, aortic, mitral, tricuspid in that order from above downwards (18 to 21).
• Because of the overlying bone and cartilage and the direction of blood flow, the sites where the sounds of the valves closing are best heard are not usually over the valves themselves, except for the tricuspid valve (21). For pulmonary valve (18) sounds, the stethoscope is placed over the second left intercostal space at the costal margin (below 16), for the aortic valve (19) over the second right interspace (above 15), and for the mitral valve (20) near the apex of the heart (11).

B

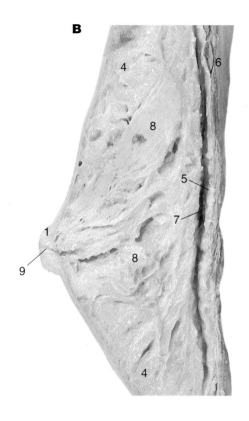

Female breast (mammary gland), B median sagittal section, C dissection of lower part, from the front and below, D xeromammogram

The glandular elements in B have been consolidated by cancerous change, emphasizing the surrounding unaffected fat. The section has passed through a lactiferous duct. The loose tissue in front of the fascia over pectoralis major (5) has been opened up to emphasize the retromammary space. In C the fatty and glandular tissue has been dissected away to show the irregular network of fibrous tissue septa which pass from the overlying skin to the underlying fascia. Xeromammography, as illustrated in D, is a radiographic technique which better shows soft-tissue detail

C

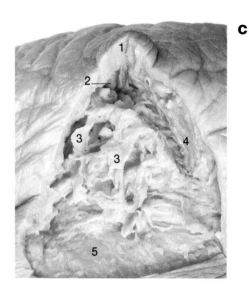

1 Nipple
2 Ampulla of lactiferous duct
3 Fibrous septum
4 Fat
5 Fascia over pectoralis major
6 Pectoralis major
7 Retromammary space
8 Condensed glandular tissue
9 Lactiferous duct

D

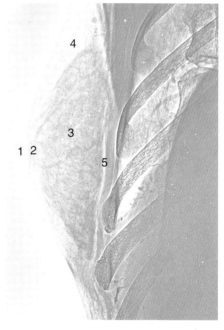

E

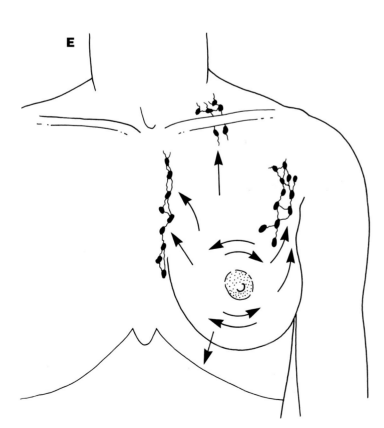

E Diagram of lymph drainage of the breast

There is a diffuse network of anastomosing lymphatic channels within the breast, including the overlying skin, and *lymph in any part may travel to any other part.* Larger channels drain most of the lymph to axillary nodes, but some from the medial part pass through the thoracic wall near the sternum to parasternal nodes adjacent to the internal thoracic vessels. These are the commonest and initial sites for cancerous spread, but other nodes may be involved (especially in the later spread of disease); these include infraclavicular and supraclavicular (deep cervical) nodes, nodes in the mediastinum, and nodes in the abdomen (via the diaphragm and rectus sheath). Spread to the opposite breast may also occur

A Right side of the thorax, from behind with the arm abducted

With the arm fully abducted, the medial (vertebral) border of the scapula (9) comes to lie at an angle of about 60° to the vertical, and indicates approximately the line of the oblique fissure of the lung (interrupted line)

1	Spinous process of third thoracic vertebra
2	Trapezius
3	Spine of scapula
4	Deltoid
5	Teres major
6	Inferior angle of scapula
7	Latissimus dorsi
8	Fifth intercostal space
9	Medial border of scapula

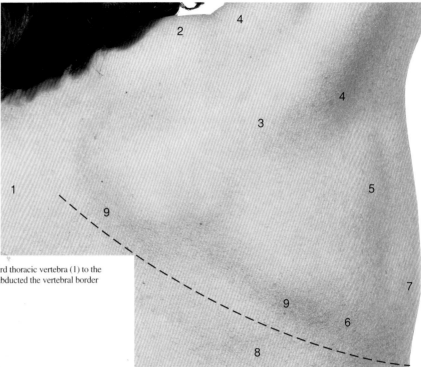

• The line of the oblique fissure of the lung runs from the level of the spine of the third thoracic vertebra (1) to the sixth costal cartilage at the lateral border of the sternum (see B). With the arm fully abducted the vertebral border of the scapula (9) is a good guide to the direction of this fissure.

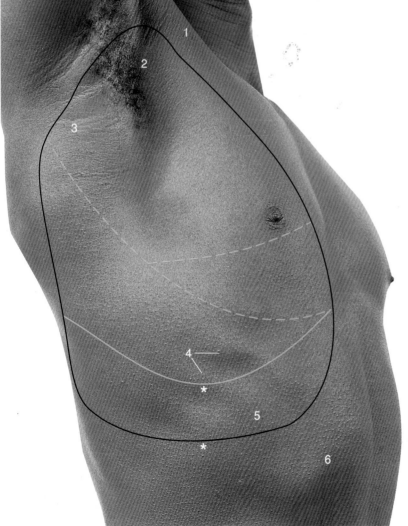

B Surface markings of the right side of the thorax, from the right, with the arm abducted

The black line indicates the extent of the pleura, and the solid green line the lower limit of the lung; note the gap between the two at the lower part of the thorax, indicating the costodiaphragmatic recess of pleura, which does not contain any lung. The transverse and oblique fissures of the lung are represented by the interrupted green lines

1	Pectoralis major
2	Floor of axilla
3	Latissimus dorsi
4	Digitations of serratus anterior
5	External oblique
6	Costal margin

• The transverse fissure of the right lung is represented by a line drawn horizontally backwards from the fourth costal cartilage until it meets the line of the oblique fissure (described in A) running forwards to the sixth costal cartilage. The triangle so outlined indicates the middle lobe of the lung, with the superior lobe above it and the inferior lobe below and behind it.
• On the left side where the lung has only two lobes, superior and inferior, there is no transverse fissure; the surface marking for the oblique fissure is similar to that on the right.
• The asterisks represent the places where the lower edges of the lung and pleura cross the eighth and tenth ribs respectively in the midaxillary line.

C Muscles of the thorax. Left external and internal intercostal muscles, from the front

Pectoral and abdominal muscles have been removed, together with all vessels and nerves and the anterior intercostal membranes, to show the external and internal intercostal muscles (as at 4 and 5)

1 Sternal angle
2 Second costal cartilage
3 Second rib
4 External intercostal
5 Internal intercostal
6 Xiphoid process
7 Seventh ⎫
8 Eighth ⎬ costal cartilage
9 Ninth   ⎪
10 Tenth ⎭

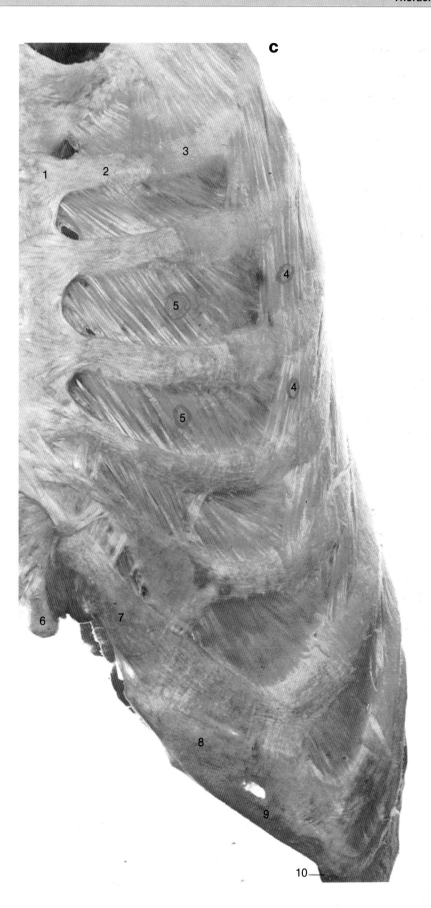

c

• The fibres of the external intercostal muscles (4) run downwards and medially, and near the costochondral junctions (as between 2 and 3) give place to the anterior intercostal membrane (here removed); these are thin sheets of connective tissue through which the underlying internal intercostal muscles (5) can be seen.

• The fibres of the internal intercostal muscles (5) run downwards and laterally. At the front they are covered by the anterior intercostal membranes, and at the back of the thorax they give place to the posterior intercostal membranes. The different directions of the muscle fibres enable the two muscle groups to be distinguished—down and medially for the externals (4), down and laterally for the internals (5).

• The seventh costal cartilage (7) is the lowest to join the sternum and together with the eighth, ninth and tenth cartilages (8 to 10) forms the costal margin.

Muscles of the thorax. Right intercostal muscles, A from the outside, B from the inside

In A each intercostal space has been dissected to a different depth, showing from above downwards an external intercostal muscle (2), internal intercostal (4), innermost intercostal (7) and pleura (9). The main intercostal vessels and nerve lie between the internal and innermost muscles; the nerve (6) is seen in the sixth interspace immediately below the sixth rib (5) and lying on the outer surface of the innermost intercostal (7), but the artery and vein are under cover of the costal groove. The vessels as well as the nerve are seen in the fifth intercostal space when this is dissected from the inside of the thorax, as in B; here the pleura and innermost intercostal muscle have been removed, and the vessels (11 and 12) and fifth intercostal nerve (13) lie against the inner surface of the internal intercostal (4)

1	Fourth rib
2	External intercostal
3	Fifth rib
4	Internal intercostal
5	Sixth rib
6	Sixth intercostal nerve
7	Innermost intercostal
8	Seventh rib
9	Pleura
10	Eighth rib
11	Fifth posterior intercostal vein
12	Fifth posterior intercostal artery
13	Fifth intercostal nerve

C Muscles of the thorax. Levator costae muscles, left side, from behind

The left erector spinae and latissimus dorsi have been removed from the left side of the vertebral column and adjacent ribs to show the levator costae muscles (as at 3) and the medial ends of the external intercostals (as at 2)

1	Seventh rib
2	External intercostal
3	Levator costae
4	Lateral costotransverse ligament
5	Transverse process of eighth thoracic vertebra
6	Lamina of eighth thoracic vertebra
7	Tubercle of ninth rib
8	Angle of ninth rib

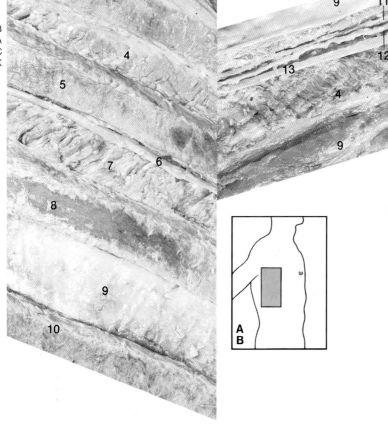

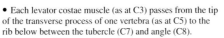

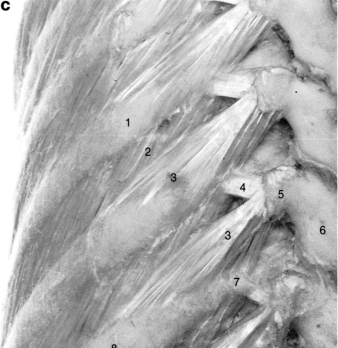

• Each levator costae muscle (as at C3) passes from the tip of the transverse process of one vertebra (as at C5) to the rib below between the tubercle (C7) and angle (C8).
• The internal intercostal muscles are continuous posteriorly with the posterior intercostal membranes which are covered up by the medial ends of the external intercostals (as at C2).

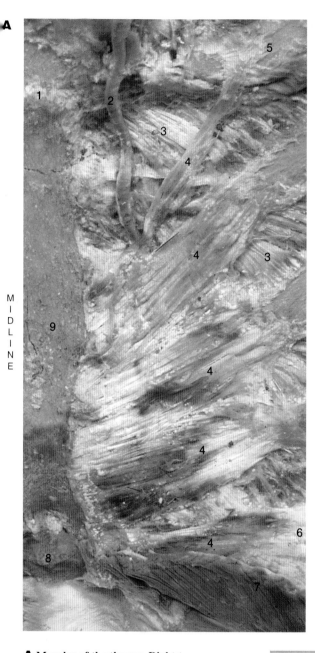

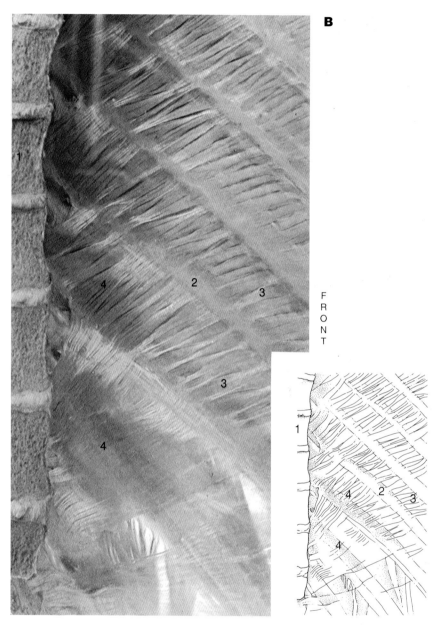

A Muscles of the thorax. Right transversus thoracis, from behind

This view of the internal surface of the thoracic wall shows the posterior surface of the right half of the sternum and adjacent wall, with the pleura removed. The internal thoracic artery (2) is seen passing deep to the slips of transversus thoracis (4, previously called sternocostalis)

- Transversus thoracis (A4) is in the same plane as the innermost intercostal muscles at the lateral side of the thoracic wall (B3) and the subcostal muscles on the posterior part (B4).
- The subcostal muscles (B4) span more than one rib. They and the innermost intercostals (B3, intercostales intimi) are often poorly developed or absent in the upper part of the thorax.

1	Sternal angle
2	Internal thoracic artery
3	Internal intercostal
4	Slips of transversus thoracis muscle
5	Second rib
6	Sixth rib
7	Diaphragm
8	Xiphoid process
9	Body of sternum

B Muscles of the thorax. Left lower subcostal and innermost intercostal muscles

This view of the lower left hemithorax is seen from the right and in front, with vertebral bodies (as at 1) sectioned and the pleura, vessels and nerves removed, and shows part of the innermost layer of thoracic wall muscles (3 and 4)

1	Eighth thoracic vertebra
2	Eighth rib
3	Innermost intercostal
4	Subcostal

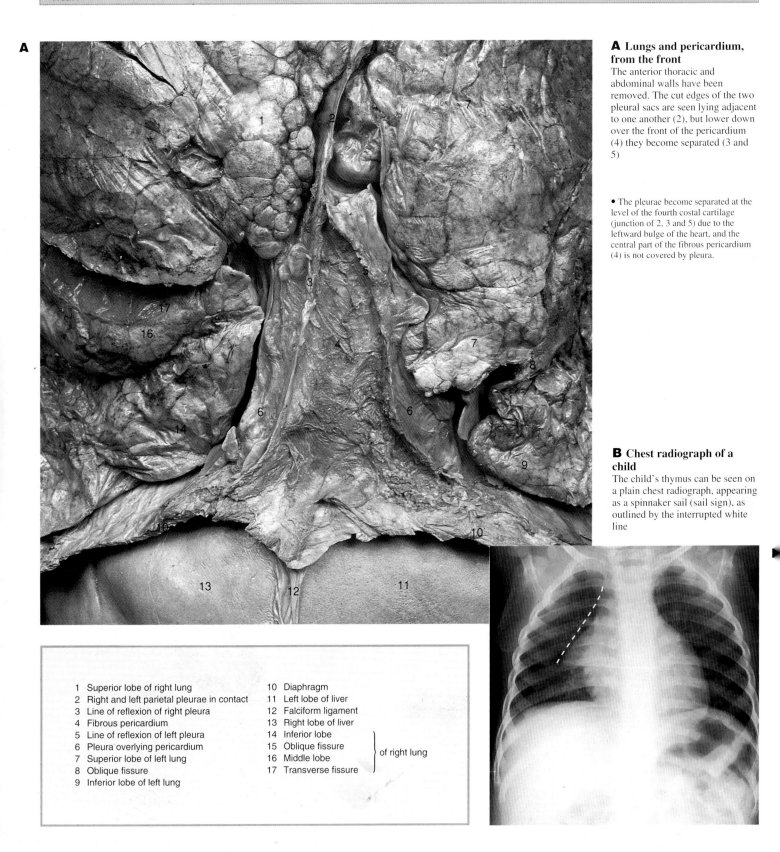

A Lungs and pericardium, from the front

The anterior thoracic and abdominal walls have been removed. The cut edges of the two pleural sacs are seen lying adjacent to one another (2), but lower down over the front of the pericardium (4) they become separated (3 and 5)

• The pleurae become separated at the level of the fourth costal cartilage (junction of 2, 3 and 5) due to the leftward bulge of the heart, and the central part of the fibrous pericardium (4) is not covered by pleura.

B Chest radiograph of a child

The child's thymus can be seen on a plain chest radiograph, appearing as a spinnaker sail (sail sign), as outlined by the interrupted white line

1 Superior lobe of right lung	10 Diaphragm	
2 Right and left parietal pleurae in contact	11 Left lobe of liver	
3 Line of reflexion of right pleura	12 Falciform ligament	
4 Fibrous pericardium	13 Right lobe of liver	
5 Line of reflexion of left pleura	14 Inferior lobe	
6 Pleura overlying pericardium	15 Oblique fissure	} of right lung
7 Superior lobe of left lung	16 Middle lobe	
8 Oblique fissure	17 Transverse fissure	
9 Inferior lobe of left lung		

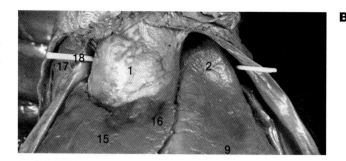

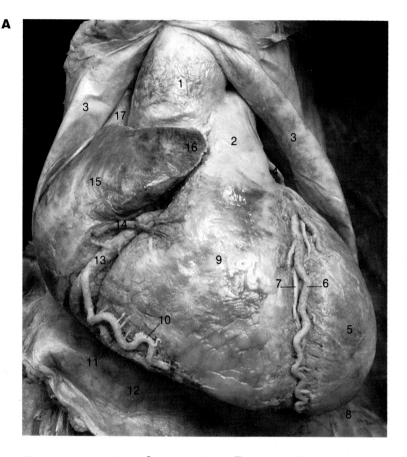

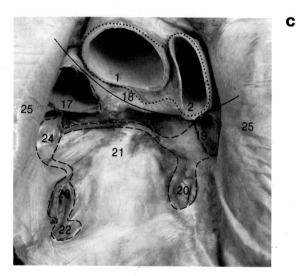

Heart and pericardium, **A** from the front, **B** with marker in the transverse sinus, **C** oblique sinus after removal of the heart

In A the pericardium has been incised and turned back (3) to display the anterior surface of the heart. The pulmonary trunk (2) leaves the right ventricle (9) in front and to the left of the ascending aorta (1), which is overlapped by the auricle (16) of the right atrium (15). The superior vena cava (17) is to the right of the aorta and still largely covered by pericardium. The anterior interventricular branch (6) of the left coronary artery and the great cardiac vein (7) lie in the interventricular groove between the right and left ventricles (9 and 5), and the right coronary artery (13) is in the atrioventricular groove between the right ventricle (9) and right atrium (15). In B only the upper part of another heart is shown, with a marker in the transverse sinus, the space behind the aorta (1) and pulmonary trunk (2). In C the heart has been removed from the pericardium, leaving the orifices of the great vessels. The dotted line indicates the attachment of the single sleeve of serous pericardium surrounding the aorta (1) and pulmonary trunk (2). The interrupted line indicates the attachment of another more complicated but still single sleeve of serous pericardium surrounding all the other six great vessels (the four pulmonary veins, 19, 20, 23 and 24, and the superior and inferior venae cavae, 17 and 22). The narrow interval between the two sleeves is the transverse sinus; the solid line in C indicates the path of the marker in B. The area of the pericardium (21) between the pulmonary veins and limited above by the reflexion of the serous pericardium on to the back of the heart is the oblique sinus

• The right border of the heart is formed by the right atrium (A15).
• The left border is formed mostly by the left ventricle (A5) with at the top the uppermost part (infundibulum) of the right ventricle (A9) and the tip of the left auricle (A4).
• The inferior border is formed by the right ventricle (A9) with a small part of the left ventricle at the apex (page 168, A9).

 1 Ascending aorta
 2 Pulmonary trunk
 3 Serous pericardium overlying fibrous pericardium (turned laterally)
 4 Auricle of left atrium
 5 Left ventricle
 6 Anterior interventricular branch of left coronary artery
 7 Great cardiac vein
 8 Diaphragm
 9 Right ventricle
10 Marginal branch of right coronary artery
11 Small cardiac vein
12 Pericardium fused with tendon of diaphragm
13 Right coronary artery
14 Anterior cardiac vein
15 Right atrium
16 Auricle of right atrium
17 Superior vena cava
18 Marker in transverse sinus
19 Left superior pulmonary vein
20 Left inferior pulmonary vein
21 Posterior wall of pericardial cavity and oblique sinus
22 Inferior vena cava
23 Right inferior pulmonary vein
24 Right superior pulmonary vein
25 Pericardium turned laterally over lung

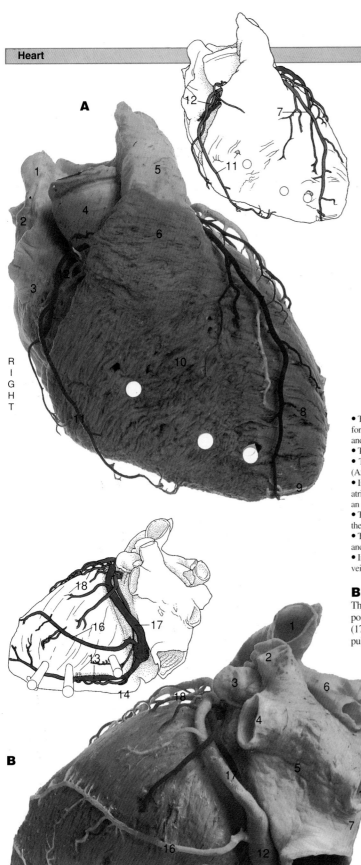

A

R
I
G
H
T

A Heart, from the front, with blood vessels injected

The coronary arteries have been injected with red latex and the cardiac veins with grey latex. The pulmonary trunk (5) passes upwards from the infundibulum (6) of the right ventricle (10), and at its commencement it is just in front and to the left of the ascending aorta (4)

1	Superior vena cava
2	Right atrium
3	Auricle of right atrium (displaced laterally)
4	Ascending aorta
5	Pulmonary trunk
6	Infundibulum of right ventricle
7	Anterior interventricular branch of left coronary artery and great cardiac vein in interventricular groove
8	Left ventricle
9	Apex
10	Right ventricle
11	Marginal branch of right coronary artery
12	Right coronary artery in anterior atrioventricular groove

- The *sternocostal* surface of the heart is the *anterior* surface (as seen in A on page 167 and A above) formed mainly by the right ventricle (A10, D2), with parts of the left ventricle (A8,) and right atrium (A2 and D11).
- The *apex* of the heart (A9) is formed by the left ventricle.
- The infundibulum (A6) is the part of the right ventricle (A10) from which the pulmonary trunk arises (A5).
- In A the anterior atrioventricular groove has been opened up by displacing the auricle (A3) of the right atrium to show the right coronary artery (A12) more clearly. The marginal branch (11) of this vessel has an unusually high origin.
- The *base* of the heart is the *posterior* surface, formed mainly by the left atrium (B5) with a small part of the right atrium (B7).
- The *inferior* surface is the *diaphragmatic* surface, formed by the two ventricles (mainly the left) (B15 and 14).
- In B there is a large ventricular branch of the left coronary artery passing superficial to the great cardiac vein (B17).

B Heart, from behind, with blood vessels injected

This posterior view of the same specimen as in A shows the coronary sinus (12) in the posterior atrioventricular groove and three large tributaries entering it—the great cardiac vein (17), the posterior vein of the left ventricle (16) and the middle cardiac vein (13). The four pulmonary veins (2, 4, 9 and 10) enter the left atrium (5)

B

R
I
G
H
T

1	Left pulmonary artery
2	Superior left pulmonary vein
3	Auricle of left atrium
4	Inferior left pulmonary vein
5	Left atrium
6	Right pulmonary artery
7	Right atrium
8	Superior vena cava
9	Superior right pulmonary vein
10	Inferior right pulmonary vein
11	Inferior vena cava
12	Coronary sinus in posterior atrioventricular groove
13	Middle cardiac vein and posterior interventricular branch of right coronary artery in posterior interventricular groove
14	Right ventricle
15	Left ventricle
16	Posterior vein of left ventricle
17	Great cardiac vein and circumflex branch of left coronary artery
18	Great cardiac vein and anterior interventricular branch of left coronary artery

C Right atrium, from the front and right

The anterior wall has been incised near its left margin and reflected to the right, showing on its internal surface the vertical crista terminalis (2) and horizontal pectinate muscles (1). The fossa ovalis (11) is on the interatrial septum, and the opening of the coronary sinus (7) is to the left of the inferior vena caval opening (10)

1	Pectinate muscles	8	Valve of coronary sinus
2	Crista terminalis	9	Valve of inferior vena cava
3	Superior vena cava	10	Inferior vena cava
4	Auricle	11	Fossa ovalis
5	Tricuspid valve	12	Limbus
6	Position of atrioventricular node	13	Position of intervenous tubercle
7	Opening of coronary sinus		

- The intervenous tubercle, which is rarely detectable in the human heart (13), may have served in the embryo to direct blood from the superior vena cava towards the tricuspid orifice.
- The fossa ovalis (11) forms part of the interatrial septum, and is part of the embryonic primary septum.
- The limbus (12), which forms the margin of the fossa ovalis (11), represents the lower margin of the embryonic secondary septum. Before the primary and secondary septa fuse (at birth), the gap between them forms the foramen ovale.
- The sinuatrial node (SA node, not illustrated) is embedded in the anterior wall of the atrium at the upper end of the crista terminalis, just below the opening of the superior vena cava.
- The atrioventricular node (AV node, 6) is embedded in the interatrial septum, just above and to the left of the opening of the coronary sinus (7).

D Right ventricle, from the front

Most of the anterior wall has been removed, but the part to which the anterior papillary muscle (5) is attached remains. The septomarginal trabecula (4) joins the anterior papillary muscle (5), and the anterior cusp of the tricuspid valve (7) largely obscures the other cusps (they are shown in D on page 171)

1	Pulmonary trunk
2	Infundibulum of right ventricle
3	Trabeculae on interventricular septum
4	Septomarginal trabecula
5	Anterior ⎫ papillary
6	Posterior ⎬ muscle
7	Anterior cusp of tricuspid valve
8	Chordae tendineae
9	Ascending aorta
10	Auricle of right atrium
11	Right atrium
12	Inferior vena cava
13	Superior vena cava

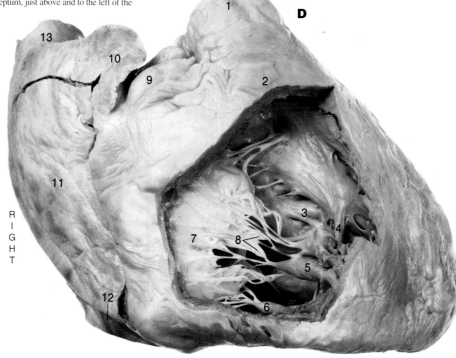

- The septomarginal trabecula (4), which conducts part of .the right limb of the atrioventricular bundle from the interventricular septum (3) to the anterior papillary muscle (5), was formerly known as the moderator band.
- The chordae tendineae (8) connect the cusps of the tricuspid valve to the papillary muscles. The usual arrangement of the connexions is given in the following notes.
- The anterior papillary muscle (5) is large and connected to the anterior (7) and posterior cusps.
- The posterior papillary muscle (6) is small and connected to the posterior and septal cusps.
- Several small septal papillary muscles are connected to the septal and anterior cusps.
- The posterior papillary muscle (6) is so called because it is *behind* the anterior cusp (7), but it might be better named *inferior* because it is on the *floor* of the ventricle.

A

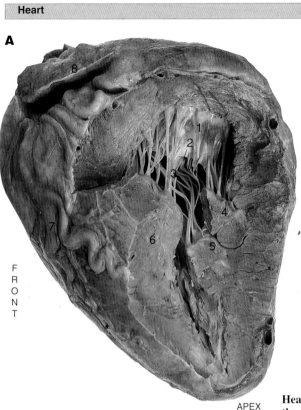

FRONT

APEX

B

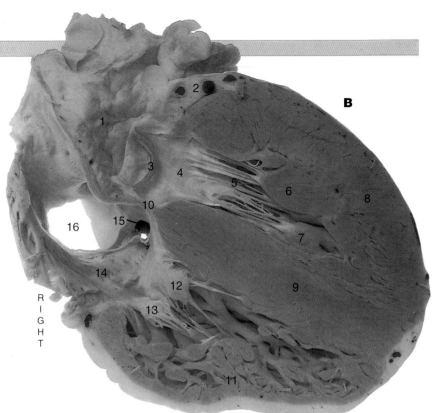

RIGHT

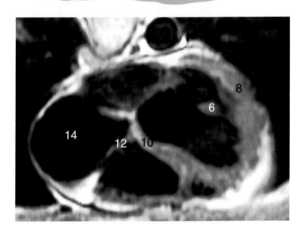

C

A Left ventricle, from the left and below

The ventricle has been opened by removing much of the left, anterior and posterior walls, and is viewed from below, looking upwards to the under-surface of the cusps of the mitral valve (1 and 2) which are anchored to the anterior and posterior papillary muscles (4 and 5) by chordae tendineae (3). The posterior cusp (2) is largely hidden by the anterior cusp (1) in this view

Heart, B coronal section of the ventricles, C axial MR image

In B the heart has been cut in two in the coronal plane, and this is the posterior section seen from the front, looking towards the back of both ventricles. The section has passed immediately in front of the anterior cusp of the mitral valve (4) and the posterior cusp of the aortic valve (3). Compare features seen in the MR image with the section

1 Anterior ⎫
2 Posterior ⎬ cusp of mitral valve
3 Chordae tendineae
4 Anterior ⎫
5 Posterior ⎬ papillary muscle
6 Anterior ventricular wall
7 Anterior interventricular branch of left coronary artery
8 Auricle of left atrium

• The wall of the left ventricle (8) is normally three times as thick as the wall of the right ventricle (11).
• The mitral orifice (which is immediately behind the anterior cusp of the mitral valve, 4) and aortic orifice (whose posterior cusp is at 3) are adjacent to one another and separated from each other only by the anterior cusp of the mitral valve (4).

1 Ascending aorta
2 Left coronary artery branches and great cardiac vein
3 Posterior cusp of aortic valve
4 Anterior cusp of mitral valve
5 Chordae tendineae
6 Anterior papillary muscle
7 Posterior papillary muscle
8 Left ventricular wall
9 Muscular ⎫
10 Membranous ⎬ part of interventricular septum
11 Right ventricular wall
12 Septal ⎫
13 Posterior ⎬ cusp of tricuspid valve
14 Right atrium
15 Opening of coronary sinus
16 Inferior vena cava

• The anterior and posterior papillary muscles (4 and 5) are both connected by chordae tendineae (3) to both valve cusps (1 and 2).

• The cusps of the aortic and pulmonary valves are here given their official names but some English texts use slightly different alternatives, as follows:

		Official	English
Aortic		Right	Anterior
		Left	Left posterior
		Posterior	Right posterior
Pulmonary		Left	Posterior
		Anterior	Left anterior
		Right	Right anterior

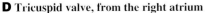

D Tricuspid valve, from the right atrium

The atrium has been opened by incising the anterior wall (3) and turning the flap outwards so that the atrial surface of the atrioventricular orifice is seen, guarded by the three cusps of the tricuspid valve—anterior (4), posterior (5) and septal (6)

1	Superior vena cava	7	Interatrial septum
2	Auricle of right atrium	8	Crista terminalis
3	Anterior wall of right atrium	9	Pectinate muscles
4	Anterior ⎫ cusp of		
5	Posterior ⎬ tricuspid		
6	Septal ⎭ valve		

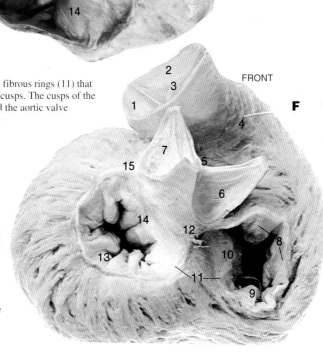

D

FRONT

• The posterior cusp (5) of the tricuspid valve is the smallest.

E Pulmonary, aortic and mitral valves, from above

The pulmonary trunk (1) and ascending aorta (5) have been cut off immediately above the three cusps of the pulmonary and aortic valves (2 to 4, 7 to 9). The upper part of the left atrium (14) has been removed to show the upper surface of the mitral valve cusps (15 and 16)

1	Pulmonary trunk
2	Left ⎫
3	Anterior ⎬ cusps of pulmonary valve
4	Right ⎭
5	Ascending aorta
6	Marker in ostium of right coronary artery
7	Right ⎫
8	Posterior ⎬ cusp of aortic valve
9	Left ⎭
10	Ostium of left coronary artery
11	Auricle of right atrium
12	Right atrium
13	Superior vena cava
14	Left atrium
15	Posterior ⎫ cusp of mitral valve
16	Anterior ⎭

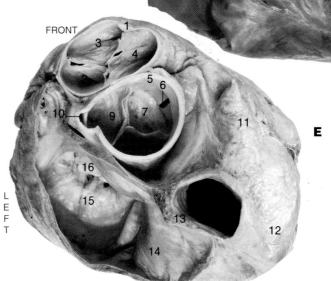

FRONT

LEFT

E

F Fibrous framework of the heart

The heart is seen from the right and behind after removing both atria, looking down on to the fibrous rings (11) that surround the mitral and tricuspid orifices and form the attachments for the bases of the valve cusps. The cusps of the pulmonary valve (1 to 3) are seen at the top of the infundibulum of the right ventricle (4), and the aortic valve cusps (5 to 7) have been dissected out from the beginning of the ascending aorta

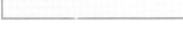

1	Left ⎫ cusps of	8	Anterior ⎫ cusps of	
2	Anterior ⎬ pulmonary	9	Posterior ⎬ tricuspid	
3	Right ⎭ valve	10	Septal ⎭ valve	
4	Infundibulum of right ventricle	11	Fibrous ring	
		12	Right fibrous trigone	
5	Right ⎫ cusps of	13	Posterior ⎫ cusps of	
6	Posterior ⎬ aortic	14	Anterior ⎭ mitral valve	
7	Left ⎭ valve	15	Left fibrous trigone	

FRONT

F

LEFT

• The fibrous framework of the heart consists of the fibrous rings which form a figure-of-eight round the atrioventricular orifices, and which extend round the pulmonary and aortic orifices.
• The red marker is in the right fibrous trigone (12) at the junction of the mitral, tricuspid and aortic orifices; it is continuous below with the membranous part of the interventricular septum, through which the atrioventricular bundle passes.

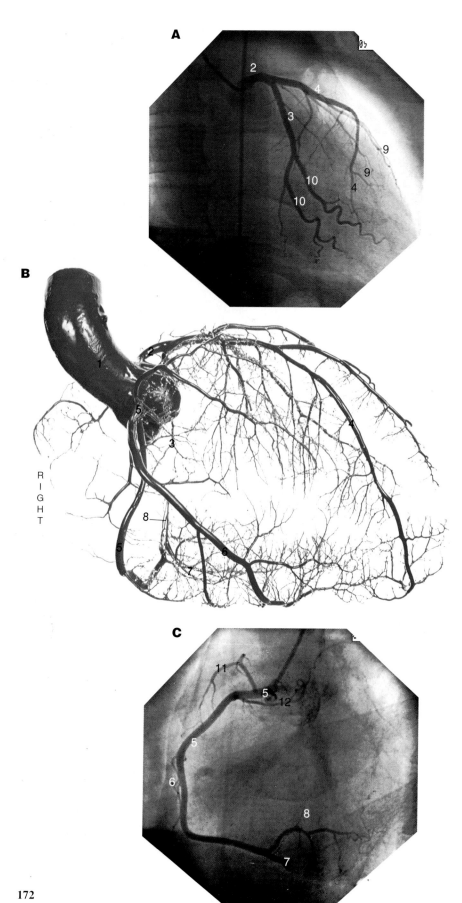

A Left coronary arteriogram, right anterior oblique projection. B Cast of the coronary arteries, from the front. C Right coronary arteriogram, left anterior oblique projection

Compare the cast B with the arteriograms A and C, with the dissection A on page 167, and with the combined dissection and cast A on page 168

1	Ascending aorta
2	Left coronary artery
3	Circumflex } branch of left
4	Anterior interventricular } coronary artery
5	Right coronary artery
6	Marginal } branch of right
7	Posterior interventricular } coronary artery
8	Atrioventricular nodal artery
9	Diagonal artery
10	Obtuse marginal artery
11	Conal artery
12	Sinuatrial nodal artery

• The left coronary artery (B2 and A2) gives off two main branches—the circumflex (B3 and A3) which is really the continuation of the main vessel into the posterior atrioventricular groove, and the anterior interventricular (B4 and A4) which runs down the front of the heart in the interventricular groove. Many other atrial and ventricular vessels are given off from these branches, including septal branches to the interventricular septum, which are the only branches to penetrate deeply into the myocardium, and frequently the sinuatrial nodal artery (see the page opposite).

• The right coronary artery (B5) gives off two main branches—the marginal (B6) which runs along the lower border of the heart but which frequently has a high origin (as on page 168, A11), and the posterior interventricular (B7) which runs in the interventricular groove on the under-surface of the heart. Many other atrial and ventricular vessels are given off from these branches, including the sinuatrial nodal artery (see the page opposite) and septal branches to the interventricular septum, which like their fellows from the anterior interventricular artery penetrate deeply into the septum. One of them is the atrioventricular nodal artery (B8).

• The interventricular branches are often called by clinicians the descending branches (anterior interventricular = left anterior descending; posterior interventricular = posterior descending).

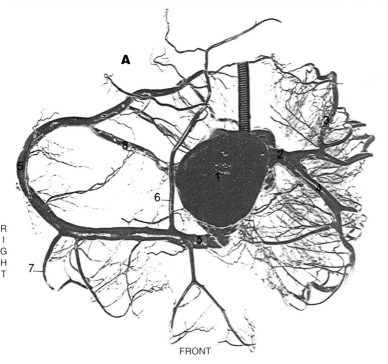

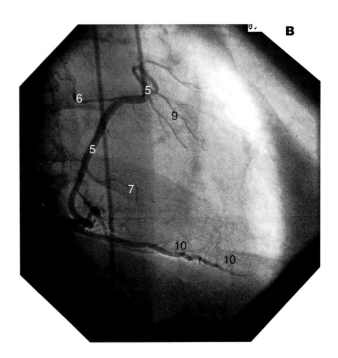

A Cast of the coronary arteries, from above. The sinuatrial nodal artery.
B Right coronary arteriogram, right anterior oblique projection
The largest *atrial* branch of the right coronary artery (5) is the sinuatrial nodal artery (6). See notes below

1	Ascending aorta	7	Marginal branch
2	Left coronary artery	8	Posterior interventricular
3	Circumflex branch		branch
4	Anterior interventricular branch	9	Conal branches
5	Right coronary artery	10	Septal arteries
6	Sinuatrial nodal artery		

C Cast of the coronary arteries, from above
This cast illustrates the origin of the sinuatrial nodal artery (4) from the circumflex branch of the left coronary (3); it passes behind the ascending aorta (1). See notes below

1	Ascending aorta	5	Anterior interventricular branch
2	Left coronary artery		
3	Circumflex branch	6	Right coronary artery
4	Sinuatrial nodal artery	7	Marginal branch

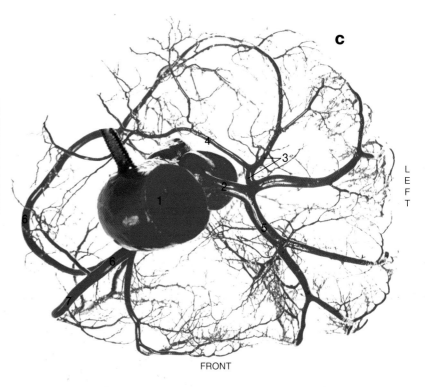

• In about 55 per cent of hearts the sinuatrial nodal artery arises from the right coronary; in 45 per cent it comes from the circumflex branch of the left coronary.
• From either origin the artery penetrates the wall of the right atrium and makes an arterial ring within the atrial wall just below the entry of the superior vena cava. The node is in the front of the atrial wall at the top of the crista terminalis (page 169, C2).

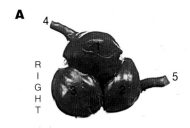

A Cast of the aortic sinuses, from below

The ascending aorta has been filled with resin, so outlining the aortic sinuses (the dilatations above the cusps of the aortic valve), which are seen here as when looking upwards through the aortic valve

1 Right	} aortic sinus	4 Right coronary artery
2 Left		5 Left coronary artery
3 Posterior		

- Strictly speaking, there is only one aortic sinus, with right, left and posterior parts, but the parts are commonly called the right, left and posterior sinuses.
- The aortic and pulmonary valve cusps (and sinuses) are named from their approximate positions in the fetal heart (see the note on page 170), before rotation to their adult positions.
- The right coronary artery (A4) arises from the right aortic sinus (A1) (alternatively named 'anterior').
- The left coronary artery (A5) arises from the left aortic sinus (A2) (alternatively named 'left posterior').

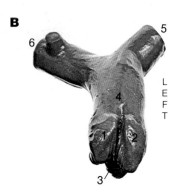

B Cast of the pulmonary trunk and arteries, from the front

As with the aorta shown in A, the filling of the pulmonary trunk (4) with resin has outlined the position of the cusps of the pulmonary valve and sinuses

1 Right	} pulmonary sinus	5 Left pulmonary artery
2 Anterior		6 Right pulmonary artery and branch to
3 Left		superior lobe of right lung
4 Pulmonary trunk		

- Clinicians often call the pulmonary trunk *the* pulmonary artery; strictly it is the pulmonary *trunk* that divides into *right* and *left* pulmonary arteries.

Colour Doppler echocardiographs, C apical long axis – left ventricle, D suprasternal notch view of aortic arch

- This technique enables both anatomy and pathology of blood vessels to be visualized in the living subject without exposure to radiation.

1	Left ventricle
2	Left atrium
3	Mitral valve
4	Ascending aorta
5	Aortic arch
6	Descending aorta
7	Brachiocephalic artery
8	Left common carotid artery
9	Left subclavian artery
10	Site of transducer

- Colour code: red = blood coming towards transducer, blue = away from the transducer

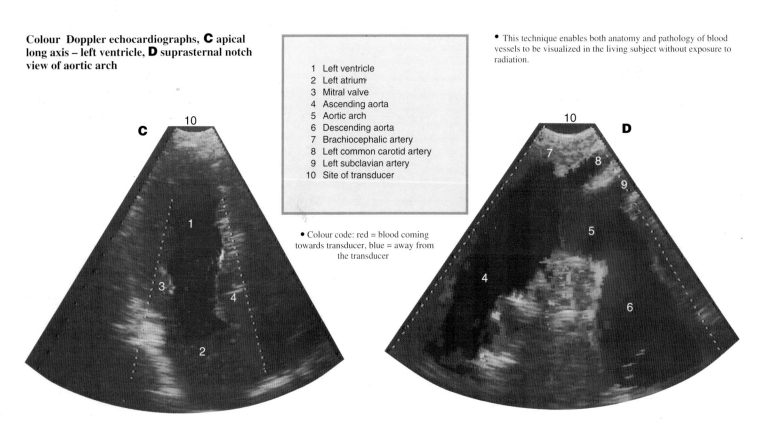

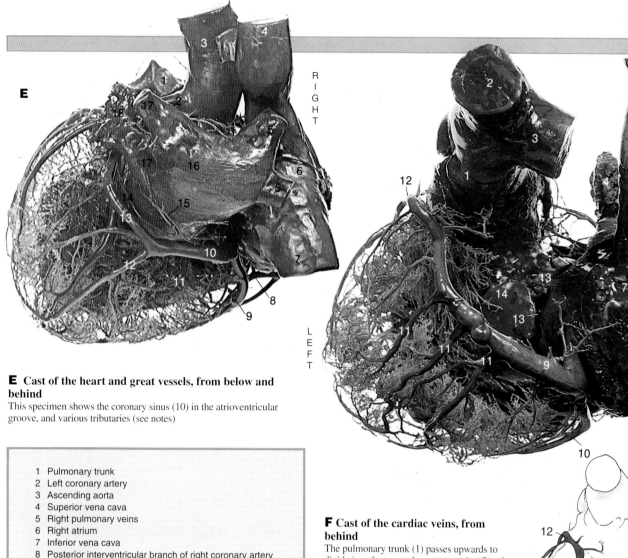

R
I
G
H
T

L
E
F
T

E Cast of the heart and great vessels, from below and behind

This specimen shows the coronary sinus (10) in the atrioventricular groove, and various tributaries (see notes)

1	Pulmonary trunk
2	Left coronary artery
3	Ascending aorta
4	Superior vena cava
5	Right pulmonary veins
6	Right atrium
7	Inferior vena cava
8	Posterior interventricular branch of right coronary artery
9	Middle cardiac vein
10	Coronary sinus
11	Left ventricle
12	Posterior vein of left ventricle
13	Great cardiac vein
14	Circumflex branch of left coronary artery
15	Oblique vein of left atrium
16	Left atrium
17	Left pulmonary veins
18	Auricle of left atrium

F Cast of the cardiac veins, from behind

The pulmonary trunk (1) passes upwards to divide into the two pulmonary arteries (2 and 3). The azygos vein (5) is seen running into the back of the superior vena cava (6) which enters the right atrium (7), with the inferior vena cava (8) entering the atrium from below. Numerous large veins from the left ventricle (11) join the coronary sinus (9) as well as the great (12) and middle (10) cardiac veins seen here

1	Pulmonary trunk	9	Coronary sinus
2	Left pulmonary artery	10	Middle cardiac vein
3	Right pulmonary artery	11	Various veins of left ventricle
4	Auricle of right atrium	12	Great cardiac vein
5	Azygos vein	13	Position of right atrioventricular (tricuspid) valve
6	Superior vena cava	14	Right ventricle
7	Right atrium		
8	Inferior vena cava		

• The *base* of the heart (like the base of the prostate) is its *posterior* surface, formed largely by the left atrium (E16). Note that the base is not the part of the heart which joins the superior vena cava, aorta and pulmonary trunk; this part has no special name.

• The very small oblique vein of the left atrium (E15) marks the point where the great cardiac vein (E13) becomes the coronary sinus (E10), but in E the junction is unusually far to the right so that the posterior vein of the left ventricle (E12) joins the great cardiac vein (E13) instead of the coronary sinus itself.

• The coronary sinus (E10), which receives most of the venous blood from the heart, lies in the posterior part of the atrioventricular groove between the left atrium and left ventricle (page 168, B12), and opens into the right atrium (page 169, C7).

• The coronary sinus normally receives as tributaries the great cardiac vein (E13), middle cardiac vein (E9), and the small cardiac vein, the posterior vein of the left ventricle (E12) and the oblique vein of the left atrium (E15).

• The small cardiac vein frequently drains directly into the right atrium and not into the coronary sinus.

• Like the veins of the brain, the veins of the heart do not usually have the same names as those of the arteries.
• The great cardiac vein accompanies the anterior interventricular and circumflex branches of the left coronary artery.
• The middle cardiac vein accompanies the posterior interventricular branch of the right coronary artery.
• The small cardiac vein accompanies the marginal branch of the right coronary artery.
• The above veins normally all drain into the coronary sinus (see the notes on the left).

A

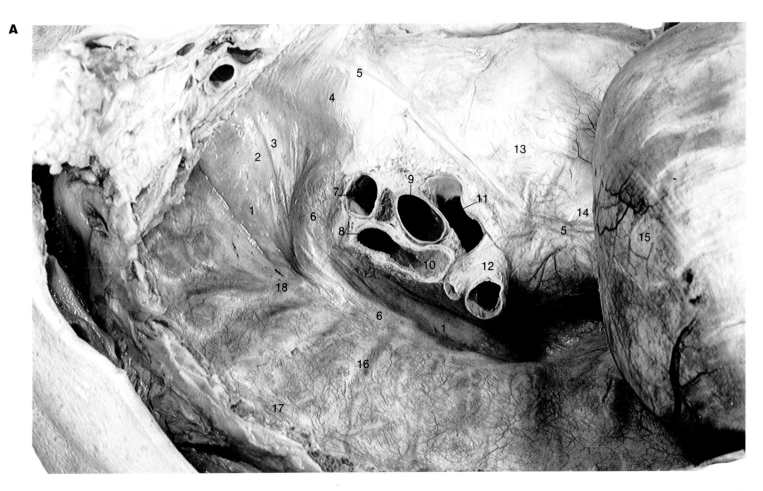

A Right lung root and mediastinal pleura

This is the view of the right side of the mediastinum after removing the lung but with the parietal pleura still intact (with the body lying on its back, head towards the left). Compare the features seen here with those in the dissection opposite (a different specimen), from which the pleura has been removed

1	Oesophagus	10	Right principal bronchus
2	Trachea	11	Right superior pulmonary vein
3	Right vagus nerve	12	Right inferior pulmonary vein
4	Superior vena cava	13	Mediastinal pleura and pericardium
5	Right phrenic nerve and		overlying right atrium
	pericardiacophrenic vessels	14	Inferior vena cava
6	Azygos vein	15	Diaphragm
7	Branch of right pulmonary artery to superior	16	Posterior intercostal vessels under parietal
	lobe		pleura
8	Superior lobe bronchus	17	Sympathetic trunk
9	Right pulmonary artery	18	Right superior intercostal vein

• The right vagus nerve (A3 and B10) passes obliquely downwards and backwards under the mediastinal pleura across the side of the trachea (A2 and B11).
• The right phrenic nerve (A5 and B7) passes downwards under the mediastinal pleura on the side of the superior vena cava (A4 and B8), the pericardium over the right atrium (A13 and B25) and the inferior vena cava (A14 and B26).
• The pleura on the right is in close contact with the side of the trachea (A2) above the arch of the azygos vein (A6), but on the left above the arch of the aorta (page 178) the left common carotid and subclavian arteries intervene between the trachea and pleura.
• The order of the main structures in the right lung root from front to back is: vein, artery, bronchus (A11, 9 and 10, and B19, 18 and 17). The lowest structure is the inferior pulmonary vein (A12 and B20). The highest structures are the branches of the artery and bronchus to the superior lobe (A7 and 8, B15 and 16).

B Right lung root and mediastinum ▷

In a similar specimen to that on the opposite page, most of the pleura has been removed to display the underlying structures seen in A. The azygos vein (13) arches over the structures forming the lung root to enter the superior vena cava (8). The highest structures in the lung root are the artery (15) and bronchus (16) to the superior lobe of the lung. The right superior pulmonary vein (19) is in front of the right pulmonary artery, with the right inferior pulmonary vein (20) the lowest structure in the root. Above the arch of the azygos vein the trachea (11), with the right vagus nerve (10) in contact with it, lies in front of the oesophagus (12). Part of the first rib has been cut away to show the structures lying in front of its neck (5)—the sympathetic trunk (2), supreme intercostal vein (3), superior intercostal artery (4) and the ventral ramus of the first thoracic nerve (6). The right recurrent laryngeal nerve (9) hooks underneath the right subclavian artery (1). The right phrenic nerve (7) runs down over the superior vena cava (8) and the pericardium overlying the right atrium (25), and pierces the diaphragm (27) beside the inferior vena cava (26). Contributions from the sympathetic trunk (23) pass over the sides of vertebral bodies superficial to posterior intercostal arteries and veins (as at 21 and 22) to form the greater splanchnic nerve. The lower part of the oesophagus (12) behind the lung root and heart has the azygos vein (13) on its right side

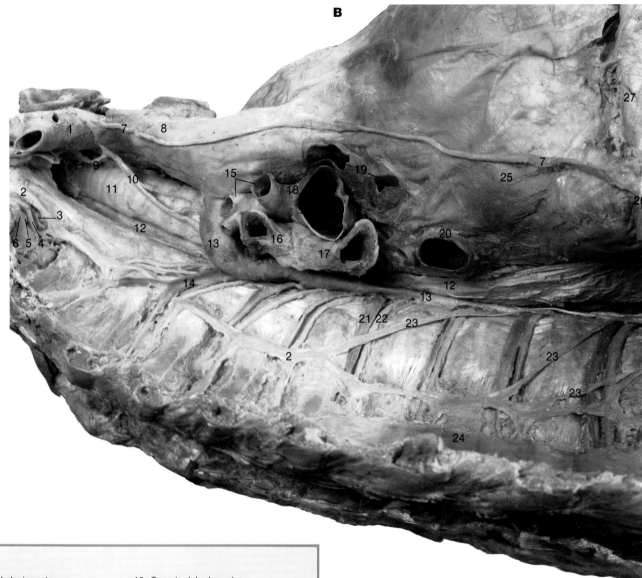

B

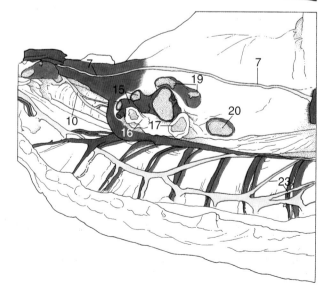

1 Right subclavian artery	16 Superior lobe bronchus
2 Sympathetic trunk and ganglion	17 Right principal bronchus
3 Supreme intercostal vein	18 Right pulmonary artery
4 Superior intercostal artery	19 Right superior pulmonary vein
5 Neck of first rib	20 Right inferior pulmonary vein
6 Ventral ramus of first thoracic nerve	21 Sixth right posterior intercostal vein
7 Right phrenic nerve	22 Sixth right posterior intercostal artery
8 Superior vena cava	23 Branches of sympathetic trunk to greater splanchnic nerve
9 Right recurrent laryngeal nerve	24 Pleura (cut edge)
10 Right vagus nerve	25 Pericardium over right atrium
11 Trachea	26 Inferior vena cava
12 Oesophagus	27 Diaphragm
13 Azygos vein	
14 Superior intercostal vein	
15 Branch of right pulmonary artery to superior lobe	

A

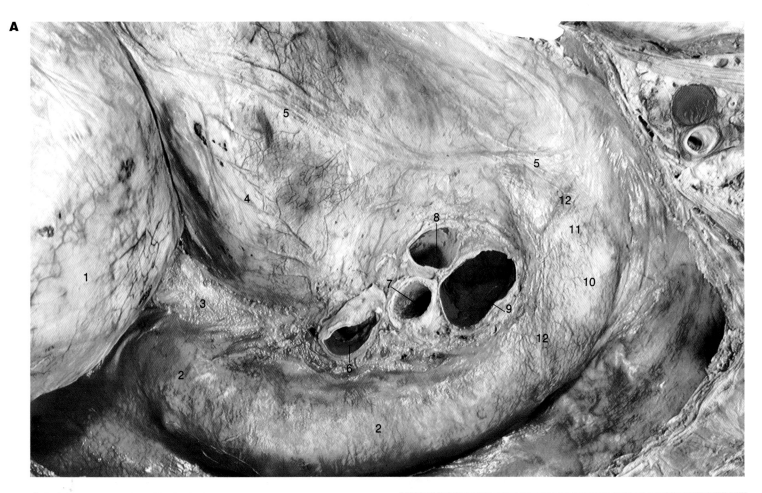

A Left lung root and mediastinal pleura

This is the view of the left side of the mediastinum after removing the lung but with the parietal pleura still intact (with the body lying on its back, head towards the right). Compare the features seen here with those in the dissection opposite (a different specimen), from which the pleura has been removed

1	Diaphragm	6	Left inferior pulmonary vein
2	Thoracic aorta	7	Left principal bronchus
3	Oesophagus	8	Left superior pulmonary vein
4	Mediastinal pleura and pericardium overlying left ventricle	9	Left pulmonary artery
		10	Arch of aorta
5	Left phrenic nerve and pericardiacophrenic vessels	11	Left vagus nerve
		12	Left superior intercostal vein

• The left vagus nerve (A11 and B9) and the left phrenic nerve (A5 and B2) pass downwards over the arch of the aorta (A10 and B10), the phrenic in front of the vagus.

• The left superior intercostal vein (A12 and B11) crosses the upper part of the arch of the aorta transversely, passing over the vagus (B9) and under the phrenic (B2).

• The order of the main structures in the left lung root from front to back is: vein, artery, bronchus (A8, 9 and 7, B4, 6 and 5). The lowest structure is the inferior pulmonary vein (A6 and B3), and the highest structure the pulmonary artery (A9 and B6).

• On the left side above the diaphragm the lower end of the oesophagus lies in a triangle bounded by the diaphragm below (A1), the heart in front (A4 and B1) and the descending aorta behind (A2 and B26).

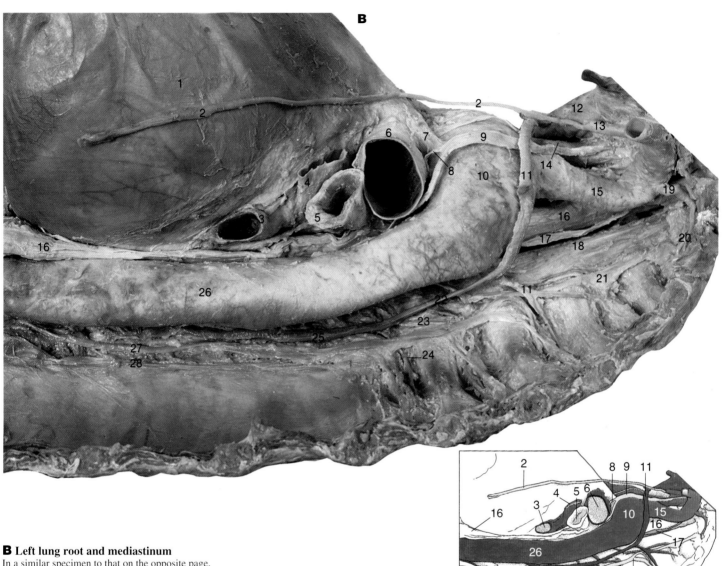

B

B Left lung root and mediastinum

In a similar specimen to that on the opposite page, most of the pleura has been removed to show the underlying structures seen in A. The left vagus nerve (9) crosses the arch of the aorta (10) with the left phrenic nerve (2) anterior to it; the superior intercostal vein (11) runs over the vagus and under the phrenic. The left recurrent laryngeal nerve (8) hooks round the ligamentum arteriosum (7) while the vagus nerve continues behind the structures forming the lung root. The left pulmonary artery (6) is the highest structure in the root, and the inferior pulmonary vein (3) the lowest. The left superior pulmonary vein (4) is in front of the principal bronchus. The thoracic duct (17) is seen behind the left edge of the oesophagus, and the origin of the left superior intercostal artery (20) from the costocervical trunk (19) of the subclavian artery (15) is shown. In this specimen there is an uncommon communication (22) between the left superior intercostal vein (11) and the accessory hemi-azygos vein (25). Above the diaphragm (not shown, having been pushed beyond the edge of the picture with the lower end of the phrenic nerve, 2) the oesophagus (16) bulges towards the left between the heart and pericardium (1) in front and the descending aorta (26) behind

1	Pericardium overlying left ventricle	15	Left subclavian artery
2	Left phrenic nerve	16	Oesophagus
3	Left inferior pulmonary vein	17	Thoracic duct
4	Left superior pulmonary vein	18	Anterior longitudinal ligament
5	Left principal bronchus	19	Costocervical trunk
6	Left pulmonary artery	20	Left superior intercostal artery
7	Ligamentum arteriosum	21	Sympathetic trunk and ganglion
8	Left recurrent laryngeal nerve	22	Communication between 11 and 25
9	Left vagus nerve	23	Fourth left posterior intercostal artery
10	Arch of aorta	24	Fifth left posterior intercostal vein
11	Left superior intercostal vein	25	Accessory hemi-azygos vein
12	Left brachiocephalic vein	26	Thoracic aorta
13	Left internal thoracic artery	27	Hemi-azygos vein
14	Left common carotid artery	28	Pleura (cut edge)

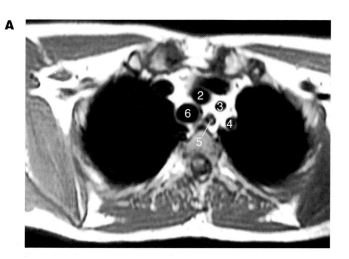

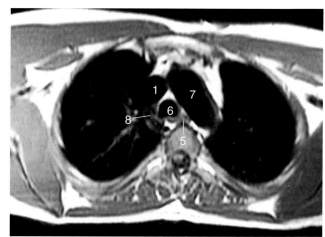

Mediastinum, A and B axial MR images

The section in B is at the level of the arch of the aorta (7), while that in A is higher and shows the three large branches of the arch (2, 3 and 4)

1	Superior vena cava	5	Oesophagus
2	Brachiocephalic trunk	6	Trachea
3	Left common carotid artery	7	Arch of aorta
4	Left subclavian artery	8	Azygos vein

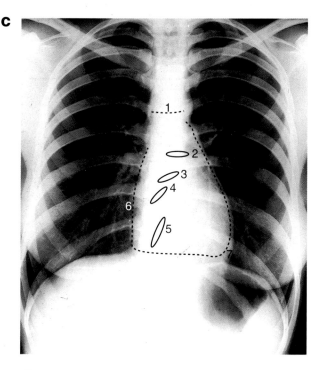

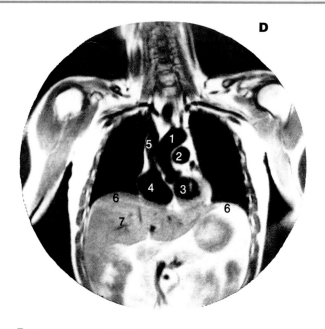

D Thorax, coronal MR image

The section shows the heart and great vessels in the mediastinum, above the domes of the diaphragm (6) and liver (7). The plane of the image is through the left ventricle (3) and right atrium (4)

1	Arch of aorta	5	Superior vena cava
2	Pulmonary trunk	6	Dome of diaphragm
3	Left ventricle	7	Liver
4	Right atrium		

C Chest radiograph

The surface markings of the heart valves are outlined by the dotted lines

1	Site of manubriosternal joint	4	Mitral valve
2	Pulmonary valve	5	Tricuspid valve
3	Aortic valve	6	Right atrium
		7	Apex of heart

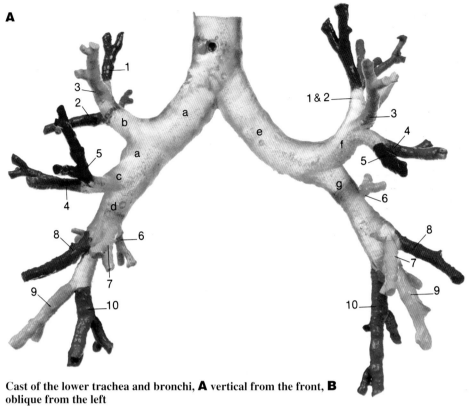

A

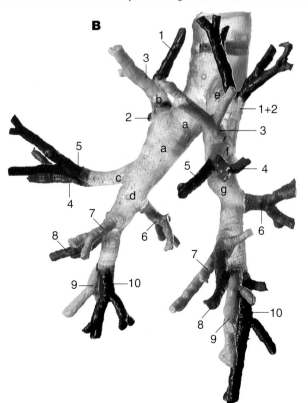

B

Cast of the lower trachea and bronchi, A vertical from the front, B oblique from the left

The main bronchi and lobar bronchi are labelled with letters; the segmental bronchi are labelled with their conventional numbers. In the side view in B the cast has been tilted to avoid overlap, and the right side is more anterior than the left

• The trachea divides into right and left principal bronchi (a and e).

• The right principal bronchus (a) is shorter, wider and more vertical than the left (e).

• The left principal bronchus (e) is longer and narrower and lies more transversely than the right. Foreign bodies are therefore more likely to enter the right principal bronchus than the left.

• The right principal bronchus (a) gives off a superior lobe bronchus (b) and then enters the hilum of the right lung before dividing into middle and inferior lobe bronchi (c and d).

• The left principal bronchus (e) enters the hilum of the lung before dividing into superior and inferior lobe bronchi (f and g).

• The branches of the lobar bronchi are called segmental bronchi and each supplies a segment of lung tissue— bronchopulmonary segment. The segmental bronchi and the bronchopulmonary segments have similar names, and the ten segments of each lung are officially numbered (as here and page 182) as well as being named.

• The segmental bronchi of the left and right lungs are essentially similar except that the apical and posterior bronchi of the superior lobe of the left lung arise from a common stem, thus called the apicoposterior bronchus and labelled here as 1 and 2; also there is no middle lobe of the left lung, and so the corresponding segments bear similar numbers; and the medial basal bronchus (7) of the left lung usually arises in common with the anterior basal (8).

• The apical (superior) bronchus of the inferior lobe (6) of both lungs is the first or highest bronchus to arise from the *posterior* surface of the bronchial tree, as illustrated in B. When lying on the back fluid may therefore gravitate into this bronchus.

RIGHT LUNG	LEFT LUNG
Lobar bronchi	
a Principal	e Principal
b Superior lobe	f Superior lobe
c Middle lobe	g Inferior lobe
d Inferior lobe	
Segmental bronchi	
Superior lobe	**Superior lobe**
1 Apical	1 & 2 Apicoposterior
2 Posterior	3 Anterior
3 Anterior	4 Superior lingular
	5 Inferior lingular
Middle lobe	
4 Lateral	
5 Medial	
	Inferior lobe
	6 Apical (superior)
Inferior lobe	7 Medial basal (cardiac)
6 Apical (superior)	8 Anterior basal
7 Medial basal	9 Lateral basal
8 Anterior basal	10 Posterior basal
9 Lateral basal	
10 Posterior basal	

Cast of the bronchial tree

The bronchi and bronchopulmonary segments have been coloured and labelled with their conventional numbers

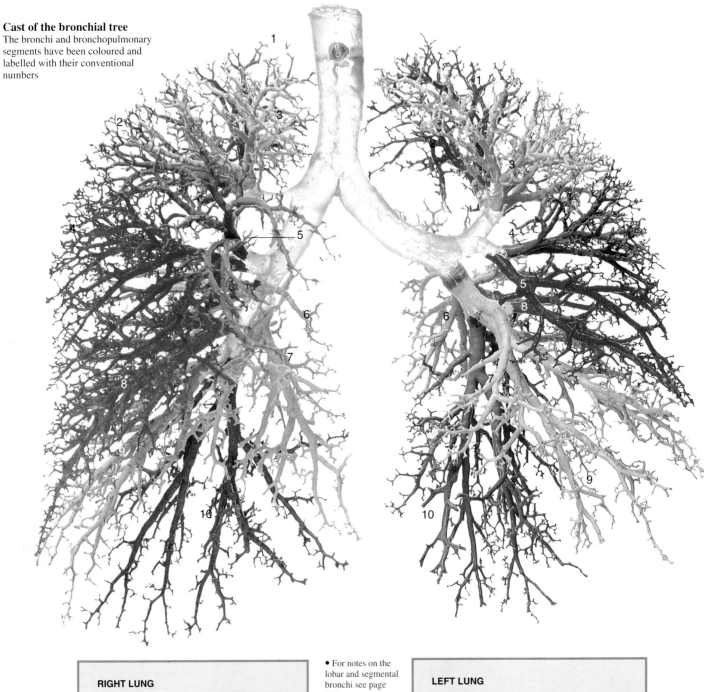

● For notes on the lobar and segmental bronchi see page 181.

RIGHT LUNG

Superior lobe	Inferior lobe
1 Apical	6 Apical (superior)
2 Posterior	7 Medial basal
3 Anterior	8 Anterior basal
	9 Lateral basal
Middle lobe	10 Posterior basal
4 Lateral	
5 Medial	

LEFT LUNG

Superior lobe	Inferior lobe
1 Apical	6 Apical (superior)
2 Posterior	7 Medial basal
3 Anterior	(cardiac)
4 Superior lingular	8 Anterior basal
5 Inferior lingular	9 Lateral basal
	10 Posterior basal

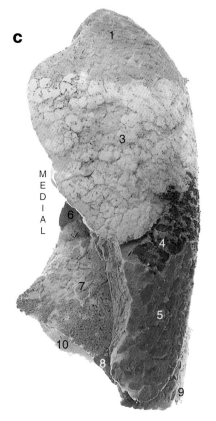

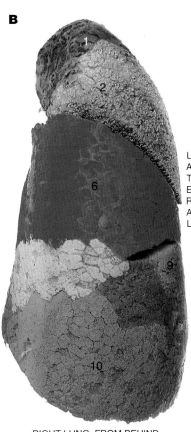

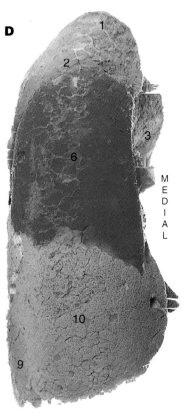

A

L
A
T
E
R
A
L

RIGHT LUNG, FROM THE FRONT

B

L
A
T
E
R
A
L

RIGHT LUNG, FROM BEHIND

C

M
E
D
I
A
L

LEFT LUNG, FROM THE FRONT

D

M
E
D
I
A
L

LEFT LUNG, FROM BEHIND

Bronchopulmonary segments of the right lung, A from the front, B from behind

Superior lobe
1 Apical
2 Posterior
3 Anterior

Middle lobe
4 Lateral
5 Medial

Inferior lobe
6 Apical (superior)
7 Medial basal
8 Anterior basal
9 Lateral basal
10 Posterior basal

• A subapical (subsuperior) segmental bronchus and bronchopulmonary segment are present in over 50 per cent of lungs; in this specimen this additional segment is shown in white.
• The posterior basal segment (10) is coloured with two different shades of green.

Bronchopulmonary segments of the left lung, C from the front, D from behind

Superior lobe
1 Apical
2 Posterior
3 Anterior
4 Superior lingular
5 Inferior lingular

Inferior lobe
6 Apical (superior)
7 Medial basal (cardiac)
8 Anterior basal
9 Lateral basal
10 Posterior basal

• The apical and posterior segments (1 and 2) are both coloured green, having been filled from the common apicoposterior bronchus (see page 181).

A Bronchopulmonary segments of the right lung, from the lateral side, **B** Right bronchogram

Superior lobe
1 Apical
2 Posterior
3 Anterior

Middle lobe
4 Lateral
5 Medial

Inferior lobe
6 Apical (superior)
7 Medial basal
8 Anterior basal
9 Lateral basal
10 Posterior basal

A

LATERAL

RIGHT LUNG

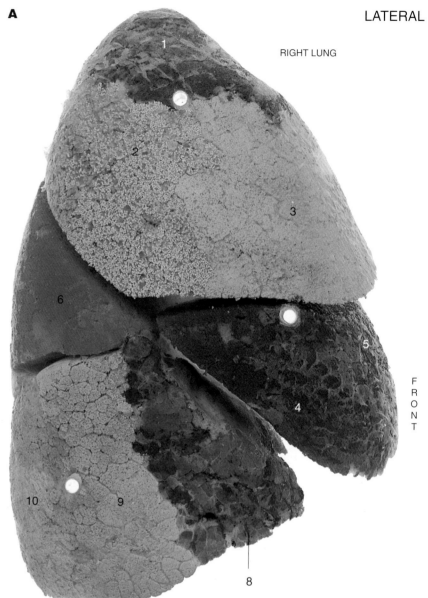

FRONT

• The medial basal segment (7) is not seen in the view in A.
• The posterior basal segment in A (10) is coloured with two different shades of green.

B

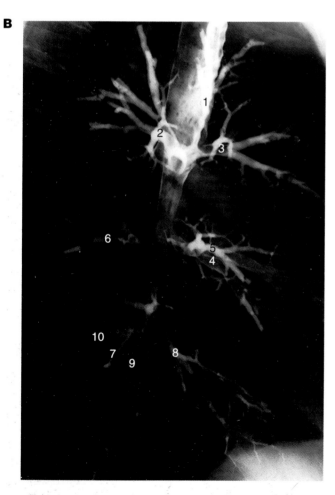

VIEWS

LEFT LUNG

C

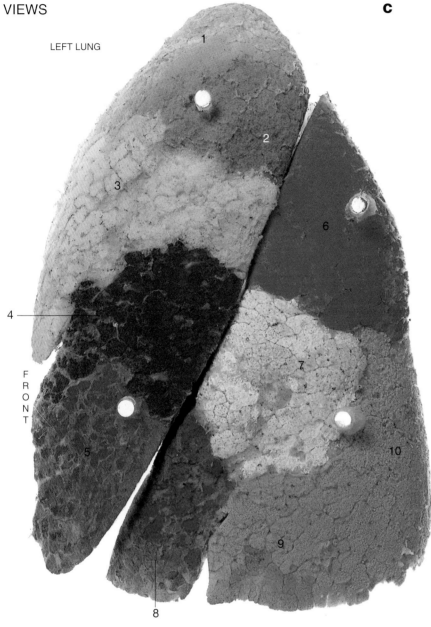

F
R
O
N
T

C Bronchopulmonary segments of the left lung, from the lateral side, **D** Left bronchogram

Superior lobe
1 Apical
2 Posterior
3 Anterior
4 Superior lingular
5 Inferior lingular

Inferior lobe
6 Apical (superior)
7 Medial basal (cardiac)
8 Anterior basal
9 Lateral basal
10 Posterior basal

D

• The apical and posterior segments (1 and 2) are both coloured green, having been filled from the common apicoposterior bronchus (see page 181).
• The medial basal segment (7) is not seen in this view.
• See note on page 183 for the white segment.

A

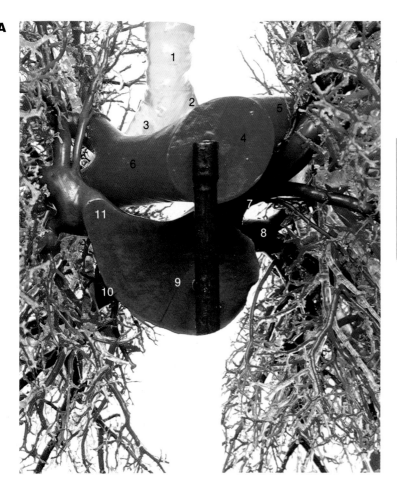

A Cast of the bronchial tree and pulmonary vessels, from the front

The pulmonary trunk (4) divides into the left and right pulmonary arteries (5 and 6), and these vessels have been injected with red resin. The four pulmonary veins (7, 8, 10 and 11) which drain into the left atrium (9) have been filled with blue resin. Note that in the living body the pulmonary veins are filled with oxygenated blood from the lungs and would normally be represented by a red colour; similarly the pulmonary arteries contain deoxygenated blood and should be represented by a blue colour

1	Trachea	7	Superior } left pulmonary
2	Left } principal	8	Inferior } vein
3	Right } bronchus	9	Left atrium
4	Pulmonary trunk	10	Inferior } right pulmonary
5	Left } pulmonary	11	Superior } vein
6	Right } artery		

C Cast of the pulmonary arteries and bronchi, from the front, **D** ▷
Pulmonary arteriogram

The upper part of the pulmonary trunk (5) is seen end-on after cutting off the lower part, and the bifurcation of the trunk into the left (6) and right (10) pulmonary arteries is in front of the beginning of the left main bronchus (7). In the living body these pulmonary vessels contain deoxygenated blood and would normally be represented by a blue colour, but here they have been filled with red resin. Compare the vessels in the cast with those in the arteriogram D

1	Branch of right pulmonary artery to superior lobe	7	Left principal bronchus
		8	Superior lobe bronchus
2	Superior lobe bronchus	9	Inferior lobe bronchus
3	Right principal bronchus	10	Right pulmonary artery
4	Trachea	11	Middle lobe bronchus
5	Pulmonary trunk	12	Inferior lobe bronchus
6	Left pulmonary artery		

FRONT

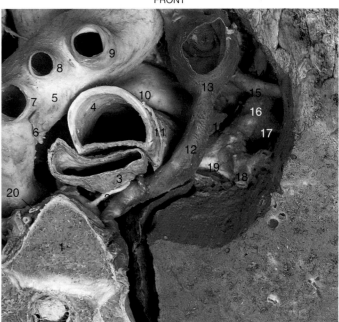

B Lung roots and bronchial arteries, right side from above

In B the thorax has been sectioned transversely at the level of the third thoracic vertebra (1), just above the arch of the aorta (5) whose three larger branches have been removed (7, 8 and 9), and lung tissue at the hilum has been dissected away from above. The oesophagus (3) and trachea (4) have been tilted forwards to show one of the bronchial arteries (2)

1	Third thoracic vertebra	12	Azygos vein
2	Right bronchial artery	13	Superior vena cava
3	Oesophagus	14	Inferior lobe artery
4	Trachea	15	Tributary of inferior pulmonary vein
5	Arch of aorta		
6	Left recurrent laryngeal nerve	16	Inferior lobe bronchus
7	Left subclavian artery	17	Middle lobe bronchus
8	Left common carotid artery	18	Superior lobe bronchus
9	Brachiocephalic trunk	19	Right principal bronchus
10	Right pulmonary artery	20	Thoracic duct
11	Right vagus nerve		

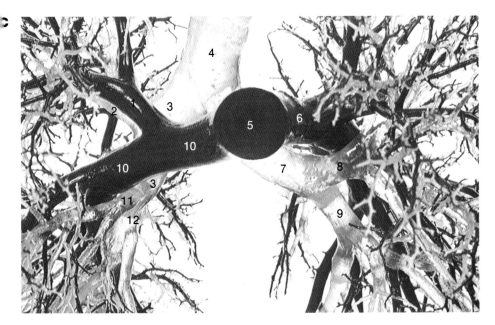

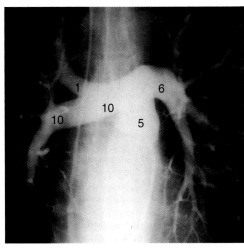

E Cast of the bronchi and bronchial arteries, from the front

Part of the aorta (4 and 5) has been injected with red resin to fill the bronchial arteries. These vessels normally run behind the bronchi and their branches but in this specimen they are in front

1	Trachea
2	Left principal bronchus
3	Right principal bronchus
4	Arch of aorta
5	Thoracic aorta
6	Origin of upper left bronchial artery
7	Origin of lower left bronchial artery
8	Origin of right bronchial artery
9	Superior lobe bronchus
10	Inferior lobe bronchus
11	Superior lobe bronchus
12	Middle lobe bronchus
13	Inferior lobe bronchus

• Compare the order of the main structures in the lung roots and casts on these two pages with the mediastinal dissections on pages 176 and 178. Note for example the order vein, artery, bronchus from front to back in the cast of the right lung root (A11, 6 and 3).
• The left pulmonary artery (C6) hooks over the left principal bronchus (C7) and descends behind the lobar bronchi.
• The right pulmonary artery (C10) passes below the bifurcation of the trachea (C4) and hooks over the right principal bronchus (C3), but its branch to the superior lobe (C1) remains in front of the superior lobe bronchus (C2).
• The pulmonary trunk (C5) divides into the two pulmonary arteries in front of the left principal bronchus (C7).
• There are usually two left bronchial arteries (from the aorta) and one right bronchial artery (from the third right posterior intercostal or upper left bronchial artery; B2). The cast E is unusual in that the vessels run in front of the bronchi rather than behind them, and the upper left artery (E6) arises from the right bronchial artery (E8).

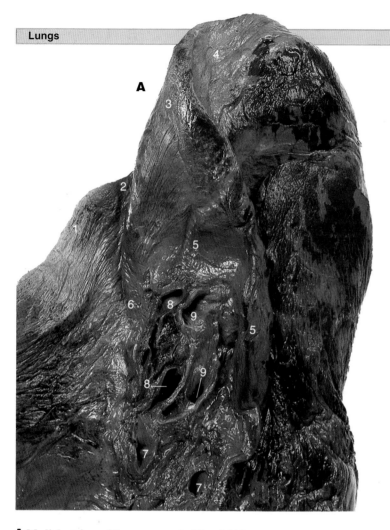

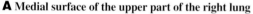

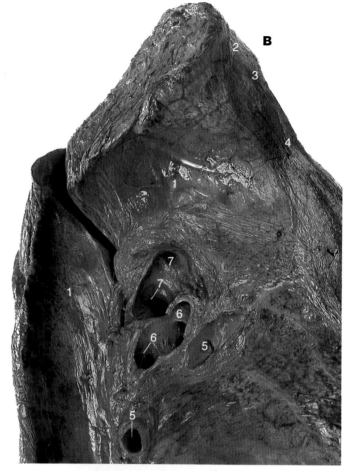

A Medial surface of the upper part of the right lung

In the hardened dissecting room specimen, adjacent structures make impressions on the medial surface of the lung. The most prominent feature on the right side is the groove for the azygos vein (5), above and behind the structures of the lung root (7 to 9)

1 Groove for first rib	6 Groove for superior vena cava
2 Groove for subclavian vein	7 Right pulmonary veins
3 Groove for subclavian artery	8 Branches of right pulmonary
4 Oesophageal and tracheal	artery
area	9 Branches of right principal
5 Groove for azygos vein	bronchus

• The upper end of the medial surface of the right lung lies against the the oesophagus and trachea (A4) with only the pleura intervening, but on the left the subclavian artery (B2) (and the left common carotid in front of it) keep the lung further away from these structures.

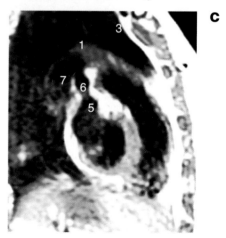

Left lung, B medial surface of the upper part , C hilum, sagittal MR image

Compare with the right lung in A, and note the large size of the impression made by the aorta on the left lung (B1), in contrast to the smaller azygos groove on the right (A5). The MR image shows the main structures in the hilum (5, 6 and 7)

1 Groove for aorta	6 Branches of left principal
2 Groove for left subclavian artery	bronchus
3 Groove for left subclavian and	7 Branches of left pulmonary
brachiocephalic vein	artery
4 Groove for first rib	
5 Left pulmonary veins	

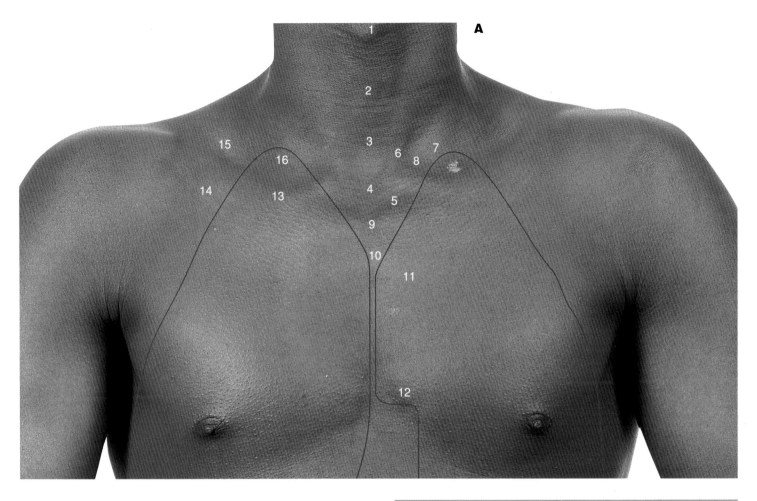

A

A Lower neck and upper thorax. Surface markings

The magenta line indicates the extent of the pleura and lung on each side; the apices of the pleura and lung (16) rise into the neck for about 3 cm above the medial third of the clavicle. The lower end of the internal jugular vein (8) lies behind the interval between the sternal (6) and clavicular (7) heads of sternocleidomastoid. Behind the sternoclavicular joint (5) the internal jugular and subclavian veins unite to form the brachiocephalic vein. The trachea (3) is felt in the midline above the jugular notch (4), and the arch of the cricoid cartilage (2) is 4 to 5 cm below the notch. The joint is at the level of the second costal cartilage (11) and opposite the lower border of the body of the fourth thoracic vertebra, and the horizontal plane through these points indicates the junction between the superior and inferior parts of the mediastinum. The left brachiocephalic vein passes behind the upper half of the manubrium to unite with the right brachiocephalic at the lower border of the right first costal cartilage (to form the superior vena cava. The midpoint of the manubrium (9) marks the highest level of the arch of the aorta and the origin of the brachiocephalic trunk. Compare many of the features mentioned here with the structures in dissections B and C on pages 190 and 191 respectively

1 Laryngeal prominence
2 Cricoid cartilage
3 Isthmus of thyroid gland overlying trachea
4 Jugular notch
5 Sternoclavicular joint
6 Sternal head ⎱ of sternocleidomastoid
7 Clavicular head ⎰
8 Internal jugular vein
9 Midpoint of manubrium of sternum
10 Manubriosternal joint
11 Second costal cartilage
12 Fourth costal cartilage
13 Clavicle
14 Infraclavicular fossa
15 Supraclavicular fossa
16 Apex of pleura and lung

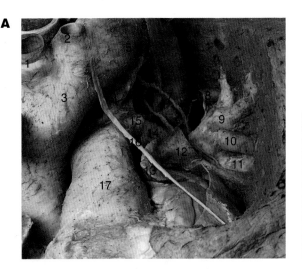

A Lung roots and bronchial arteries, left side from the front

Lung tissue has been removed from the region of the left hilum and the lung root structures are seen from the front, including a left bronchial artery (7) which ran behind the principal bronchus (14) with a branch passing on to the front of the bronchus

1	Brachiocephalic trunk	9	Superior lobe bronchus
2	Left common carotid artery	10	Inferior lobe artery
3	Arch of aorta	11	Inferior lobe bronchus
4	Ligamentum arteriosum	12	Inferior pulmonary vein
5	Left recurrent laryngeal nerve	13	Auricle of left atrium
6	Left vagus nerve	14	Left principal bronchus
7	A left bronchial artery	15	Left pulmonary artery
8	Superior lobe artery	16	Left phrenic nerve
		17	Pulmonary trunk

• For notes on the position of the main structures in the lung roots see pages 176 and 178.

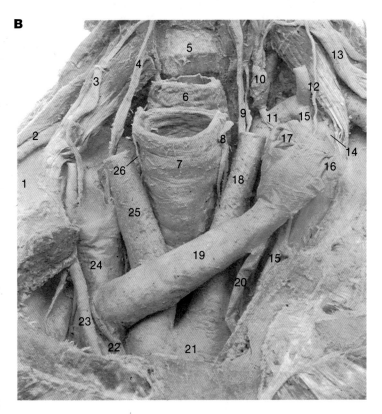

B Thoracic inlet, from the front

The manubrium and the first right costal cartilage have been removed to show the left brachiocephalic vein (19) crossing in front of the left common carotid artery (18) and the brachiocephalic trunk (25)

1	First rib	13	Upper trunk of brachial plexus
2	Lowest roots of brachial plexus	14	Apex of lung
3	Right phrenic nerve and scalenus anterior	15	Left internal thoracic artery
4	Right vagus nerve	16	Left subclavian vein
5	Cervical vertebral column	17	Left internal jugular vein
6	Oesophagus	18	Left common carotid artery
7	Trachea	19	Left brachiocephalic vein
8	Left recurrent laryngeal nerve	20	Left internal thoracic vein
9	Left vagus nerve	21	Arch of aorta
10	Middle cervical sympathetic ganglion	22	Superior vena cava
11	Ansa subclavia and left subclavian artery	23	Right internal thoracic artery
12	Left thyrocervical trunk, phrenic nerve and scalenus anterior	24	Right brachiocephalic vein
		25	Brachiocephalic trunk
		26	Right recurrent laryngeal nerve

C Thoracic inlet and mediastinum, from the front

The anterior thoracic wall and the medial ends of the clavicles have been removed, but part of the parietal pleura (14) remains over the medial part of each lung. The right internal jugular vein has also been removed, displaying the thyrocervical trunk (29) and the origin of the internal thoracic artery (12). Inferior thyroid veins (5) run down over the trachea (4) to enter the left brachiocephalic vein (15). The thymus (18) has been dissected out from mediastinal fat; thymic veins (17) enter the left brachiocephalic vein, and an unusual thymic artery (16) arises from the brachiocephalic trunk (22)

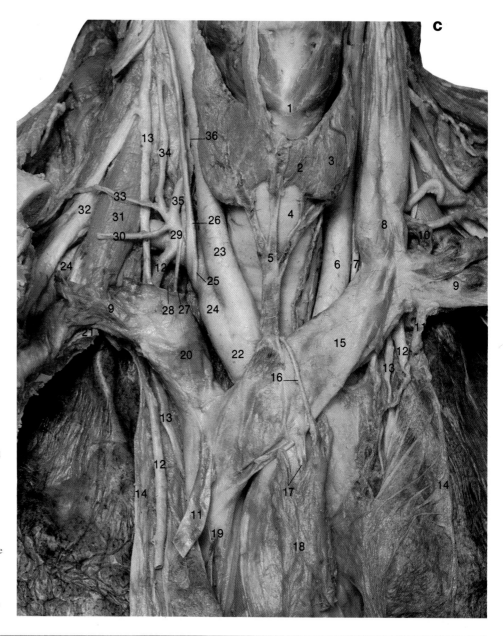

• The internal jugular (8) and subclavian (9) veins unite behind the sternoclavicular joint to form the brachiocephalic vein (left, 15, and right, 20).

• The left and right brachiocephalic veins (15 and 20) unite at the lower border of the right first costal cartilage to form the superior vena cava (19).

• The brachiocephalic trunk (22) divides into the right subclavian and common carotid arteries (24 and 23). (The left subclavian and common carotid arteries, like the brachiocephalic trunk, are direct branches from the arch of the aorta.)

• At its attachment to the first rib (21), scalenus anterior (31) has the subclavian vein (9) in front and the subclavian artery (24) behind but at a higher level, due to the obliquity of the rib.

• The remains of the thymus (18) are in front of the pericardium, but in the child, where the thymus is much larger, it may extend upwards in front of the great vessels as high as the lower part of the thyroid gland (3).

1 Arch of cricoid cartilage	13 Phrenic nerve	25 Right recurrent laryngeal nerve
2 Isthmus ⎫ of thyroid	14 Parietal pleura (cut edge) over lung	26 Right vagus nerve
3 Lateral lobe ⎭ gland	15 Left brachiocephalic vein	27 Unusual cervical tributary of 20
4 Trachea	16 A thymic artery	28 Vertebral vein
5 Inferior thyroid veins	17 Thymic veins	29 Thyrocervical trunk
6 Left common carotid artery	18 Thymus	30 Suprascapular artery
7 Left vagus nerve	19 Superior vena cava	31 Scalenus anterior
8 Internal jugular vein	20 Right brachiocephalic vein	32 Upper trunk of brachial plexus
9 Subclavian vein	21 First rib	33 Superficial cervical artery
10 Thoracic duct	22 Brachiocephalic trunk	34 Ascending cervical artery
11 Internal thoracic vein	23 Right common carotid artery	35 Inferior thyroid artery
12 Internal thoracic artery	24 Right subclavian artery	36 Sympathetic trunk

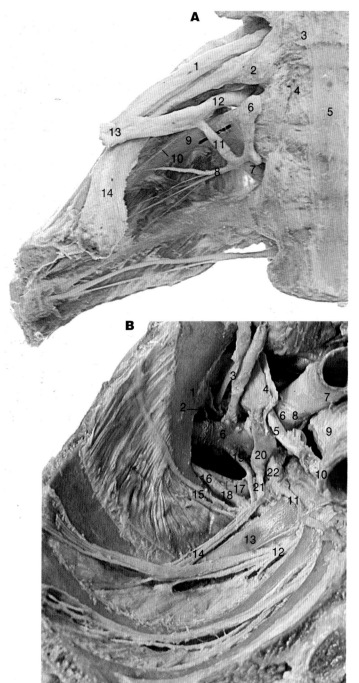

A Thoracic inlet. Right upper ribs, from the front

This dissection shows the nerves related to the first and second ribs. The ventral ramus of the first thoracic nerve (12) is joined by the ventral ramus of the eighth cervical nerve (1) to form the lower trunk of the brachial plexus (13). In this specimen there is a large communication (11) between the second and first nerves

1 Ventral ramus of eighth cervical nerve	8 Second intercostal nerve
2 Head of first rib	9 Second rib
3 Seventh cervical vertebra	10 First intercostal nerve
4 First thoracic vertebra	11 Communication with first thoracic nerve
5 Anterior longitudinal ligament	12 Ventral ramus of first thoracic nerve
6 Sympathetic trunk and ganglion	13 Lower trunk of brachial plexus
7 Ventral ramus of second thoracic nerve	14 First rib

B Thoracic inlet. Right upper ribs, from below

This is the view looking upwards into the right side of the thoracic inlet—the region occupied by the cervical pleura, here removed. The under-surface of most of the first rib (1) is seen from below, with the subclavian artery (6) passing over the top of it after giving off the internal thoracic branch (3) which runs towards the top of the picture (to the anterior thoracic wall), and the costocervical trunk whose superior intercostal branch (19) runs down over the neck of the first rib (17). The vertebral vein (20) has come down from the neck and is labelled on its posterior surface before entering the brachiocephalic vein (4, labelled at its opened cut edge). The vertebral vein receives an unusually large supreme intercostal vein (21). On its medial side is the sympathetic trunk (11) with the cervicothoracic ganglion (22). The neck of the first rib (17) has the ventral ramus of the first thoracic nerve (16) below it

1 First rib	14 Superior intercostal vein
2 Subclavian vein	15 First intercostal nerve
3 Internal thoracic vessels	16 Ventral ramus of first thoracic nerve
4 Brachiocephalic vein	17 Neck of first rib
5 Vagus nerve	18 Ventral ramus of eighth cervical nerve
6 Subclavian artery	19 Superior intercostal artery
7 Brachiocephalic trunk	20 Vertebral vein
8 Recurrent laryngeal nerve	21 Supreme intercostal vein (unusually large)
9 Trachea	22 Cervicothoracic (stellate) ganglion
10 Right principal bronchus	
11 Sympathetic trunk	
12 Second intercostal nerve	
13 Second rib	

• The neck of the first rib (17) is crossed in order from medial to lateral by the sympathetic trunk (11), supreme intercostal vein (21), superior intercostal artery (19) and the ventral ramus of the first thoracic nerve (16).

C Thoracic duct, thoracic part

All viscera and part of the pleura have been removed to show the aorta (4 and 9) in front of the vertebral column and viewed from the right, with the thoracic duct (3) lying between the aorta (4) and azygos vein (2); the lower part of the vein was overlying the duct and has been removed. The cisterna chyli (10), where the thoracic duct begins, is in the abdomen under cover of the right crus of the diaphragm (5)

1 Sympathetic trunk underlying pleura	9 Abdominal aorta
2 Azygos vein	10 Cisterna chyli
3 Thoracic duct	11 Greater splanchnic nerve
4 Thoracic aorta	12 Medial arcuate ligament
5 Right crus of diaphragm	13 Psoas major
6 Coeliac trunk	14 Diaphragm
7 Superior mesenteric artery	15 First lumbar artery and first lumbar vertebra
8 Right renal artery	16 Twelfth thoracic vertebra and subcostal artery

C

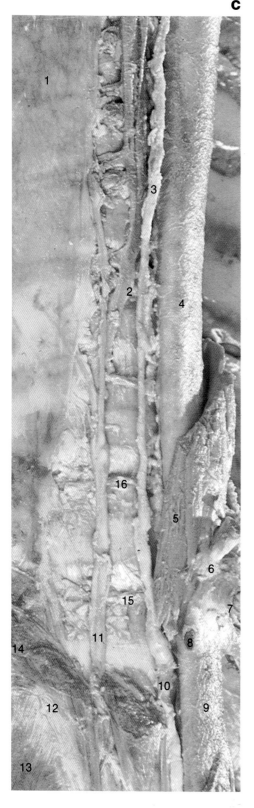

D

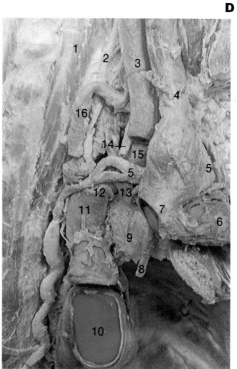

E

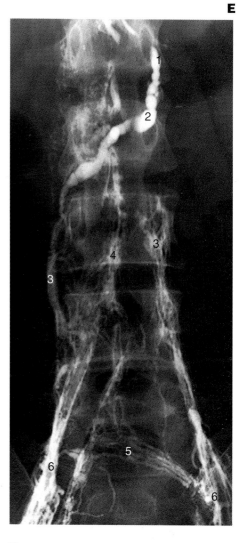

D Thoracic duct, cervical part

In this deep dissection of the left side of the root of the neck and upper thorax, the internal jugular vein (4) joins the subclavian vein (6) to form the left brachiocephalic vein (7). The thoracic duct (5) is double for a short distance just before passing in front of the vertebral artery (15) and behind the common carotid artery (3, whose lower end has been cut away to show the duct). The duct then runs behind the internal jugular vein (4) before draining into the junction of that vein with the subclavian vein (6)

1	Longus colli
2	Sympathetic trunk
3	Common carotid artery
4	Internal jugular vein
5	Thoracic duct
6	Subclavian vein
7	Brachiocephalic vein
8	Phrenic nerve
9	Pleura
10	Arch of aorta
11	Subclavian artery
12	Ansa subclavia
13	Internal thoracic artery
14	Vagus nerve
15	Origin of vertebral artery
16	Inferior thyroid artery

E First day lymphangiogram

1	Thoracic duct
2	Cysterna chyli
3	Para-aortic vessels
4	Pre-aortic vessels
5	Lumbar crossover
6	Common iliac vessels

• The cisterna chyli is usually on the right side, not on the left as here (E2).

• From the cisterna chyli (C10), situated under cover of the left margin of the right crus of the diaphragm (C5) at the level of the first and second lumbar vertebrae, the thoracic duct passes upwards (through the aortic opening in the diaphragm) on the right side of the front of the thoracic vertebral column between the aorta (C4) and azygos vein (C2), crossing to the left at the level of the fifth to sixth thoracic vertebra and ending by opening into the left side of the union of the left internal jugular (D4) and subclavian (D6) veins after passing between the common carotid artery (in front, D3) and the vertebral artery (behind, D15).

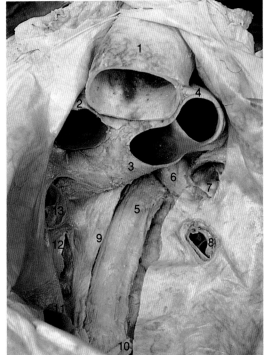

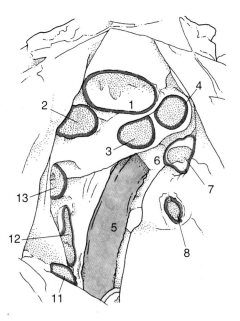

A Oesophagus, lower thoracic part, from the front

The heart has been removed from the pericardial cavity by transecting the great vessels, the pulmonary trunk being cut at the point where it divides into the two pulmonary arteries (3 and 4). Part of the pericardium (9) at the back has been removed to reveal the oesophagus (5). It is seen below the left principal bronchus (6) and is being crossed by the beginning of the right pulmonary artery (3)

1	Ascending aorta
2	Superior vena cava
3	Right pulmonary artery
4	Left pulmonary artery
5	Oesophagus
6	Left principal bronchus
7	Left superior pulmonary vein
8	Left inferior pulmonary vein
9	Pericardium (cut edge)
10	Anterior vagal trunk
11	Inferior vena cava
12	Right inferior pulmonary vein
13	Right superior pulmonary vein

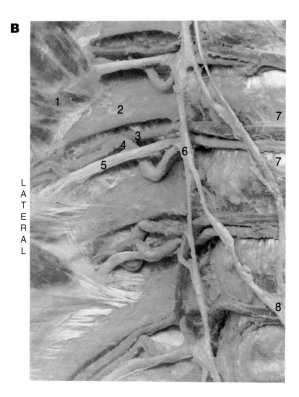

B Intercostal spaces

This dissection shows the medial ends of some intercostal spaces of the right side, viewed from the front and slightly from the right. The pleura has been removed, revealing subcostal muscles (1) laterally, the nerves and vessels (3, 4 and 5) in the intercostal spaces, and the sympathetic trunk (6) and greater splanchnic nerve (8) on the sides of the vertebral bodies (as at 7)

1	Subcostal muscle	5	Eighth intercostal nerve
2	Eighth rib	6	Sympathetic trunk and ganglia
3	Eighth posterior intercostal vein	7	Body of ninth thoracic vertebra
4	Eighth posterior intercostal artery	8	Greater splanchnic nerve

● In the medial part of an intercostal space near the vertebral column, the neurovascular structures lie in the middle of the space; only farther laterally do they take up their positions in the upper part of the space below the costal groove (as shown on page 164, A and B).

C Joints of the heads of the ribs, from the right

In this part of the right mid-thoracic region, the ribs have been cut short beyond their tubercles, and the joints that the two facets of the head of a rib make with the facets on the sides of adjacent vertebral bodies and the intervening disc are shown, as at 6 to 8, where the radiate ligament (6) covers the capsule of these small synovial joints

1	Neck of rib
2	Superior costotransverse ligament
3	Ventral ramus of spinal nerve
4	Rami communicantes
5	Sympathetic trunk
6	Radiate ligament of joint of head of rib
7	Vertebral body
8	Intervertebral disc
9	Greater splanchnic nerve

D Costotransverse joints, from behind

In this view of the right half of the thoracic vertebral column from behind, costotransverse joints between the transverse processes of vertebrae and the tubercles of ribs are covered by the lateral costotransverse ligaments (as at 5). The dorsal rami of spinal nerves (8) pass medial to the superior costotransverse ligaments (4); ventral rami (7) run in front of these ligaments

1	Spinous process	
2	Lamina	
3	Transverse process	
4	Superior	costotransverse
5	Lateral	ligament
6	Costotransverse ligament	
7	Ventral	ramus of
8	Dorsal	spinal nerve

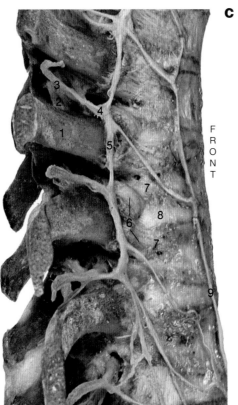

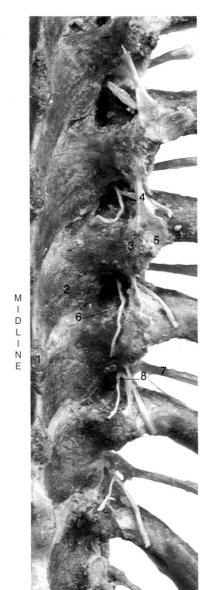

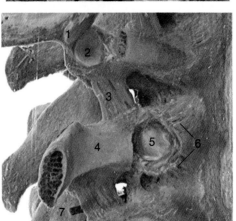

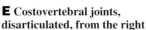

- There are two types of costovertebral joint—the joints of the heads of the ribs (C and E) with the facets on the vertebral bodies, and the costotransverse joints (D and E) between the articular facets on the tubercles of the ribs and the facets on the transverse processes.
- There are three kinds of costotransverse ligament: *the* costotransverse ligament (D6) between the back of the neck of a rib and the front of the corresponding transverse process; the *lateral* costotransverse ligament (D5), between the tip of a transverse process and the non-articular part of the tubercle of the corresponding rib; and the *superior* costotransverse ligament (D4 and E7), having anterior and posterior layers and passing from the (upper) crest of the neck of a rib to the transverse process of the vertebra above.
- The dorsal rami of spinal nerves pass backwards *medial* to the superior costotransverse ligaments (D8), dividing into medial and lateral branches.
- The ventral rami of spinal nerves (D7) pass laterally *in front of* the superior costotransverse ligaments.

E Costovertebral joints, disarticulated, from the right

In the upper part of the figure, the upper rib has been severed through its neck (4) and the part with the tubercle attached has been turned upwards after cutting through the capsule of the costotransverse joint, to show the articular facet of the tubercle (1) and the transverse process (2). The head of the lower rib has been removed after transecting the radiate ligament (6) and underlying capsule of the joint of the head of the rib (5)

1	Articular facet of tubercle of rib
2	Articular facet of transverse process
3	Superior costotransverse ligament
4	Neck of rib
5	Cavity of joint of head of rib
6	Radiate ligament
7	Marker between anterior and posterior parts of superior costotransverse ligament

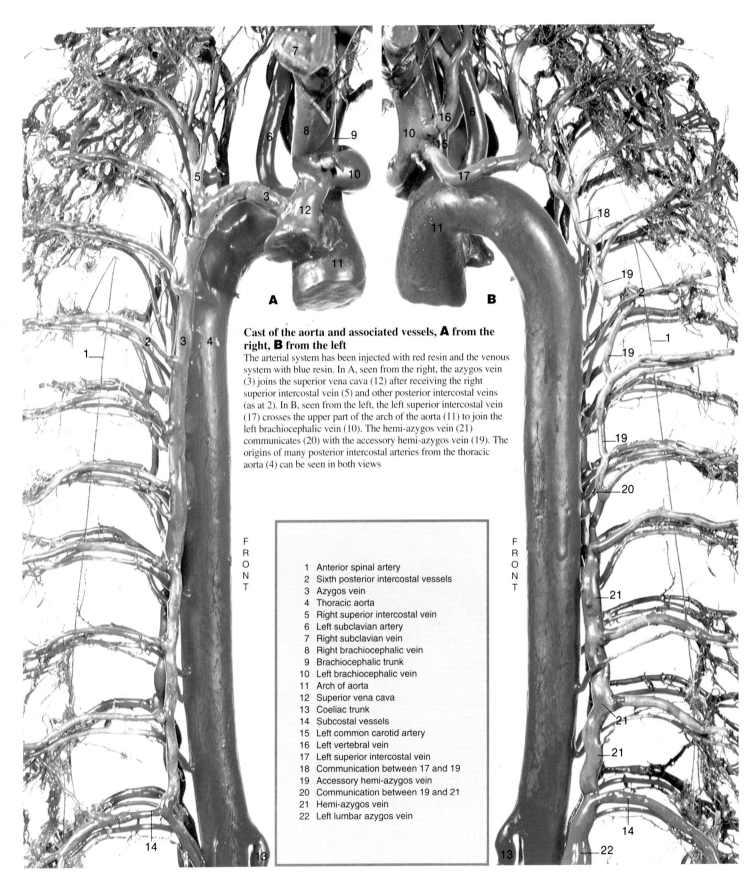

Cast of the aorta and associated vessels, A from the right, B from the left

The arterial system has been injected with red resin and the venous system with blue resin. In A, seen from the right, the azygos vein (3) joins the superior vena cava (12) after receiving the right superior intercostal vein (5) and other posterior intercostal veins (as at 2). In B, seen from the left, the left superior intercostal vein (17) crosses the upper part of the arch of the aorta (11) to join the left brachiocephalic vein (10). The hemi-azygos vein (21) communicates (20) with the accessory hemi-azygos vein (19). The origins of many posterior intercostal arteries from the thoracic aorta (4) can be seen in both views

1 Anterior spinal artery
2 Sixth posterior intercostal vessels
3 Azygos vein
4 Thoracic aorta
5 Right superior intercostal vein
6 Left subclavian artery
7 Right subclavian vein
8 Right brachiocephalic vein
9 Brachiocephalic trunk
10 Left brachiocephalic vein
11 Arch of aorta
12 Superior vena cava
13 Coeliac trunk
14 Subcostal vessels
15 Left common carotid artery
16 Left vertebral vein
17 Left superior intercostal vein
18 Communication between 17 and 19
19 Accessory hemi-azygos vein
20 Communication between 19 and 21
21 Hemi-azygos vein
22 Left lumbar azygos vein

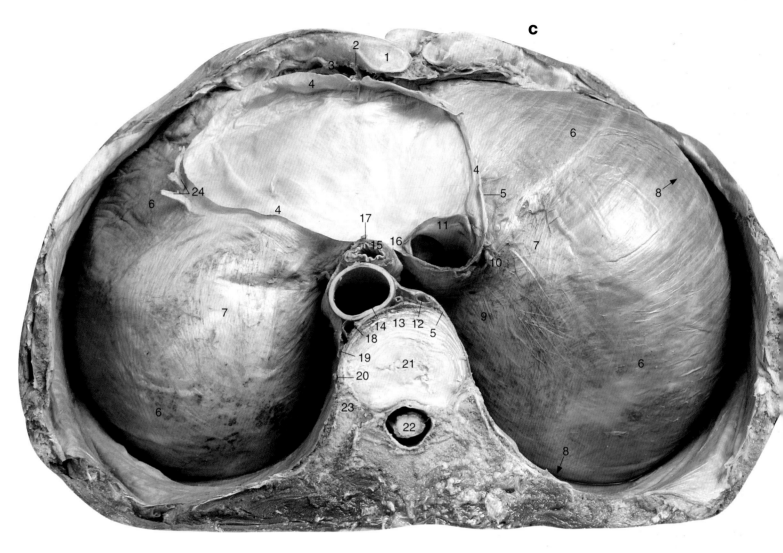

C Diaphragm, from above

The thorax has been transected at the level of the disc between the ninth and tenth thoracic vertebrae. The diaphragm is seen from above after removing the lungs and heart, but the lowest part of the fibrous pericardium (4) has been retained. The aorta (14) has the oesophagus (15) in front of it and the inferior vena cava (11) on its right. The right phrenic nerve (10) goes through the foramen for the inferior vena cava (11) in the tendinous part of the diaphragm (7, right label), while the left phrenic nerve (24) pierces the muscular part (6, left label) in front of the left part of the tendon (7, left label)

1	Seventh left costal cartilage	13	Thoracic duct
2	Left internal thoracic artery	14	Thoracic aorta
3	Left musculophrenic artery	15	Oesophagus
4	Fibrous pericardium (cut edge)	16	Posterior vagal trunk
5	Pleura (cut edge)	17	Anterior vagal trunk
6	Muscle of diaphragm	18	Hemi-azygos vein
7	Tendon of diaphragm	19	Left greater splanchnic nerve
8	Costodiaphragmatic recess	20	Left sympathetic trunk
9	Costomediastinal recess	21	Intervertebral disc
10	Right phrenic nerve	22	Spinal cord
11	Inferior vena cava	23	Head of left ninth rib
12	Azygos vein	24	Left phrenic nerve

• After forming the oesophageal plexus behind the lower part of the oesophagus, the two vagus nerves become reconstituted as the anterior and posterior vagal trunks (17 and 16) which enter the abdomen with the oesophagus (15; see also page 220).
• According to the standard textbook description, the foramen for the vena cava is at the level of the disc between the eighth and ninth thoracic vertebrae, the oesophageal opening at the level of the tenth thoracic vertebra and the aortic opening opposite the twelfth thoracic vertebra. However, it is common for the oesophageal opening to be nearer the midline, as in this specimen (15), and the vena caval foramen (11) is lower than usual.
• The vena caval foramen is in the tendinous part of the diaphragm and the oesophageal opening in the muscular part. The so-called aortic opening is not *in* the diaphragm but behind it (page 241).
• The central tendon of the diaphragm has the shape of a trefoil leaf and has no bony attachment.
• The right phrenic nerve (10) passes through the vena caval foramen, i.e. through the tendinous part, but the left phrenic nerve (24) pierces the muscular part in front of the central tendon just lateral to the overlying pericardium.
• The phrenic nerves are the *only motor* nerves to the diaphragm, including the crura. The supply from lower thoracic (intercostal and subcostal) nerves is purely afferent. Damage to one phrenic nerve completely paralyses its own half of the diaphragm.

A

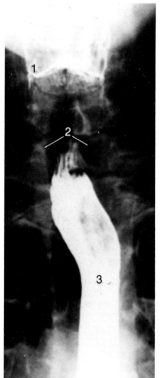

B

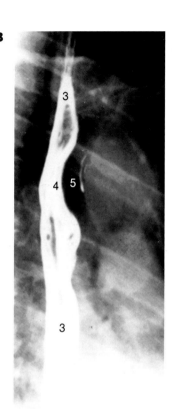

C

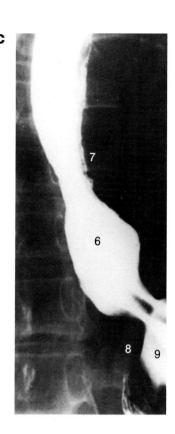

Radiographs of the oesophagus during a barium swallow, A lower pharynx and upper oesophagus, B middle part, C lower end

In A, viewed from the front, some of the barium paste adheres to the pharyngeal wall, outlining the piriform recesses (1), but most of it has passed into the oesophagus (3). In B, viewed obliquely from the left, the oesophagus is identified by the arch of the aorta (5) which shows some calcification in its wall—a useful aid to its identification. In C there is some dilatation at the lower end of the thoracic oesophagus (6) and it is constricted where it passes through the diaphragm (8) to join the stomach (9). The left atrium of the heart (7) lies in front of the lower thoracic oesophagus (page 194, A5), but only when enlarged does the atrium cause an indentation in the oesophagus

1	Piriform recess in laryngeal part of pharynx
2	Margins of trachea (translucent with contained air)
3	Barium in oesophagus
4	Aortic impression in oesophagus
5	Arch of aorta with plaque of calcification
6	Lower thoracic oesophagus
7	Position of left atrium
8	Diaphragm
9	Stomach

D

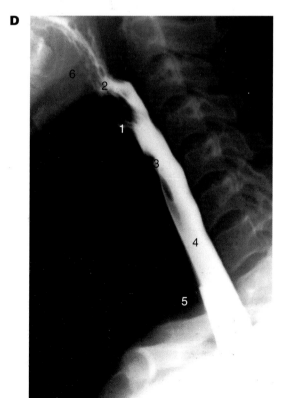

E

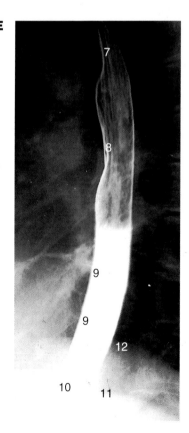

Radiograpghs of the oesophagus, D cervical part, E thoracic part

In these lateral views, note in D the impression of the postcricoid venous plexus, and in E the impressions made by the arch of the aorta (7), left bronchus (8) and left atrium (9)

1	Vallecula
2	Oropharynx
3	Postcricoid venous plexus impression
4	Oesophagus
5	Trachea
6	Base of tongue
7	Aortic arch impression
8	Left principal bronchus impression
9	Left atrium impression
10	Gastro-oesophageal junction
11	Left hemidiaphragm
12	Right hemidiaphragm

A

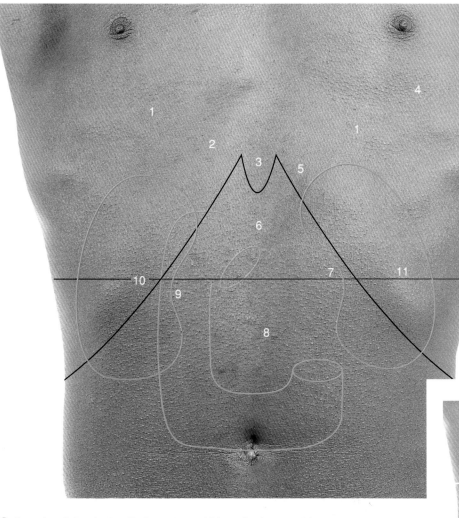

- The nipple in the male normally lies over the fourth intercostal space.
- The umbilicus normally lies at the level of the disc between the third and fourth lumbar vertebrae.
- The transpyloric plane (11) lies midway between the jugular notch of the sternum and the upper border of the pubic symphysis, or approximately a hand's breadth below the xiphisternal joint (3), and level with the lower part of the body of the first lumbar vertebra.
- The foramen for the inferior vena cava in the diaphragm (2) is about 2.5 cm from the midline at the level of the disc between the eighth and ninth thoracic vertebrae.
- The oesophageal opening in the diaphragm (5) is at the level of the tenth thoracic vertebra about 2.5 cm from the midline (but is often near or in the midline).
- The aortic opening in the diaphragm (6) is in the midline at the level of the twelfth thoracic vertebra.
- The hilum of each kidney is about 5 cm from the midline, that of the left (7) being just above the transpyloric plane and that of the right (9) just below it.
- In life the duodenum and the head of the pancreas (8) may lie at one or more vertebral levels lower than in the standard textbook or cadaveric position, shown here.
- The fundus of the gall bladder (10) lies behind the point where the lateral border of the right rectus sheath meets the costal margin at the ninth costal cartilage.

A Anterior abdominal wall above the umbilicus. Surface markings
The solid black line indicates the costal margin. The magenta line indicates the transpyloric plane. The C-shaped duodenum is outlined in blue, and the kidneys in green

1 Dome of diaphragm and upper margin of liver	7 Hilum of left kidney
2 Foramen for inferior vena cava in diaphragm	8 Head of pancreas and level of second lumbar vertebra
3 Xiphisternal joint	9 Hilum of right kidney
4 Apex of heart in fifth intercostal space	10 Fundus of gall bladder, and junction of ninth costal cartilage and lateral border of rectus sheath
5 Oesophageal ⎫ opening	
6 Aortic ⎬ in diaphragm	11 Transpyloric plane

B Regions of the abdomen
The abdomen may be divided into regions by two vertical and two horizontal lines. The vertical lines (VL) pass through the midinguinal points: the upper horizontal line corresponds to the transpyloric plane (TP, A11), the lower line is drawn between the tubercles of the iliac crests (transtubercular plane, TT)

1 Right hypochondrium	7 Right iliac region or iliac fossa
2 Epigastric region	
3 Left hypochondrium	8 Hypogastrium or suprapubic
4 Right lumbar region	
5 Umbilical region	9 Left iliac region or iliac fossa
6 Left lumbar region	

A

A Anterior abdominal wall, right upper quadrant

In this right upper quadrant of the anterior abdominal wall, above the umbilicus (12), part of the rectus sheath (3) has been removed to show the upper part of rectus abdominis (4) and two of its tendinous intersections (5). The lateral cutaneous branches of intercostal nerves (as at 13, with their anterior ends removed with the overlying skin and fascia) run round on the muscle fibres of the external oblique, which becomes aponeurotic (2) before taking part in the formation of the anterior wall of the rectus sheath (3). The anterior cutaneous branches of intercostal nerves pierce the rectus muscle (as at 6) and then pierce the anterior wall of the sheath (as at 10 and 11)

1	External oblique muscle
2	External oblique aponeurosis
3	Rectus sheath
4	Rectus abdominis
5	Tendinous intersection
6	Anterior cutaneous nerve (eighth intercostal)
7	Linea alba
8	Posterior layer } of internal
9	Anterior layer } oblique aponeurosis
10	Anterior cutaneous nerve (ninth intercostal)
11	Anterior cutaneous nerve (tenth intercostal)
12	Umbilicus
13	Lateral cutaneous nerve (eighth intercostal)

• The rectus sheath (A3) is formed by the internal oblique aponeurosis (B16) which splits at the lateral border of the rectus muscle (B4) into two layers. The posterior (B12) passes behind the muscle to blend with the aponeurosis of transversus abdominis (B7) to form the posterior wall of the sheath (B6), and the anterior layer (B13) passes in front of the muscle to blend with the external oblique aponeurosis (A2) as the anterior wall (B3).

• The anterior and posterior walls of the sheath unite at the medial border of the rectus muscle to form the midline linea alba (A7, B2).

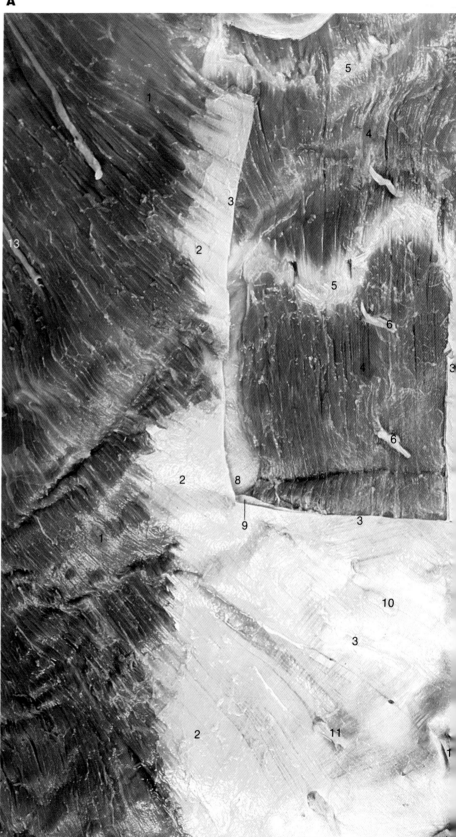

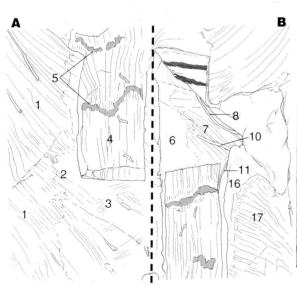

B

Anterior abdominal wall, B left upper quadrant, C axial MR image

The anterior wall of the rectus sheath and most of the external oblique muscle (1) and aponeurosis have been removed, together with a segment of the rectus muscle (4), whose upper end has been turned upwards to show branches of the superior epigastric vessels (5) on its deep surface. The aponeurosis (16) of the internal oblique muscle (17) splits at the lateral border of the rectus muscle into anterior (13) and posterior (12) layers which, when fused with the external oblique and transversus abdominis aponeurosis respectively, become the anterior (3) and posterior (6) walls of the rectus sheath. Below the costal margin (as at 9) the muscle fibres of transversus abdominis (7) run for some distance behind the rectus muscle before becoming aponeurotic. The seventh intercostal nerve (8) runs upwards parallel with the costal margin under the rectus muscle; other intercostal nerves (as at 11) are seen piercing the posterior layer (12) of the internal oblique aponeurosis before entering the rectus muscle (4). The MR image in C shows the muscles in transverse section (4, 1, 17 and 7)

1	External oblique muscle
2	Linea alba
3	Anterior wall of rectus sheath
4	Rectus abdominis
5	Superior epigastric vessels
6	Posterior wall of rectus sheath
7	Transversus abdominis
8	Seventh intercostal nerve
9	Ninth costal cartilage
10	Eighth intercostal nerve
11	Ninth intercostal nerve
12	Posterior layer } of internal
13	Anterior layer } oblique aponeurosis
14	Tendinous intersection
15	Anterior cutaneous nerve (ninth intercostal)
16	Internal oblique aponeurosis
17	Internal oblique muscle
18	Umbilicus

• The tendinous intersections of the rectus muscle (A5, B14) are irregular and usually incomplete fibrous bands which adhere to the anterior wall of the rectus sheath but not to the posterior wall. There are usually three—one below the xiphoid process, one at umbilical level and one between these two—but there may be others (as on page 203, B, unlabelled below the umbilicus).

C

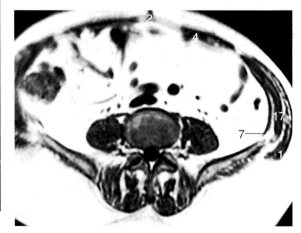

A Anterior abdominal wall, right lower quadrant

The external oblique muscle (1) and aponeurosis (2) and the
rectus sheath (3) remain intact. Over the inguinal region parts of
the fatty layer (7) and fibrous layer (8) of the superficial fascia
have been preserved. As the fibrous layer passes down below the
level of the upper margin of the pubic symphysis (14) it becomes
the superficial perineal fascia (15)

1	External oblique muscle
2	External oblique aponeurosis
3	Anterior wall of rectus sheath
4	Anterior cutaneous nerve (eleventh intercostal)
5	Anterior superior iliac spine
6	Inguinal ligament
7	Fatty layer ⎫ of superficial
8	Fibrous layer ⎭ fascia
9	Superficial circumflex iliac artery
10	Superficial epigastric artery
11	A superficial inguinal lymph node
12	Position of saphenous opening
13	Suspensory ligament of penis
14	Level of pubic symphysis
15	Superficial perineal fascia
16	Umbilicus

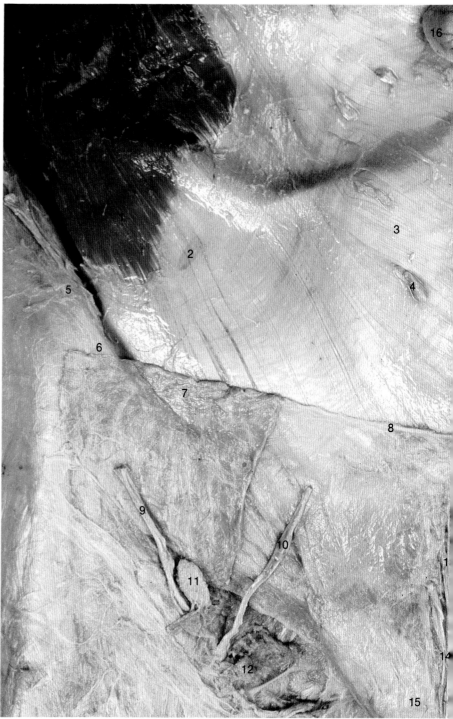

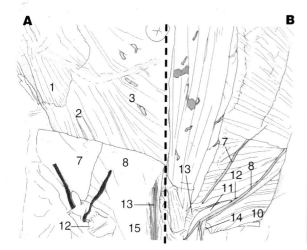

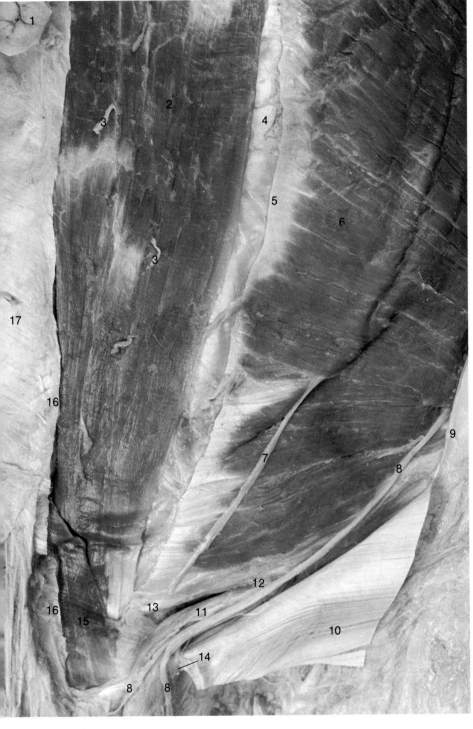

B

Anterior abdominal wall, B left lower quadrant, C axial MR image

The anterior wall of the rectus sheath and most of the external oblique have been removed but a small part of the external oblique aponeurosis has been turned down (10) to show the spermatic cord (11) and ilio-inguinal nerve (8) in the inguinal canal. The iliohypogastric nerve (7) is at a higher level and does not enter the inguinal canal. Compare features seen in B with those in the MR image

1	Umbilicus
2	Rectus abdominis
3	Anterior cutaneous nerve (eleventh intercostal)
4	Eleventh intercostal nerve
5	Lateral border of rectus sheath
6	Internal oblique
7	Iliohypogastric nerve
8	Ilio-inguinal nerve
9	Anterior superior iliac spine
10	External oblique aponeurosis
11	Spermatic cord
12	Margin of deep inguinal ring
13	Conjoint tendon
14	External spermatic fascia and margin of superficial inguinal ring
15	Pyramidalis
16	Medial border of rectus sheath
17	Linea alba

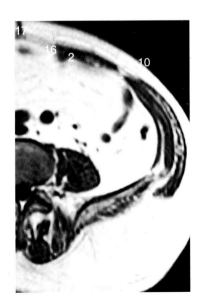

C

• For further details of the inguinal canal in the male see pages 204 and 246, and in the female page 247.

- McBurney's point (4) lies at the junction of the lateral and middle thirds of a line drawn from the anterior superior iliac spine (3) to the umbilicus. It is usually taken to indicate the level of the *opening* of the appendix into the caecum, though the opening is often somewhat lower.
- The superficial inguinal ring (9, at the medial end of the inguinal canal) lies 1 cm above the pubic tubercle (8).
- The deep inguinal ring (15, at the lateral end of the inguinal canal) lies 1 cm above the midpoint of the inguinal ligament.
- The femoral artery (12, whose pulsation should normally be palpable) enters the thigh midway between the pubic symphysis (7) and the anterior superior iliac spine (3). This is often referred to as the 'femoral' point or the midinguinal point.
- Note the slight difference between the surface markings of the midpoint of the inguinal ligament (used to find the deep ring, 15) and the midinguinal point (used to locate the femoral artery, 12).

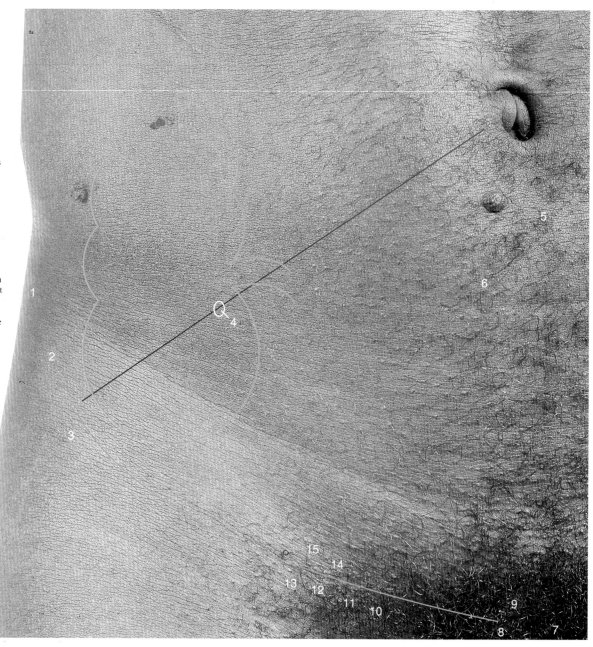

A Anterior abdominal wall, right lower quadrant. Surface markings

The caecum with the ileum opening into it from the left and the ascending colon continuing upwards from it are indicated by the blue line. McBurney's point (4; see notes) overlies the opening of the appendix into the caecum, and is on the line (magenta) from the anterior superior iliac spine (3) to the umbilicus. The inguinal ligament, between the anterior superior iliac spine (3) and the pubic tubercle (8), is indicated by the green line. The femoral artery (12) has the femoral vein (11) on its medial side and the femoral nerve (13) on its lateral side. The femoral canal (10) is on the medial side of the vein. The deep inguinal ring (15) and inferior epigastric vessels (14) are above the artery, while the superficial inguinal ring (9) is above and medial to the pubic tubercle (8)

1 Tubercle of iliac crest	8 Pubic tubercle
2 Iliac crest	9 Superficial inguinal ring
3 Anterior superior iliac spine	10 Femoral canal
4 McBurney's point	11 Femoral vein
5 Bifurcation of aorta (fourth lumbar vertebra)	12 Femoral artery
	13 Femoral nerve
6 Lower end of inferior vena cava (fifth lumbar vertebra)	14 Inferior epigastric vessels
	15 Deep inguinal ring
7 Pubic symphysis	

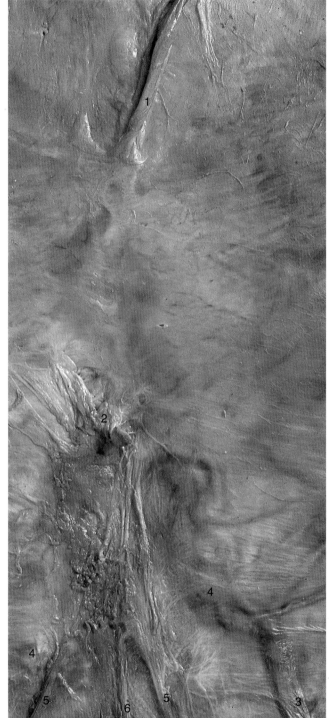

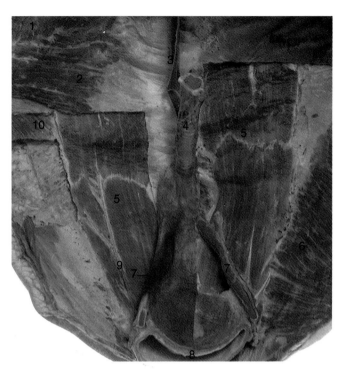

C Fetal anterior abdominal wall, from behind

In this full-term fetus the peritoneum and extraperitoneal tissues have been removed from the anterior abdominal wall to show the umbilical arteries (7) and left umbilical vein (4) converging at the back of the (unlabelled) umbilicus

1	Diaphragm	6	Internal oblique
2	Transversus abdominis	7	Umbilical artery
3	Falciform ligament	8	Urinary bladder
4	Left umbilical vein	9	Inferior epigastric vessels
5	Rectus abdominis	10	External oblique

B Anterior abdominal wall, from behind. Umbilical folds

This view of the peritoneal surface of the central region of the anterior abdominal wall shows the peritoneal folds raised by underlying structures. There is one fold above the umbilicus—the falciform ligament (1)—and there are five below it: the median umbilical fold (6) in the midline, and a pair of medial and lateral umbilical folds on each side (5 and 3). See the notes for the contents of the folds

1	Falciform ligament	4	Arcuate line
2	Umbilicus	5	Medial umbilical fold
3	Lateral umbilical fold	6	Median umbilical fold

• The falciform ligament (B1) contains the ligamentum teres, which is the obliterated remains of the left umbilical vein (C4). In B the ligamentum teres has not raised a fold until some distance above the umbilicus.
• The median umbilical fold (B6) contains the median umbilical ligament, which is the obliterated remains of the urachus (formed from the allantois, the embryonic connexion between

the bladder and umbilicus).
• The medial umbilical fold (B5) contains the medial umbilical ligament, which is the obliterated remains of the umbilical artery (C7).
• The lateral umbilical fold (B3) contains the inferior epigastric vessels, conducting them from the external iliac vessels to the rectus sheath. Although called an umbilical fold, it does not

extend as far as the umbilicus, since the vessels enter the rectus sheath by passing beneath the arcuate line (B4), which is the lower border of the posterior wall of the sheath. Below this level the three aponeuroses that form the sheath (page 200) all pass in front of the rectus muscle.

A

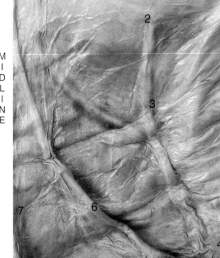

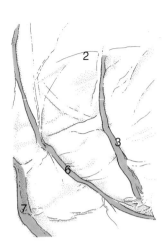

A Anterior abdominal wall, right side, from behind

This view shows the posterior surface of the anterior abdominal wall to the right of the midline and above the pelvic brim (5), with the peritoneum intact. The medial umbilical fold (6) is prominent, and the inferior epigastric vessels (3) are seen passing deep to the arcuate line (2)

---

1 Posterior layer of rectus sheath
2 Arcuate line
3 Inferior epigastric vessels in lateral umbilical fold
4 Position of deep inguinal ring
5 Pelvic brim
6 Medial umbilical fold
7 Median umbilical fold

• The arcuate line (A2, B3) is sometimes called the semicircular fold (not to be confused with the semilunar line, which is the name sometimes given to the lateral border of the rectus sheath, nor with the arcuate line of the ilium—page 263, 12).
• The umbilicus is a midline scar in the anterior abdominal wall at the level of the disc between the third and fourth lumbar vertebrae (page 199). It contains on its deep (posterior) surface the obliterated remains of the two umbilical arteries (page 205, C7), the left umbilical vein (page 205, C4), the urachus and perhaps the remains of the vitello-intestinal duct. This duct normally disappears completely; in early fetal life it connected the yolk sac to the intestine. If the intestinal end persists it forms the ileal or Meckel's diverticulum which when present is about 60 cm from the ileocaecal junction.
• The right umbilical vein disappears very early in development; it is the left one which persists and eventually becomes the ligamentum teres within the falciform ligament (page 205, B1).
• For notes on the peritoneal folds see previous page.

B

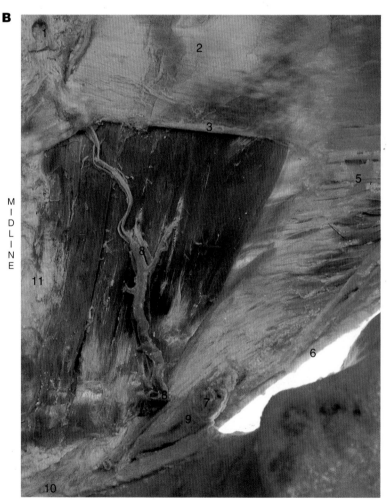

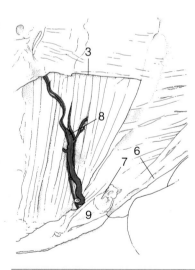

B Anterior abdominal wall, right side, from behind

In a similar specimen to that in A, the peritoneum and extraperitoneal tissues have been removed, leaving the inferior epigastric vessels (8) coursing over the back of the rectus muscle (4) to enter the rectus sheath (2) beneath the arcuate line (3)

1	Umbilicus	6	Inguinal ligament
2	Posterior wall of rectus sheath	7	Spermatic cord
3	Arcuate line	8	Inferior epigastric vessels
4	Rectus abdominis	9	Position of deep inguinal ring
5	Transversus abdominis	10	Pubic crest
		11	Linea alba

C Upper abdominal viscera, in transverse section

This section through the upper abdomen at the level of the first lumbar vertebra, seen from below looking towards the thorax, shows the general disposition of some of the viscera. The vertebral column (22) bulges forwards into the abdominal cavity, with the kidneys (14 and 28) lying in the trough on either side. The bulk of the liver (29) is on the right side, extending towards the left (3) to overlap part of the stomach (8), and the pancreas (5) lies centrally, also extending towards the left (but on a deeper plane) to overlap part of the left kidney (14). Parts of the colon (9 and 13) are adjacent to the spleen (11) which lies against the part of the diaphragm attached to the thoracic wall in the region of the tenth rib (12)

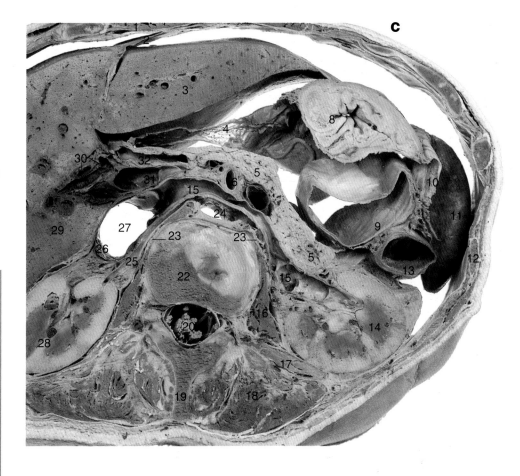

1 Right rectus abdominis	22 Body of first lumbar vertebra	26 Right renal vein	30 Hepatic ducts
2 Falciform ligament	23 Sympathetic trunk	27 Inferior vena cava	31 Portal vein
3 Left lobe of liver	24 Abdominal aorta	28 Right kidney	32 Hepatic artery
4 Lesser omentum	25 Right renal artery	29 Right lobe of liver	
5 Pancreas			
6 Superior mesenteric artery			
7 Splenic vein			
8 Stomach			
9 Transverse colon			
10 Greater omentum (gastrosplenic ligament)			
11 Spleen			
12 Tenth rib			
13 Descending colon			
14 Left kidney			
15 Left renal vein			
16 Psoas major			
17 Quadratus lumborum			
18 Erector spinae			
19 Spine of first lumbar vertebra			
20 Conus medullaris of spinal cord			
21 Nerve roots of cauda equina			

D CT scan of the upper abdomen, at the level of the coeliac trunk

All CT (computerized tomography) scans of the trunk are, by convention, viewed from below (as with the body lying on the back and the viewer looking towards the head). In D both oral and intravenous contrast media have been used (to emphasize the outlines of the gut and vascular system). To avoid too many labels, only some key features have been numbered, and the various parts of the alimentary tract are unlabelled. The coeliac trunk arising from the aorta (9) is seen to divide as a Y into the splenic artery running towards the left behind the pancreas (5) and the common hepatic artery passing to the right near the portal vein (3). On the left side the spleen (6) and the upper pole of the kidney (7) are shown, but on the right the plane of the scan is too high to show the right kidney

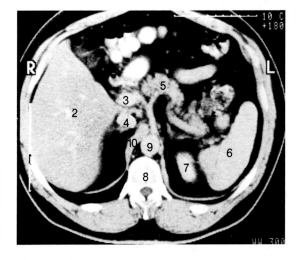

1 Gall bladder	5 Pancreas	8 Twelfth thoracic vertebra
2 Liver	6 Spleen	9 Abdominal aorta
3 Portal vein	7 Left kidney	10 Right crus of diaphragm
4 Inferior vena cava		

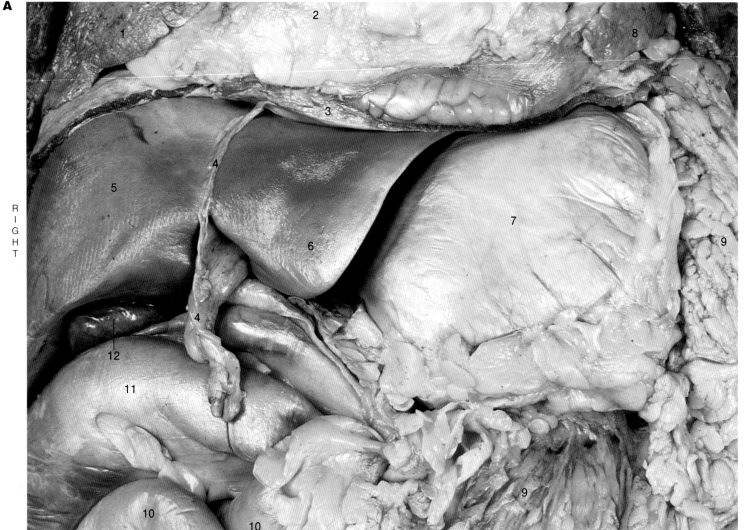

A Upper abdominal viscera, from the front
The thoracic and abdominal walls and the anterior part of the diaphragm have been
removed to show the undisturbed viscera. The liver (5 and 6) and stomach (7) are
immediately below the diaphragm (3). The greater omentum (9) hangs down from
the greater curvature (lower margin) of the stomach (7), overlying much of the
small and large intestine but leaving some of the transverse colon (11) and small
intestine (10) uncovered. The fundus (tip) of the gall bladder (12) is seen between
the right lobe of the liver (5) and transverse colon (11)

B Upper abdominal viscera, from the front
In this view of the undisturbed abdomen the upper part of the greater omentum (as
at 5) overlies much of the transverse colon and mesocolon (with the right part of the
transverse colon seen at 11). The lower part of the omentum (6) covers coils of
small intestine, some of which (7) are visible beyond the right margin of the
omentum. The caecum (8) is at the lower end of the ascending colon (9) which
continues upwards into the right colic flexure (hepatic flexure, 10) and then
becomes the transverse colon (11)

1	Inferior lobe of right lung	7	Stomach
2	Pericardial fat	8	Inferior lobe of left lung
3	Diaphragm	9	Greater omentum
4	Falciform ligament	10	Small intestine
5	Right lobe of liver	11	Transverse colon
6	Left lobe of liver	12	Gall bladder

1	Right lobe of liver	7	Small intestine
2	Falciform ligament	8	Caecum
3	Left lobe of liver	9	Ascending colon
4	Stomach	10	Right colic flexure
5	Greater omentum overlying transverse colon and mesocolon	11	Transverse colon
6	Greater omentum overlying coils of small intestine	12	Fundus of gall bladder

• For an explanation of peritoneal structures see the diagrams on page 214.

B

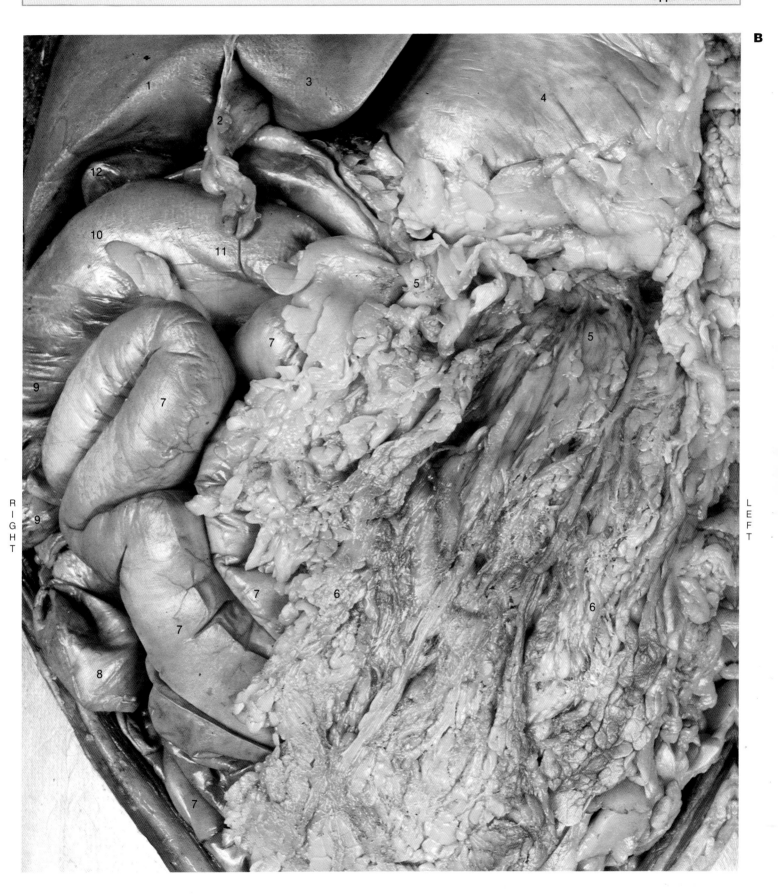

RIGHT

LEFT

A Upper abdominal viscera, from the front

In this view of the same specimen as on pages 208 and 209, the greater omentum (4) has been lifted upwards to show its adherence to the transverse colon (5) (see page 214)

1 Right lobe of liver
2 Falciform ligament
3 Left lobe of liver
4 Posterior surface of greater omentum
5 Transverse colon
6 Appendices epiploicae
7 Small intestine
8 Gall bladder (fundus)

• For further details of the peritoneum and greater omentum in a less obese subject, see pages 212 and 213.

• The appendices epiploicae (A6) are fat-filled appendages of peritoneum on the various parts of the colon (ascending, transverse, descending and sigmoid). They are not present on the small intestine or the rectum, and may be rudimentary on the caecum and appendix. In abdominal operations they are one feature that helps to distinguish colon from other parts of the intestine.

• In strict anatomical nomenclature the term 'small intestine' includes the duodenum, jejunum and ileum, but clinically it is frequently used to mean jejunum and ileum, with the duodenum being referred to by its own name.

• The parts of the duodenum are properly called superior, descending, horizontal and ascending, but are more commonly known as the first, second, third and fourth parts respectively.

A

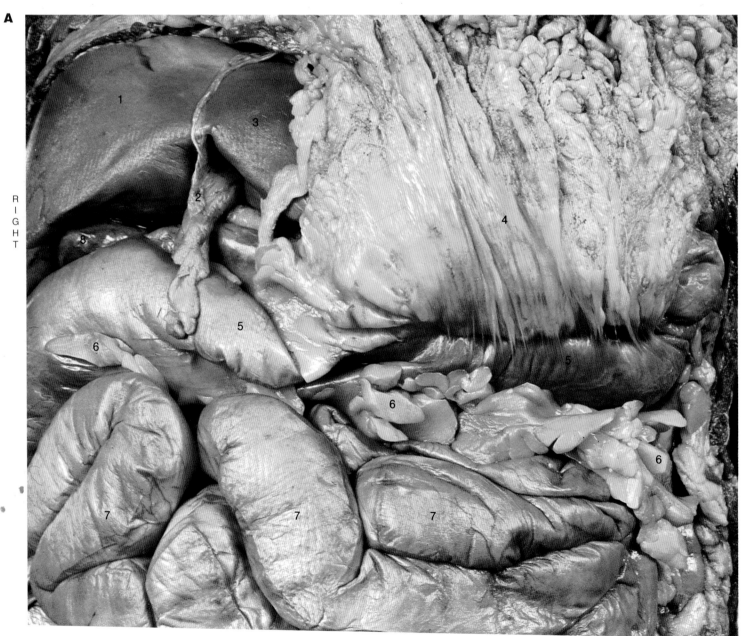

B

FRONT

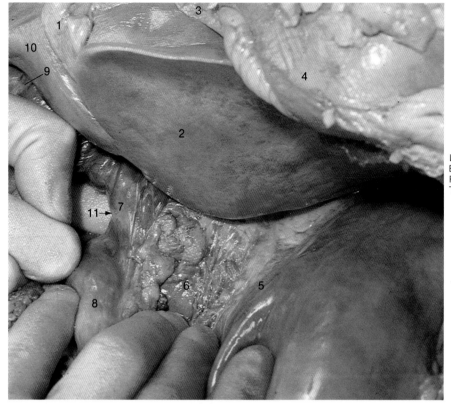

LEFT

C

HEAD

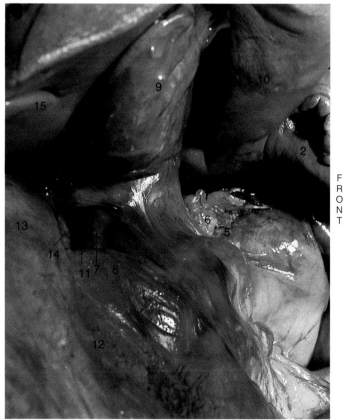

FRONT

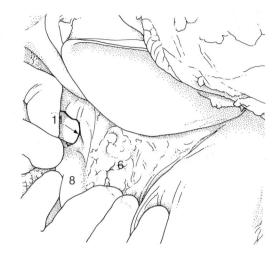

1 Falciform ligament
2 Left lobe of liver
3 Diaphragm
4 Pericardium
5 Lesser curvature of stomach
6 Lesser omentum
7 Right free margin of lesser omentum
8 Superior (first) part of duodenum
9 Gall bladder
10 Quadrate lobe of liver
11 Epiploic foramen
12 Descending (second) part of duodenum
13 Upper pole of right kidney
14 Inferior vena cava
15 Right lobe of liver

Lesser omentum and epiploic foramen, B from the front, C from the front and the right

In B a finger has been placed in the epiploic foramen (11) behind the right free margin of the lesser omentum (7), and the tip can be seen in the lesser sac, through the transparent lesser omentum (6) which stretches between the liver (2) and the lesser curvature of the stomach (5). In the more lateral view in C, looking into the foramen from the right, the foramen (11) is identified between the right free margin of the lesser omentum (7) in front and the inferior vena cava (14) behind, above the first part of the duodenum (8)

• The epiploic foramen (of Winslow, B11 and C11) is the communication between the general peritoneal cavity (sometimes called the greater sac) and the lesser sac (omental bursa), a space lined by peritoneum behind the stomach (B5 and C5) and lesser omentum (B6 and B7) and in front of parts of the pancreas and left kidney.
• The epiploic foramen, the opening into the lesser sac (B11 and C11), has the following boundaries:
Behind—the inferior vena cava (C14).
In front—the right free margin of the lesser omentum (B7) which contains the portal vein, hepatic artery and bile duct (page 215, F22, 21 and 18). The portal vein is the most posterior of these structures, so the foramen may be said to lie between the two great veins—inferior vena cava and portal vein.
Below—the first part of the duodenum (B8 and C8) which passes backwards as well as to the right.
Above—the caudate process of the liver (page 224, A13).

A

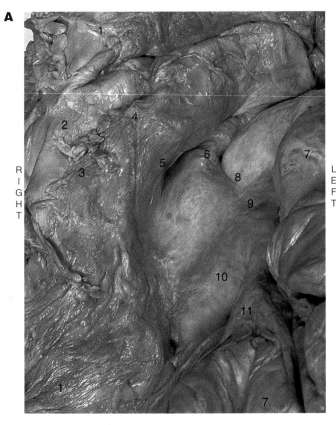

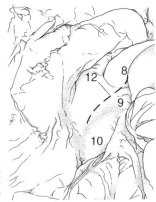

A Upper abdominal viscera, from the front

In this view the stomach (4 and 5), transverse colon (2) and greater omentum (1) have been lifted up to show the region of the duodenojejunal flexure (8). The left end of the horizontal (third) part of the duodenum (10) turns upwards as the ascending (fourth) part (9) which is continuous with the jejunum at the duodenojejunal flexure (8) below the lower border of the pancreas (6)

1 Greater omentum (posterior surface)	7 Jejunum
2 Transverse colon (posterior surface)	8 Duodenojejunal flexure
3 Transverse mesocolon (posterior surface)	9 Ascending (fourth) } part of
	10 Horizontal (third) } duodenum
4 Greater } curvature of stomach	11 Mesentery
5 Lesser	12 Line of attachment of root of mesentery
6 Lower border of pancreas	

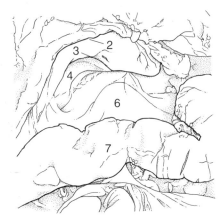

B Lesser sac and transverse mesocolon, from the front

The greater omentum (1) hanging down from the greater curvature of the stomach (2) has been separated from the underlying transverse colon (7) and mesocolon (6) and lifted upwards, and an opening made into the lesser sac (as in D on page 214). This view therefore shows the posterior surface of the greater omentum (1), stomach and lesser omentum (4), and the anterior surface of the transverse mesocolon (6)

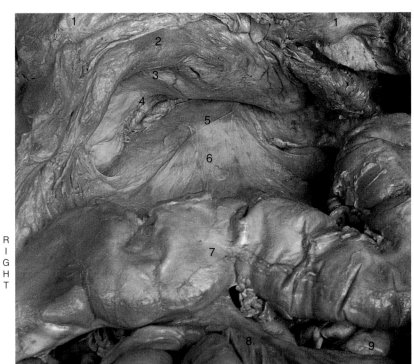

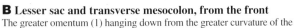

• The greater omentum hanging down from the greater curvature of the stomach overlies the transverse mesocolon and transverse colon and fuses with them, so that when the greater omentum is lifted up the transverse colon is lifted also (as in C on page 214). When the greater omentum (B1) is dissected off the transverse colon (B7) and mesocolon (B6) and lifted up (as in B, and in E on page 214), the transverse colon is left behind, suspended from the lower border of the pancreas (B5) by its mesocolon (B6).

1 Greater omentum (posterior surface)	6 Transverse mesocolon overlying horizontal (third) part of duodenum
2 Greater } curvature of stomach	7 Transverse colon
3 Lesser	8 Mesentery
4 Lesser omentum (posterior surface)	9 Coils of jejunum and ileum
5 Peritoneum of lesser sac overlying pancreas	

c

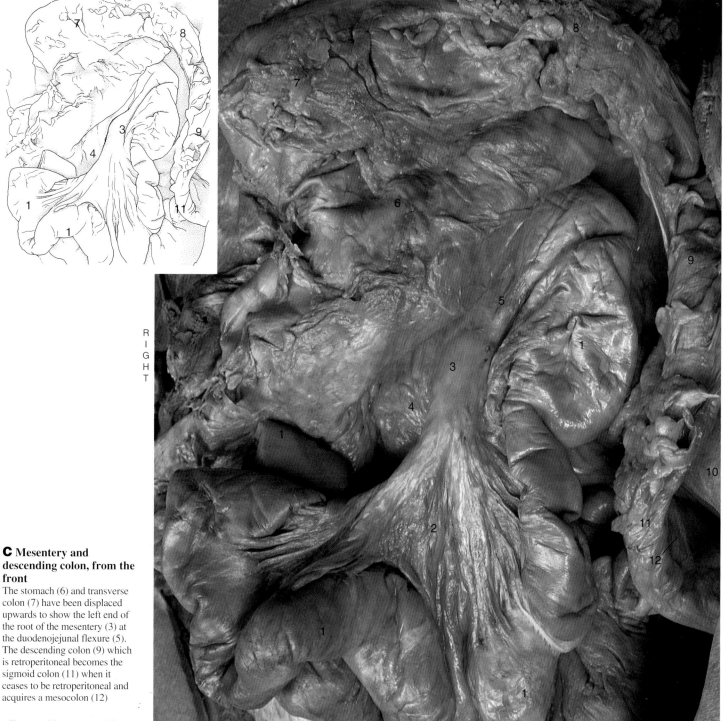

C Mesentery and descending colon, from the front

The stomach (6) and transverse colon (7) have been displaced upwards to show the left end of the root of the mesentery (3) at the duodenojejunal flexure (5). The descending colon (9) which is retroperitoneal becomes the sigmoid colon (11) when it ceases to be retroperitoneal and acquires a mesocolon (12)

• The root of the mesentery (C3) begins at the duodenojejunal flexure (C5) and passes downwards and to the right, crossing the horizontal (third) part of the duodenum (C4); the superior mesenteric vessels enter the mesentery at this point (see page 216).

• The sigmoid colon (C11), like the transverse colon, has its own mesentery, the sigmoid mesocolon (C12).

1	Coils of jejunum and ileum	6	Greater curvature of stomach
2	Mesentery	7	Transverse colon
3	Root of mesentery	8	Left colic (splenic) flexure
4	Horizontal (third) part of duodenum	9	Descending colon
5	Duodenojejunal flexure		
10	Peritoneum overlying external iliac vessels		
11	Sigmoid colon		
12	Sigmoid mesocolon		

A

FRONT

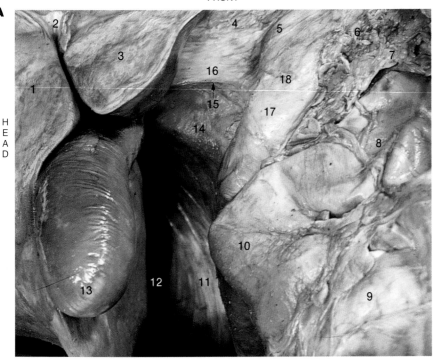

HEAD

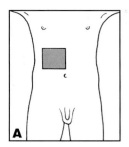

● The upper boundary of the hepatorenal pouch is the inferior layer of the coronary ligament, where the peritoneum is reflected from the lower margin of the bare area of the liver to the upper pole of the right kidney (see page 224, B19).

A Hepatorenal pouch of peritoneum, from the right and below

With the body lying on its back and seen from the right (with the head towards the left), the liver (1) has been turned upwards (towards the left) to open up the gap between the liver and upper pole of the right kidney (11)—the hepatorenal pouch of peritoneum (12, Morison's pouch or the right subhepatic compartment of the peritoneal cavity)

1	Right lobe of liver
2	Falciform ligament
3	Left lobe of liver
4	Lesser omentum overlying pancreas
5	Lesser ⎫ curvature of stomach
6	Greater ⎭
7	Greater omentum
8	Transverse colon
9	Ascending colon
10	Right colic (hepatic) flexure
11	Upper pole of right kidney
12	Hepatorenal (Morison's) pouch
13	Gall bladder
14	Inferior vena cava
15	Epiploic foramen
16	Right free margin of lesser omentum
17	Superior (first) part of duodenum
18	Gastroduodenal junction

Diagrams of peritoneum. B Normal position, C with the lower part of the greater omentum lifted up, D with the greater omentum lifted up and separated from the transverse mesocolon and colon, with an opening into the lesser sac, E with the greater omentum and transverse mesocolon and colon lifted up, with an opening into the lesser sac

These drawings of a sagittal section through the middle of the abdomen, viewed from the left, illustrate theoretically how the peritoneum forms the lesser omentum (L, passing down to the stomach, S), greater omentum (G), transverse mesocolon (TM) passing to the transverse colon (TC), and the mesentery (M) of the small intestine (SI). The layer in blue represents the peritoneum of the lesser sac. The superior mesenteric artery passes

between the head and uncinate process of the pancreas (P and U), and continues across the duodenum (D) into the mesentery (M) to the small intestine (SI), giving off the middle colic artery which runs in the transverse mesocolon (TM) to the transverse colon (TC).The greater omentum (G) is formed by four layers fused together and also fused with the front of the transverse mesocolon (TM, two layers) and transverse colon. On dissection, no separation between any layers is possible except between the greater omentum and the transverse mesocolon. The six layers between the stomach and transverse colon are sometimes collectively known as the gastrocolic omentum. B corresponds to the dissections on pages 208 and 209, C to page 210, D to page 212B, and E to page 217B. The arrows in D and E indicate the layers cut to make artificial openings into the lesser sac

B
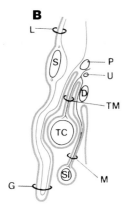

C
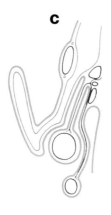

D
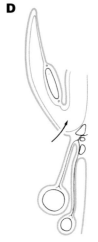

E
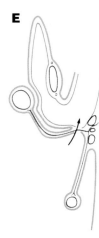

F

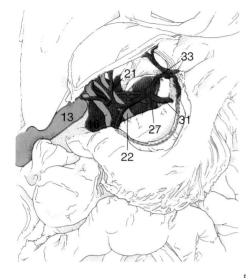

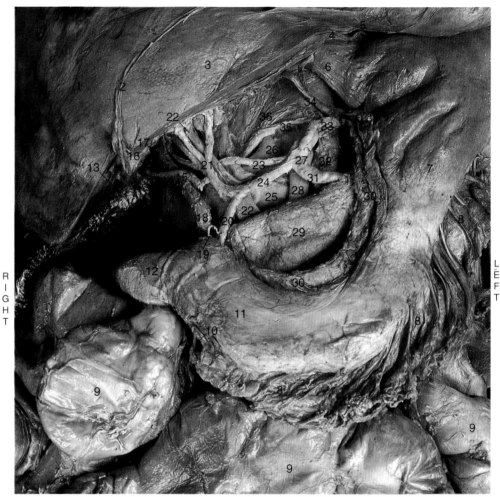

RIGHT

LEFT

F Coeliac trunk and surrounding area

Part of the left lobe of the liver (3), and most of the lesser and greater omentum (30 and 8) have been removed, together with peritoneum of the central part of the posterior abdominal wall (posterior wall of the lesser sac), to show some of the most important structures in the upper abdomen: the coeliac trunk (27) and its branches (33, 31 and 24), the portal vein (22), and the bile duct (18) formed by the union of the cystic duct (16) from the gall bladder (13) with the common hepatic duct (17) from the liver (1 and 3)

1 Right lobe of liver	20 Gastroduodenal artery
2 Falciform ligament	21 Hepatic artery and right and left
3 Left lobe of liver	branches
4 Left triangular ligament	22 Portal vein
5 Diaphragm	23 Accessory hepatic artery
6 Abdominal part of oesophagus	24 Common hepatic artery
7 Body of stomach	25 Left renal vein
8 Branches of left and right gastro-	26 Abdominal aorta
epiploic arteries in greater	27 Coeliac trunk
omentum	28 Superior mesenteric artery
9 Transverse colon	29 Body of pancreas
10 Right gastro-epiploic artery	30 Lesser omentum containing right
11 Pyloric part of stomach	and left gastric arteries
12 Superior (first) part of duodenum	31 Splenic artery
13 Gall bladder	32 Left crus of diaphragm
14 Inferior vena cava	33 Left gastric artery
15 Cystic artery	34 Oesophageal branch of left gastric
16 Cystic duct	artery
17 Common hepatic duct	35 Median arcuate ligament
18 Bile duct	36 Right crus of diaphragm
19 Right gastric artery	

- The portal vein (22), hepatic artery (21) and bile duct (18) are contained within the right free margin of the lesser omentum, the duct being the structure farthest to the right.
- The cystic artery (15) is normally derived from the right branch of the hepatic artery and passes behind the common hepatic and cystic ducts. Here it comes from the hepatic artery itself (21) and passes in front of the bile duct (18).
- If an accessory hepatic artery is present (as in this specimen, 23) it passes *behind* the portal vein (22), not in front like the normal artery.
- It is normal for the right gastric artery (19) to be much smaller than the left (33).
- The coeliac trunk (27) gives off three branches: the left gastric artery (33), the splenic artery (31) and the common hepatic artery (24).
- The left gastric artery (33) passes upwards and to the left and then turns down to run along the lesser curvature of the stomach between the two layers of peritoneum that form the lesser omentum (30). It gives off an oesophageal branch which passes up through the oesophageal opening in the diaphragm and supplies the lower part of the oesophagus (6). The accompanying veins (not shown here) drain to the left gastric vein and thence to the portal vein, making the lower end of the oesophagus one of the most important sites of portal–systemic anastomosis.
- The splenic artery (31) passes to the left along the upper border of the pancreas (29).
- The common hepatic artery (24) passes to the right, to give off the gastroduodenal artery (20) and then turns upwards in the right free margin of the lesser omentum as the hepatic artery (21) which divides into right and left branches to enter the porta hepatis of the liver.

A

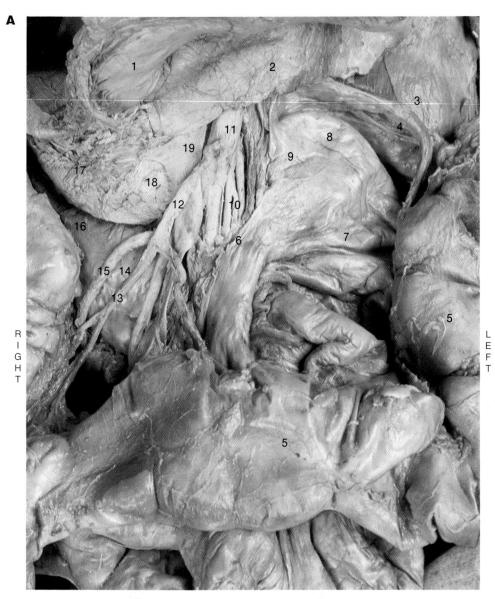

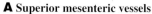

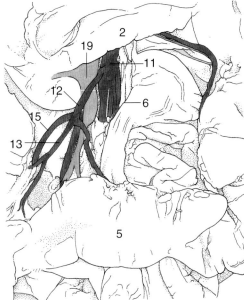

A Superior mesenteric vessels

The stomach (1) has been lifted upwards and transverse mesocolon removed, leaving the transverse colon (5) in its normal position. Part of the peritoneum of the mesentery (6) has been dissected away to show branches of the superior mesenteric artery (11)

• The right colic artery (13) is normally a branch of the superior mesenteric artery (11) but often (as here) arises from its middle colic branch (12).

• The superior mesenteric vein (19) lies on the right side of its companion artery (11). They appear at the lower border of the pancreas (2), crossing the uncinate process (18) of the head of the pancreas (17) and lower down crossing the horizontal (third) part of the duodenum (14) which is where they enter or leave the root of the mesentery (6).

1	Posterior surface of pyloric part of stomach
2	Body of pancreas
3	Lower pole of left kidney
4	Branches of left colic vessels
5	Transverse colon
6	Cut edge of peritoneum at root of mesentery
7	Jejunum
8	Duodenojejunal flexure
9	Ascending (fourth) part of duodenum
10	Jejunal and ileal arteries
11	Superior mesenteric artery
12	Middle colic artery
13	Right colic artery
14	Horizontal (third) part of duodenum
15	Ileocolic artery
16	Descending (second) part of duodenum
17	Head of pancreas
18	Uncinate process of head of pancreas
19	Superior mesenteric vein

B

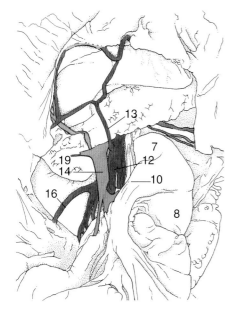

B Superior mesenteric vessels

This dissection is similar to A opposite, but here the stomach (2) and transverse colon (1) have both been lifted upwards, so lifting the middle colic artery (13) upwards also. The root of the mesentery (10) begins at the duodenojejunal flexure (7) and passes obliquely downwards to the right over the horizontal (third) part of the duodenum (15), where the superior mesenteric vessels and their branches (14, 12 and 11) become enclosed between the two layers of the peritoneum that form the mesentery (see B on page 214)

1 Transverse colon
2 Posterior surface of body of stomach
3 Body of pancreas
4 Left kidney
5 Left colic vessels
6 Descending colon
7 Duodenojejunal flexure
8 Jejunum
9 Mesentery
10 Cut edge of peritoneum at root of mesentery
11 Jejunal and ileal arteries
12 Superior mesenteric artery
13 Middle colic artery
14 Superior mesenteric vein

15 Horizontal (third) part of duodenum
16 Ileocolic artery
17 Descending (second) part of duodenum
18 Uncinate process of head of pancreas
19 Head $\Big\}$ of pancreas
20 Neck
21 Right branch of middle colic artery

• In its normal position the middle colic artery runs downwards from its superior mesenteric origin (A12), but obviously when the transverse colon is lifted upwards (as here, B1, and in E on page 214), the vessel (B13) passes upwards also. Textbook drawings of the arteries of the colon often illustrate it in this position, but it must be remembered that with the body in the normal anatomical position it runs downwards.

HEAD

A

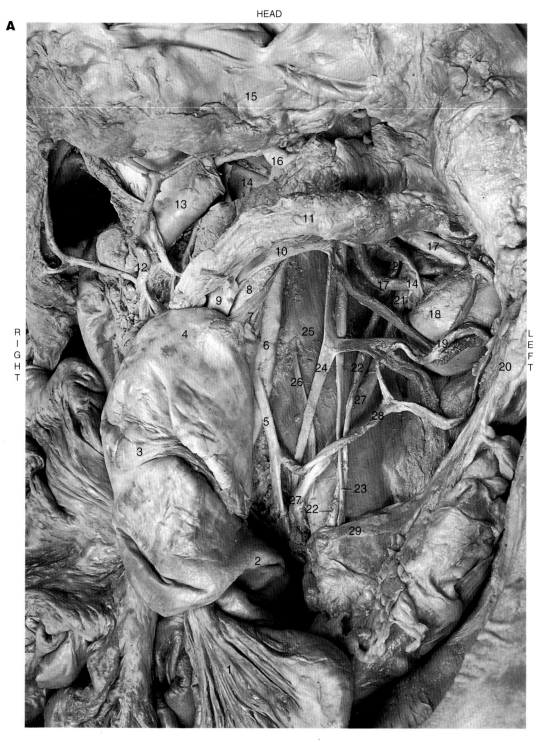

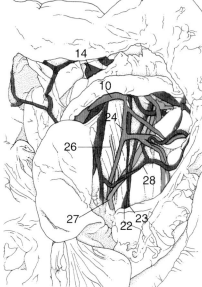

1 Mesentery
2 Horizontal (third) ⎫ part of
3 Ascending (fourth) ⎬ duodenum
4 Duodenojejunal flexure
5 Inferior mesenteric artery
6 Abdominal aorta
7 Suspensory muscle of
   duodenum (muscle of Treitz)
8 Superior mesenteric artery
9 Superior mesenteric vein
10 Splenic vein
11 Body of pancreas
12 Middle colic artery
13 Posterior surface of pyloric part
   of stomach
14 Left renal vein
15 Transverse colon
16 Splenic artery
17 Left renal artery
18 Lower pole of left kidney
19 Branches of left colic vessels
20 Descending colon
21 Pelvis of kidney
22 Gonadal artery
23 Gonadal vein
24 Inferior mesenteric vein
25 Psoas major
26 Genitofemoral nerve
27 Ureter
28 Left colic artery
29 Cut edge of peritoneum

A Inferior mesenteric vessels, from the front

The stomach (13) and transverse colon (15) are lifted upwards. The peritoneum of the posterior abdominal wall has been removed and the left-sided parts of the duodenum (3 and 4) reflected towards the right, to show the origin of the inferior mesenteric artery (5) from the aorta (6). The lower border of the pancreas (11) has been lifted up, revealing the splenic vein (10) with the inferior mesenteric (24) running into it. The ureter (27) has the gonadal vessels (22 and 23) in front of it and the genitofemoral nerve (26) behind it, lying on psoas major (25)

• In this specimen (as in D on page 241) the gonadal (testicular) artery (22) arises from the renal artery (17) and not from the aorta (6).

B **Radiograph of the large intestine**
In this double-contrast barium enema (barium and air), the sacculations (haustrations, 3) of the various parts of the colon allow it to be distinguished from the narrower terminal ileum (9), which has become partly filled by barium flowing into it through the ileocaecal junction (10)

1 Right colic (hepatic) flexure	7 Hip joint
2 Transverse colon	8 Rectum
3 Sacculations	9 Terminal ileum
4 Left colic (splenic) flexure	10 Ileocaecal junction
5 Descending colon	11 Caecum
6 Sigmoid colon	12 Ascending colon

C Small bowel enema via a tube in the duodenum

1 Stomach	3 Coils of jejunum
2 Descending (second) part of duodenum	4 Coils of ileum
	5 Valvulae conniventes

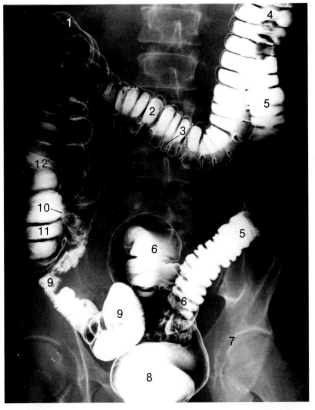

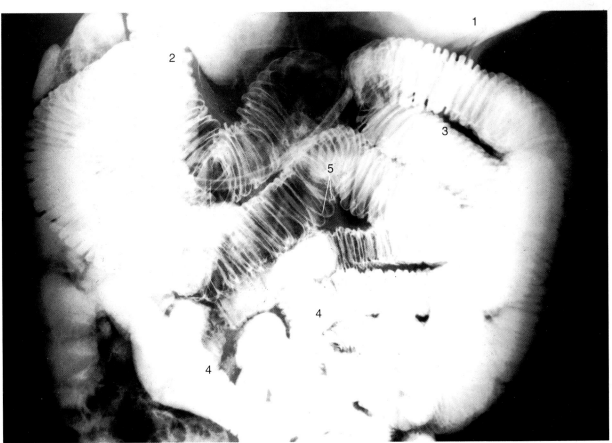

A

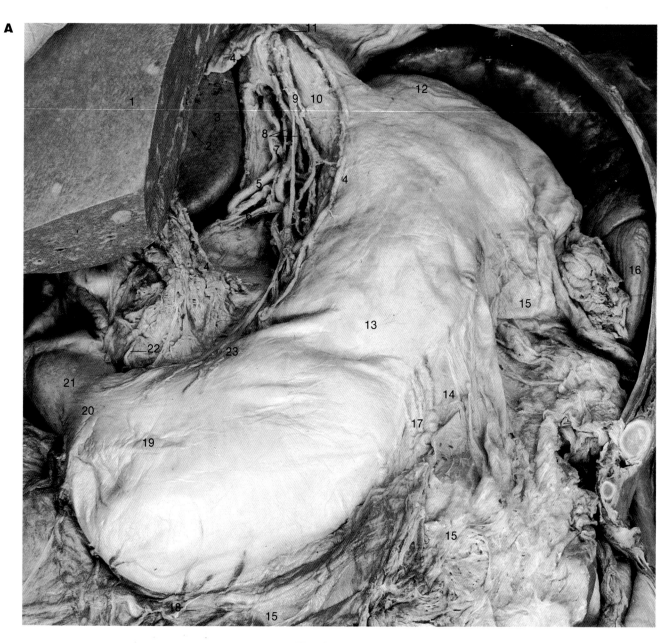

• For a diagrammatic representation of the peritoneal layers forming the omenta see page 214.

Stomach, **A** with vessels and vagus nerves, from the front, **B** radiograph after barium meal

The anterior thoracic and abdominal walls and the left lobe of the liver have been removed, with part of the lesser omentum (4), to show the stomach (12, 13, 19 and 20) in its undisturbed position. The removal of the upper part of the lesser omentum between the liver (1) and the lesser curvature of the stomach (23) has displayed the left gastric vessels (5 and 6) and branches, with the anterior and posterior vagal trunks (9 and 7) which enter the abdomen with the lower end of the oesophagus (10) through the oesophageal opening in the diaphragm (11). The greater omentum (15) remains at the greater curvature, with the gastro-epiploic vessels (17 and 18) between the layers of the omentum. In B flecks of barium adhere to the mucosa of the upper part of the stomach (13). Note the constriction of the gut lumen at the pyloric canal (20)

1 Right lobe of liver	12 Fundus ⎫
2 Fissure for ligamentum venosum	13 Body ⎬ of stomach
3 Caudate lobe of liver	14 Greater curvature ⎭
4 Lesser omentum (cut edge)	15 Greater omentum
5 Left gastric artery	16 Lower end of spleen
6 Left gastric vein	17 Branches of left gastro-epiploic vessels
7 Posterior vagal trunk	18 Right gastro-epiploic vessels and branches
8 Oesophageal branches of left gastric vessels	19 Pyloric antrum
9 Anterior vagal trunk	20 Pyloric canal
10 Oesophagus	21 Superior (first) part of duodenum
11 Oesophageal opening in diaphragm	22 Right gastric artery
	23 Lesser curvature of stomach

B

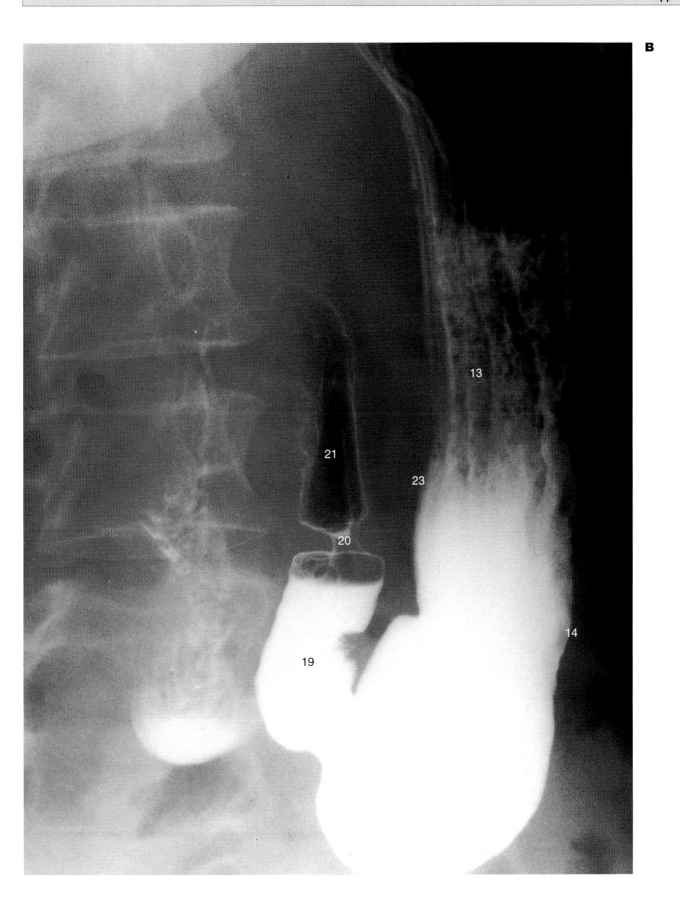

A

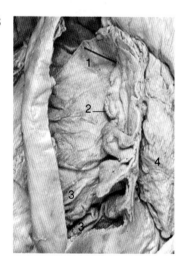

A Duodenum and pancreas

The stomach (4) has been lifted up, the colon and the peritoneum of the posterior abdominal wall removed and branches of the superior mesenteric vessels (13 and 14) cut off. The C-shaped duodenum (24, 21, 15 and 9) is seen embracing the head of the pancreas (23); the neck (5) and body (6) of the pancreas have been displaced slightly upwards to show the splenic vein (7) joining the superior mesenteric vein (14) (to form the portal vein behind the neck of the pancreas). The descending (second) part of the duodenum (21) overlaps the hilum of the right kidney (20). The superior mesenteric artery (13) and vein (14) cross the uncinate process (8) of the head of the pancreas and then the horizontal (third) part of the duodenum (15)

1 Right lobe of liver	15 Horizontal (third) part of duodenum
2 Falciform ligament	
3 Left lobe of liver	16 Abdominal aorta
4 Posterior surface of greater omentum overlying stomach	17 Inferior vena cava
	18 Gonadal vein
5 Neck } of pancreas	19 Ureter
6 Body	20 Right kidney
7 Splenic vein	21 Descending (second) part of duodenum
8 Uncinate process of head of pancreas	
	22 Branches of pancreaticoduodenal vessels
9 Ascending (fourth) part of duodenum	
	23 Head of pancreas
10 Sympathetic trunk	24 Superior (first) part of duodenum
11 Gonadal artery	
12 Psoas major	25 Gall bladder
13 Superior mesenteric artery	
14 Superior mesenteric vein	

B

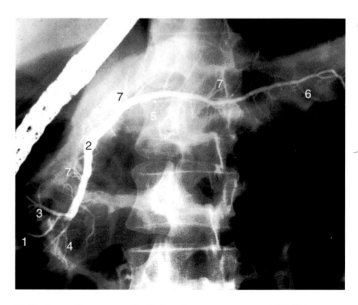

B Duodenal papillae

The anterior wall of the descending (second) part of the duodenum has been removed. A bristle has been placed in the opening of the minor duodenal papilla (1), which is about 1.5 cm above the major papilla (2)

1 Bristle in minor duodenal papilla	3 Circular folds of mucous membrane
2 Major duodenal papilla	4 Head of pancreas

C Endoscopic retrograde cholangiopancreatogram (ERCP)

See page 227 for explanation

1 Cannula in ampulla	4 Head of pancreas
2 Pancreatic duct (Wirsung)	5 Body of pancreas
3 Accessory pancreatic duct (Santorini)	6 Tail of pancreas
	7 Intralobular ducts

Liver, from above and in front

Part of the diaphragm (2 and 6) remains attached, with a portion of fibrous pericardium (5)

1 Right triangular ligament
2 Diaphragm overlying bare area
3 Superior layer of coronary ligament
4 Inferior vena cava
5 Fibrous pericardium
6 Diaphragm overlying left triangular ligament
7 Superior ⎫
8 Anterior ⎬ surface of left lobe
9 Falciform ligament
10 Anterior ⎫
11 Superior ⎬ surface of right lobe
12 Right surface

● The surfaces of the liver are named as diaphragmatic and visceral (or inferior).
● The diaphragmatic surface can be subdivided into anterior (8 and 10), superior (7 and 11), right (12), and posterior surfaces, but they merge into one another without distinct boundaries, as does the inferior or visceral surface with the posterior.

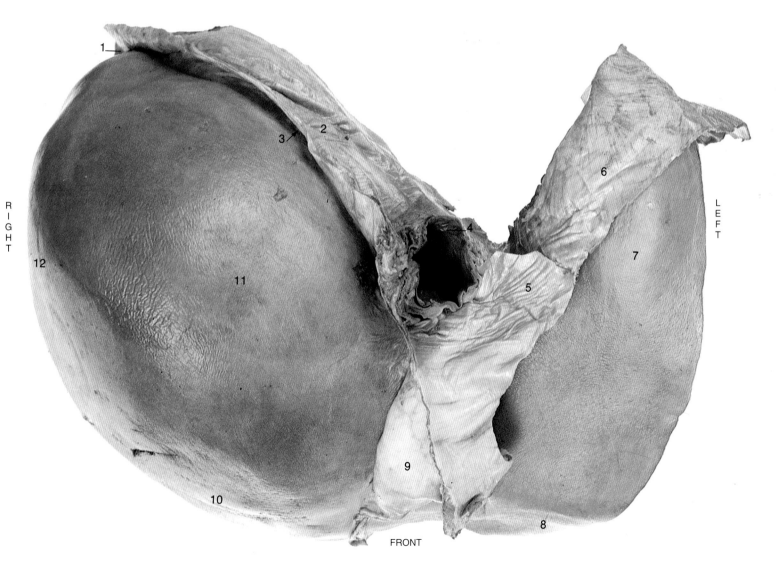

A Liver, from below and behind

Looking from below and behind with the front edge of the liver lifted, this view shows the posterior and inferior (visceral) surfaces, with no clear demarcation between them. As a general guide, note that the bare area (20) and groove for the inferior vena cava (10) are on the posterior surface, and the fossa for the gall bladder (1) and the structures of the porta hepatis (14–17) on the inferior surface. The inferior layer of the coronary ligament is here Z-shaped (at the three key-number 19s); it is normally straight

1	Gall bladder	11	Lesser omentum in fissure for ligamentum venosum
2	Quadrate lobe	12	Caudate lobe
3	Ligamentum teres and falciform ligament in fissure for ligamentum teres	13	Caudate process
4	Omental tuberosity	14	Right free margin of lesser omentum in porta hepatis
5	Gastric impression	15	Hepatic artery
6	Left lobe	16	Portal vein
7	Left triangular ligament	17	Common hepatic duct
8	Diaphragm	18	Suprarenal impression
9	Oesophageal groove	19	Inferior layer of coronary ligament
10	Inferior vena cava	20	Bare area
		21	Diaphragm on part of bare area (obstructing view of superior layer of coronary ligament)
		22	Right triangular ligament
		23	Renal impression
		24	Right lobe
		25	Colic impression
		26	Duodenal impression

• The caudate (12) and quadrate (2) lobes are classified *anatomically* as part of the right lobe (24), but *functionally* they belong to the left lobe (6), since they receive blood from the left branches of the hepatic artery and portal vein, and drain bile to the left hepatic duct.
• The caudate *process* (13) joins the caudate lobe (12) to the right lobe (24). It is the caudate process (not the caudate lobe) that forms the upper boundary of the epiploic foramen (page 211).
• The posterior surface contains the bare area (20), the groove for the inferior vena cava (10), the caudate lobe (12) and the fissure for the ligamentum venosum (11), the suprarenal impression (18) and most of the right renal impression (23).

• The inferior (visceral) surface contains the porta hepatis where the hepatic artery (15), portal vein (16) and hepatic ducts (17) enter or leave, enclosed within the peritoneum forming the right free margin of the lesser omentum (14). It also contains the quadrate lobe (2), the fossa for the gall bladder (1), the fissure for the ligamentum teres (3), and the gastric (5), duodenal (26) and colic (25) impressions.

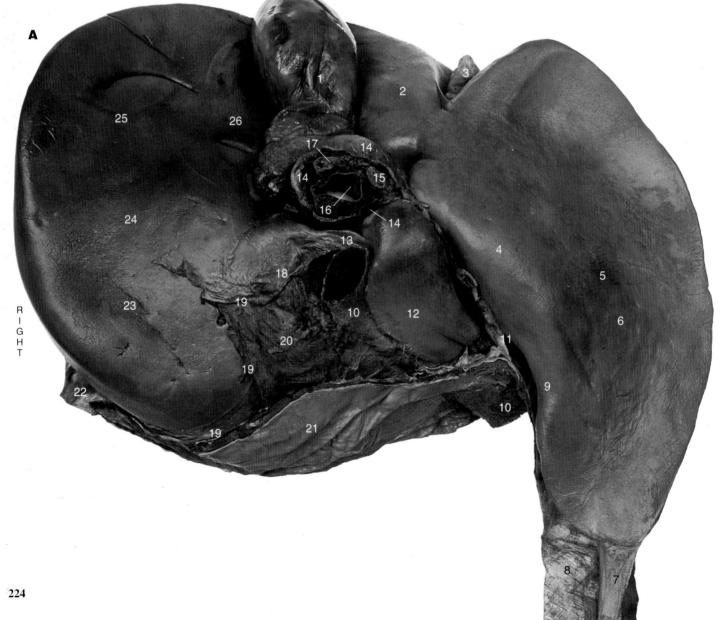

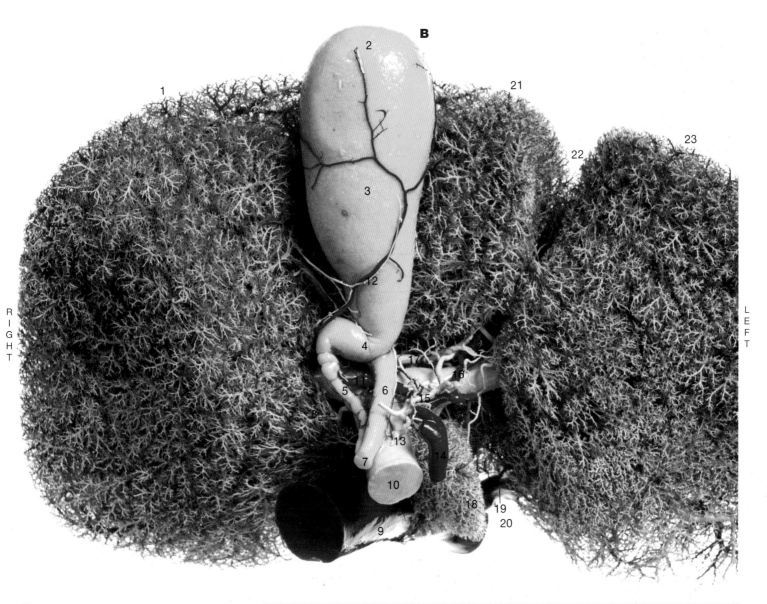

B

B Cast of the liver, extrahepatic biliary tract and associated vessels, from behind

Yellow = gall bladder and biliary tract
Red = hepatic artery and branches
Light blue = portal vein and tributaries
Dark blue = inferior vena cava, hepatic veins and tributaries

This view, like that of A opposite, shows the inferior and posterior surfaces, as when looking into the abdomen from below with the lower border of the liver pushed up towards the thorax

1	Right lobe	13	Right gastric vein
2	Fundus ⎫	14	Hepatic artery
3	Body ⎬ of gall bladder	15	Left gastric vein
4	Neck ⎭	16	Left branch of hepatic artery overlying left
5	Cystic duct		branch of portal vein
6	Common hepatic duct	17	Left hepatic duct
7	Bile duct	18	Caudate lobe
8	Caudate process	19	Left hepatic vein
9	Inferior vena cava	20	Fissure for ligamentum venosum
10	Portal vein	21	Quadrate lobe
11	Right branch of hepatic artery overlying right	22	Fissure for ligamentum teres
	branch of portal vein	23	Left lobe
12	Cystic artery and veins		

• The hepatic artery (14) divides like a Y into left (16) and right (11) branches.
• The portal vein (10) divides like a T into left (16) and right (11) branches.
• The common hepatic duct (6) is formed by the union of the left (17) and right (obscured) hepatic ducts, and is joined by the cystic duct (5) to form the bile duct (7).

FROM BEHIND

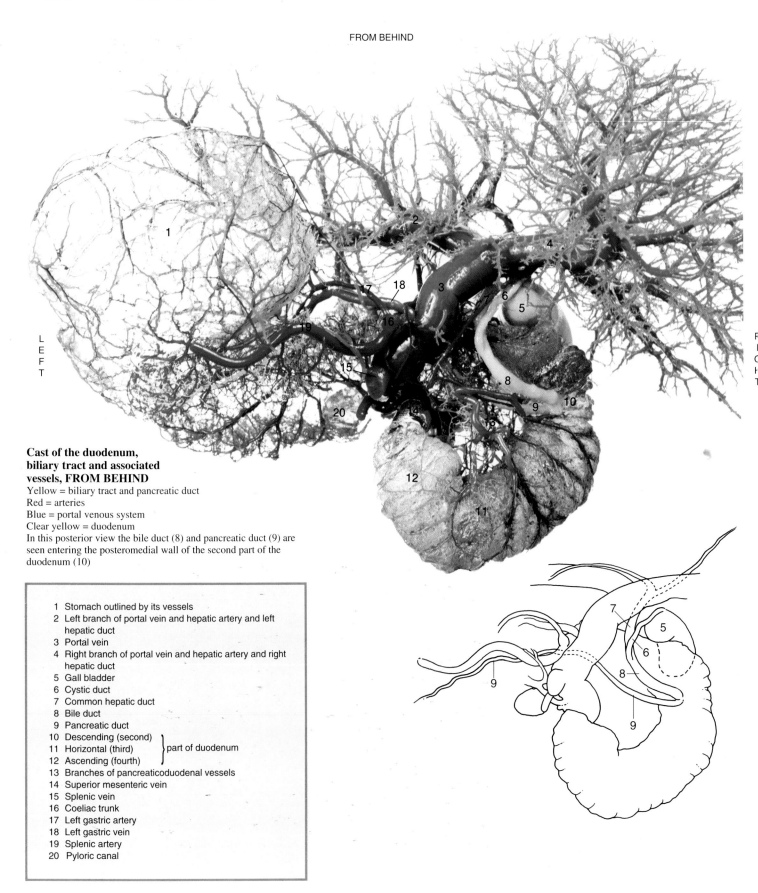

**Cast of the duodenum,
biliary tract and associated
vessels, FROM BEHIND**

Yellow = biliary tract and pancreatic duct
Red = arteries
Blue = portal venous system
Clear yellow = duodenum

In this posterior view the bile duct (8) and pancreatic duct (9) are
seen entering the posteromedial wall of the second part of the
duodenum (10)

1 Stomach outlined by its vessels
2 Left branch of portal vein and hepatic artery and left
   hepatic duct
3 Portal vein
4 Right branch of portal vein and hepatic artery and right
   hepatic duct
5 Gall bladder
6 Cystic duct
7 Common hepatic duct
8 Bile duct
9 Pancreatic duct
10 Descending (second) ⎫
11 Horizontal (third)   ⎬ part of duodenum
12 Ascending (fourth)   ⎭
13 Branches of pancreaticoduodenal vessels
14 Superior mesenteric vein
15 Splenic vein
16 Coeliac trunk
17 Left gastric artery
18 Left gastric vein
19 Splenic artery
20 Pyloric canal

A Radiography of the gall bladder. Endoscopic retrograde cholangiopancreatogram (ERCP)

In ERCP an endoscope is passed through the mouth, pharynx, oesophagus and stomach into the duodenum, and through it a cannula is introduced into the major duodenal papilla (page 222, B2) and bile duct so that contrast medium can be injected up the biliary tract. (The pancreatic duct can also be cannulated in this way—see C on page 222)

1 Liver shadow and tributaries of hepatic ducts
2 Right hepatic duct
3 Left hepatic duct
4 Common hepatic duct
5 Cystic duct
6 Gall bladder
7 Bile duct

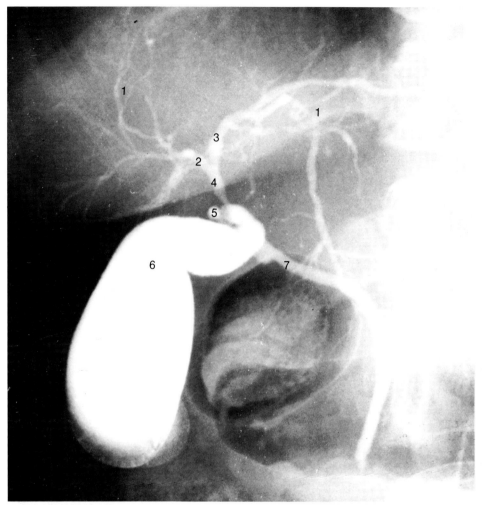

A

B Ultrasound scan of the gall bladder

To an untrained observer, ultrasound scans are difficult to interpret but here the gall bladder can be distinguished as a sausage-shaped cavity (2)

1 Liver
2 Gall bladder
3 Diaphragm

• Ultrasound scans are best interpreted by the operator on a screen.

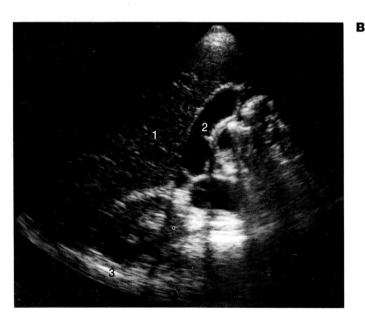

B

227

A Cast of the hepatic vessels and associated structures, FROM ABOVE AND BEHIND

Green = biliary tract
Yellow = pancreatic duct
Red = arteries
Blue = portal venous system
Clear yellow = duodenum

The areas 1 to 4 demarcated by the interrupted lines indicate the four main segments of the liver. The specimen shows an accessory left hepatic artery (19) arising from the left gastric (18), a common occurrence. The accessory pancreatic duct (7) is seen entering the duodenum (6) proximal to the entry of the bile duct (8) and pancreatic duct (9)

1 Left lateral	12 Superior mesenteric artery
2 Left medial	13 Portal vein
3 Right anterior } segments of liver	14 Left gastric vein
4 Right posterior	15 Common hepatic artery
5 Gall bladder	16 Gastroduodenal artery
6 Descending (second) part of duodenum	17 Coeliac trunk
7 Accessory pancreatic duct	18 Left gastric artery
8 Bile duct	19 Accessory hepatic artery
9 Pancreatic duct	20 Splenic artery
10 Inferior pancreaticoduodenal vessels	21 Splenic vein
11 Superior mesenteric vein	

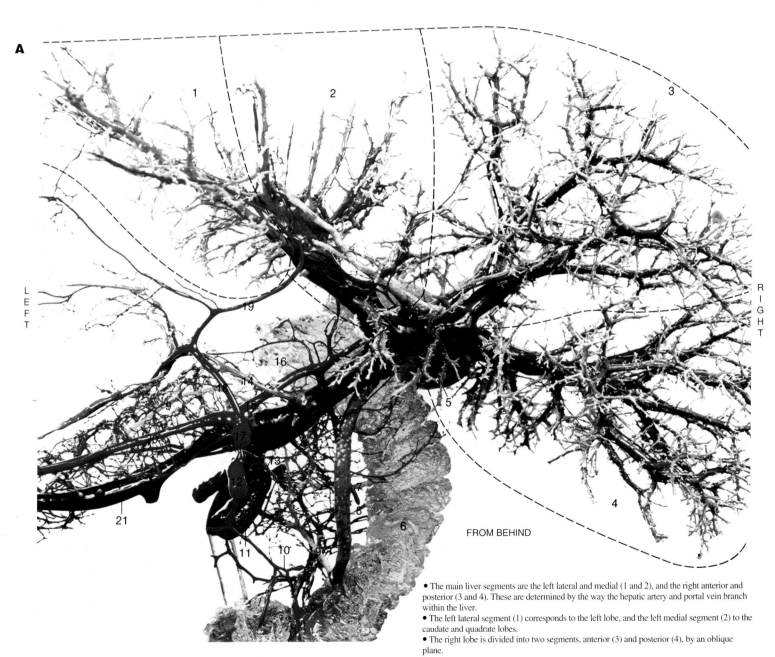

A

FROM BEHIND

• The main liver segments are the left lateral and medial (1 and 2), and the right anterior and posterior (3 and 4). These are determined by the way the hepatic artery and portal vein branch within the liver.
• The left lateral segment (1) corresponds to the left lobe, and the left medial segment (2) to the caudate and quadrate lobes.
• The right lobe is divided into two segments, anterior (3) and posterior (4), by an oblique plane.

B **Cast of the portal vein and tributaries, and the mesenteric vessels, FROM BEHIND**

Yellow = biliary tract and pancreatic ducts
Red = arteries
Blue = portal venous system

In this posterior view (chosen in preference to the anterior view, where the many very small vessels to the intestines would have obscured the larger branches), the superior mesenteric vein (22) is seen continuing upwards to become the portal vein (8) after it has been joined by the splenic vein (2). In the porta hepatis the portal vein divides into its left and right branches (9 and 10). Due to removal of the aorta, the upper part of the inferior mesenteric artery (17) has become displaced slightly to the right and appears to have given origin to the ileocolic artery (16), but this is simply an overlap of the vessels; the origin of the ileocolic from the superior mesenteric is not seen in this view

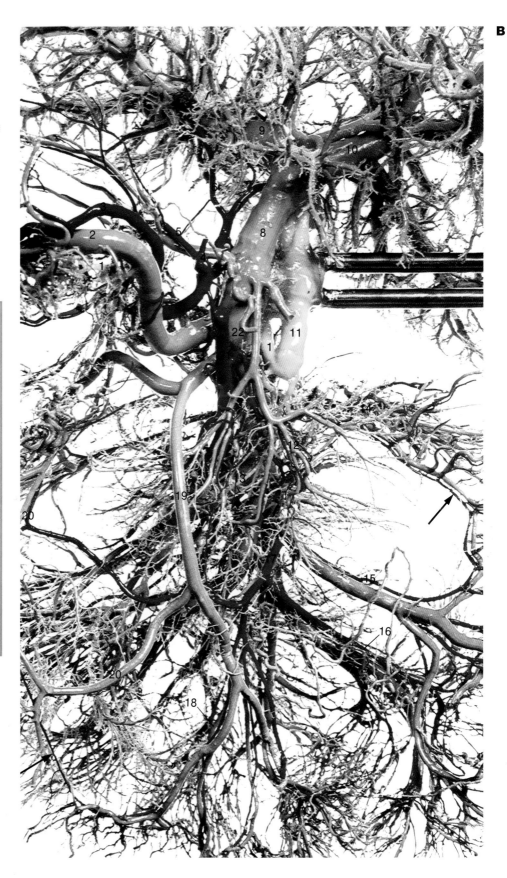

1 Pancreatic duct
2 Splenic vein
3 Splenic artery
4 Coeliac trunk
5 Left gastric artery and vein
6 Left } branch of
7 Right } hepatic artery
8 Portal vein
9 Left } branch of
10 Right } portal vein
11 Bile duct
12 Pancreaticoduodenal vessels
13 Pancreatic ducts in head of pancreas
14 Branches of middle colic vessels
15 Right colic vessels
16 Ileocolic vessels
17 Inferior mesenteric artery
18 Sigmoid vessels
19 Inferior mesenteric vein
20 Left colic vessels
21 Superior mesenteric artery
22 Superior mesenteric vein

• The inferior mesenteric vein (19) normally drains into the splenic vein (2) behind the body of the pancreas, but it may join the splenic vein nearer the union with the superior mesenteric vein or (as in this specimen) enter the superior mesenteric vein itself (22).
• The colic arteries (14, 15, 16, 20) anastomose with one another near the colonic wall forming what is often called the marginal artery (as at the arrows).

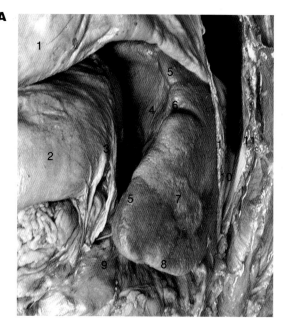

A Spleen, from the front

The left upper anterior abdominal and lower anterior thoracic walls have been removed and part of the diaphragm (1) turned upwards to show the spleen in its normal position, lying adjacent to the stomach (2) and colon (9), with the lower part against the kidney (D9 and 10, opposite)

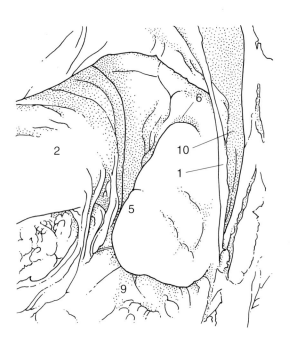

1	Diaphragm
2	Stomach
3	Gastrosplenic ligament
4	Gastric impression
5	Superior border
6	Notch
7	Diaphragmatic surface
8	Inferior border
9	Left colic flexure
10	Costodiaphragmatic recess
11	Thoracic wall

• The gastrosplenic ligament contains the short gastric and left gastro-epiploic branches of the splenic vessels.
• The lienorenal ligament contains the tail of the pancreas and the splenic vessels.

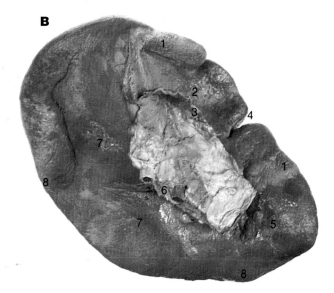

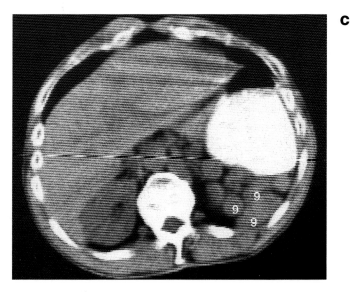

Spleen, B visceral surface, C CT scan (polysplenia)

In B the spleen has been removed and its visceral or medial surface is shown, with a small part of the gastrosplenic (3) and lienorenal (6) ligaments remaining attached. The scan of the upper abdomen shows a developmental anomaly—several small splenunculi (9) instead of a single organ

1	Superior border	5	Colic impression
2	Gastric impression	6	Tail of pancreas and splenic vessels in lienorenal ligament
3	Gastrosplenic ligament containing short gastric and left gastro-epiploic vessels	7	Renal impression
4	Notch	8	Inferior border
		9	Spleen—multiple splenunculi

D Spleen, in a transverse section of the left upper abdomen

The section is at the level of the disc (18) between the twelfth thoracic and first lumbar vertebrae, and is viewed from below looking towards the thorax. The spleen (9) lies against the diaphragm (3) and left kidney (10) but separated from them by peritoneum of the greater sac (8). The peritoneum behind the stomach (2) forming part of the gastrosplenic (4) and lienorenal (15) ligaments belongs to the lesser sac (16)

D

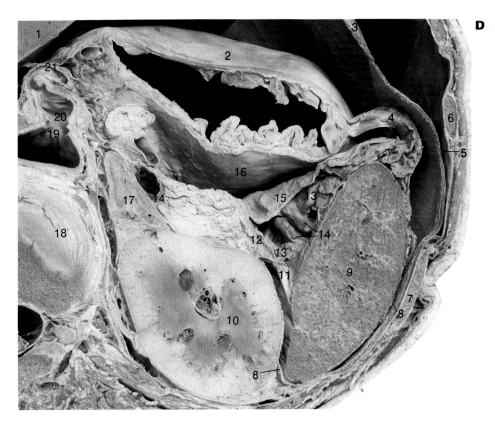

1	Left lobe of liver
2	Stomach
3	Diaphragm
4	Gastrosplenic ligament
5	Costodiaphragmatic recess of pleura
6	Ninth rib
7	Tenth rib
8	Peritoneum of greater sac
9	Spleen
10	Left kidney
11	Posterior layer of lienorenal ligament
12	Tail of pancreas
13	Splenic artery
14	Splenic vein
15	Anterior layer of lienorenal ligament
16	Lesser sac
17	Left suprarenal gland
18	Intervertebral disc
19	Abdominal aorta
20	Coeliac trunk
21	Left gastric artery

● The position of the *base* (E7) of the appendix (properly called the vermiform appendix) is constant, opening (F3) just below and behind the ileocaecal valve (F2), but the *tip* may lie in a variety of positions—over the pelvic brim, behind the caecum or ascending colon, below the caecum, or behind or in front of the terminal part of the ileum.

● The three taeniae coli of the ascending colon and caecum converge on the base of the appendix (E3 and E7), and serve as useful guides to the base.

E Caecum and appendix, from the front

The terminal ileum (5) is seen joining the large intestine at the junction of the caecum (2) and ascending colon (1), and the appendix (7) joins the caecum just below the ileocaecal junction

1	Ascending colon
2	Caecum
3	Anterior taenia coli
4	Superior ileocaecal recess
5	Terminal ileum
6	Inferior ileocaecal recess
7	Base } of appendix
8	Tip
9	Peritoneum overlying external iliac vessels
10	Retrocaecal recess

F

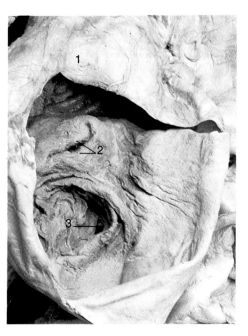

F Interior of the caecum

The anterior wall has been cut open and reflected to show the lips of the ileocaecal valve (2) and the opening of the appendix (3)

1	Ascending colon
2	Lips of ileocaecal valve
3	Opening of appendix

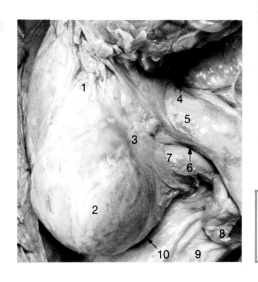

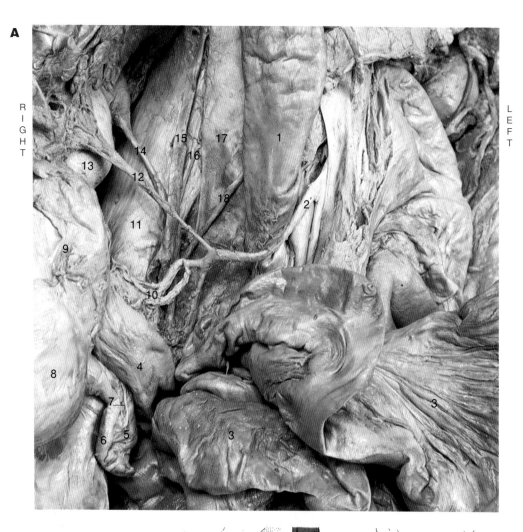

A Appendix, ileocolic artery and related structures, from the front

Most of the peritoneum of the mesentery and posterior abdominal wall have been removed, and coils of small intestine (3) have been displaced to the right of the picture, to show the ileocolic artery (2), terminal ileum (4) and appendix (6) with its appendicular artery (7)

1 Descending (second) part of duodenum
2 Ileocolic artery
3 Mesentery and coils of jejunum and ileum
4 Terminal part of ileum
5 Mesoappendix
6 Appendix
7 Appendicular artery in mesoappendix
8 Caecum
9 Ascending colon
10 Ileal and caecal vessels
11 Psoas major
12 Right colic artery
13 Lower pole of kidney
14 Ureter
15 Testicular vein
16 Genitofemoral nerve
17 Inferior vena cava
18 Testicular artery

• The appendix gets its blood supply from the appendicular artery (7), normally a branch of one of the caecal arteries (10), usually the posterior caecal. The vessel is not at first closely applied to the appendix but approaches it through the mesoappendix (5), the peritoneal fold continuous with the lower part of the mesentery of the terminal ileum (4). If this arterial supply becomes obstructed, the appendix becomes necrotic, as there is no collateral circulation.

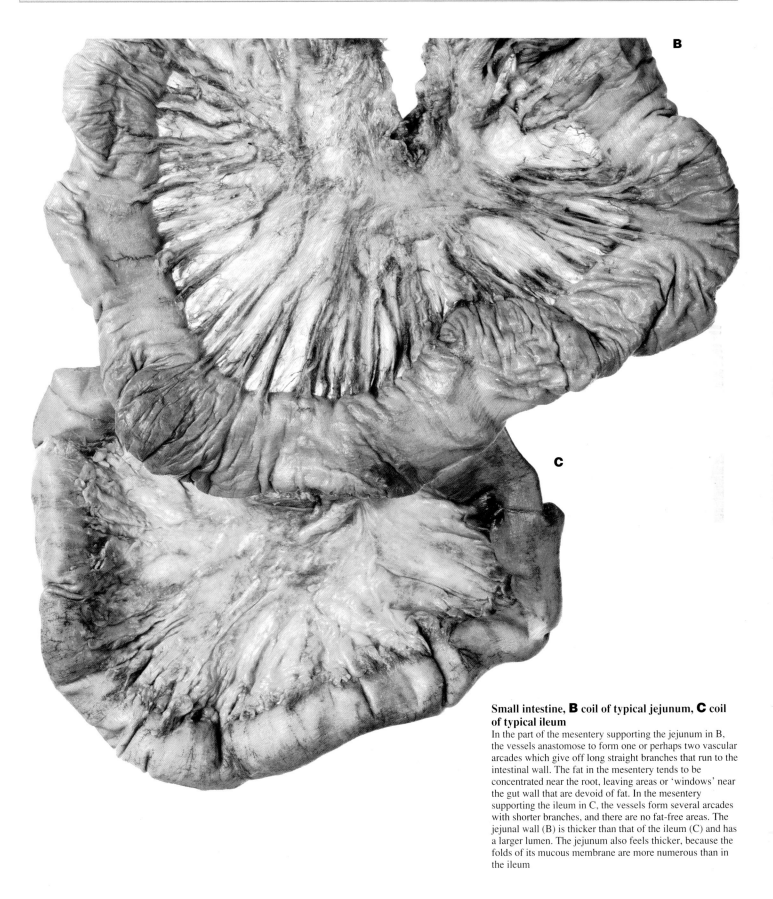

Small intestine, B coil of typical jejunum, C coil of typical ileum

In the part of the mesentery supporting the jejunum in B, the vessels anastomose to form one or perhaps two vascular arcades which give off long straight branches that run to the intestinal wall. The fat in the mesentery tends to be concentrated near the root, leaving areas or 'windows' near the gut wall that are devoid of fat. In the mesentery supporting the ileum in C, the vessels form several arcades with shorter branches, and there are no fat-free areas. The jejunal wall (B) is thicker than that of the ileum (C) and has a larger lumen. The jejunum also feels thicker, because the folds of its mucous membrane are more numerous than in the ileum

233

Kidneys and suprarenal glands, **A** dissection, **B** axial MR image

The kidneys (13 and 30) and suprarenal glands (11 and 33) are displayed on the posterior abdominal wall after the removal of all other viscera. The left renal vein (15) receives the left suprarenal (12) and gonadal (17) veins (and in this specimen an unusually large tributary from lumbar veins, 16) and then passes over the aorta (22) and deep to the superior mesenteric artery (10) to reach the inferior vena cava (24). In the hilum of the right kidney (30) a large branch of the renal artery (31) passes in front of the renal vein (32). The origins of the renal arteries from the aorta are not seen because they underlie the left renal vein (15) and inferior vena cava (24). The MR image in B passes through the kidneys but is too low to show the suprarenal glands

- Because of the forward bulge of the lumbar part of the vertebral column on the posterior abdominal wall, the kidneys do not lie flat but are tilted at an angle, each hanging down into the 'gutter' at the side of the lumbar vertebrae and the psoas major muscle (A19), as though suspended there by the renal vessels (A14 and 15) extending into the hilum from the aorta and inferior vena cava (A22 and 24).
- The hilum of the kidney (see the notes opposite) is the region at the medial border occupied by the renal vessels (as at A31 and 32) and by the renal pelvis (hidden behind the vessels) which becomes the ureter (as at A27).
- Because of the bulk of the liver on the right side, the right kidney lies at a slightly lower level than the left (see the surface markings on page 199).
- The right suprarenal gland (A33) overlaps the top of the upper pole of the right kidney (A30).
- The left suprarenal gland (A11) lies along the medial border of the upper pole of the left kidney (A13).

1	Right crus of diaphragm	19	Left psoas major
2	Common hepatic artery	20	Left gonadal artery
3	Left gastric artery	21	Left sympathetic trunk
4	Splenic artery	22	Abdominal aorta and aortic plexus
5	Left crus of diaphragm	23	Inferior mesenteric artery
6	Left inferior phrenic artery	24	Inferior vena cava
7	Left inferior phrenic vein	25	Right gonadal artery
8	Coeliac trunk	26	Right gonadal vein
9	Left coeliac ganglion	27	Right ureter
10	Superior mesenteric artery	28	Right ilio-inguinal nerve
11	Left suprarenal gland	29	Right iliohypogastric nerve
12	Left suprarenal vein	30	Right kidney
13	Left kidney	31	Right renal artery
14	Left renal artery	32	Right renal vein
15	Left renal vein	33	Right suprarenal gland
16	Lumbar tributary of renal vein	34	Right inferior phrenic artery
17	Left gonadal vein	35	Right coeliac ganglion
18	Left ureter	36	A hepatic vein

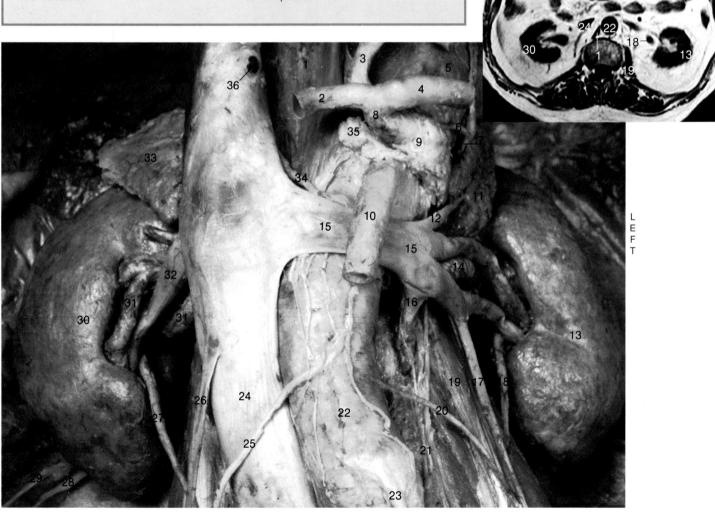

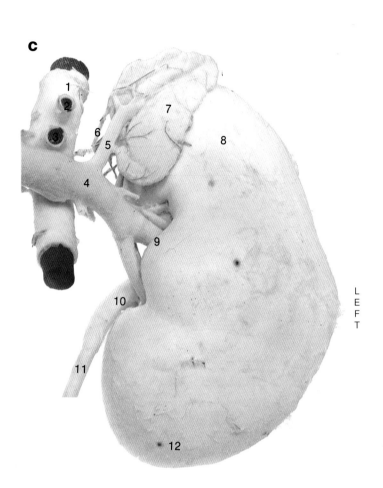

C Left kidney, suprarenal gland and related vessels, from the front

The vessels have been distended by injection of resin, and all fascia has been removed, but the suprarenal gland (7) has been retained in its normal position, lying against the medial side of the upper pole of the kidney (8)

D Right kidney, suprarenal gland and related vessels, from behind

Similar to B, but note that this is the right kidney from behind, not the left; the hilum of each kidney faces medially

1	Abdominal aorta	7	Suprarenal gland
2	Coeliac trunk	8	Upper pole of kidney
3	Superior mesenteric artery	9	Hilum of kidney
4	Left renal vein overlying renal artery	10	Pelvis of kidney
5	Left suprarenal vein	11	Ureter
6	Suprarenal arteries	12	Lower pole of kidney

1	Right renal artery	6	Hilum of kidney
2	Right inferior phrenic artery	7	Pelvis of kidney
3	Suprarenal arteries	8	Lower pole of kidney
4	Suprarenal gland	9	Ureter
5	Upper pole of kidney	10	Inferior vena cava

● The ureter (C11, D9) is the constricted downward continuation of the pelvis of the kidney (C10, D7). Note that the correct term is pelvis of the kidney or renal pelvis, not pelvis of the ureter.

● In the hilum of the kidney, the order of the principal structures from front to back is usually remembered as vein, artery, ureter (strictly speaking, pelvis—see note above), although small branches of the vessels may sometimes get out of order. Compare with vein, artery, bronchus in the hilum of the lung (page 178).

● Each suprarenal gland receives arteries from three sources—the inferior phrenic artery, the aorta and the renal artery—but there are not just three arteries; there are several from each source, perhaps up to a total of 20, and only some of the larger ones are shown (as at D3).

● There is usually only one suprarenal vein on each side. On the left (C5) it drains into the renal vein (C4); on the right it is very short and runs directly into the inferior vena cava (in D it is hidden by the gland itself, but is shown in the cast on page 237, D2).

● For details of the renal arteries see pages 236 and 237.

235

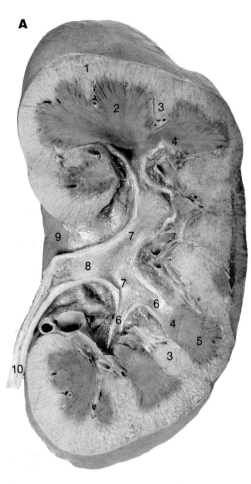

A Kidney. Internal structure in longitudinal section

The section is through the centre of the kidney and has included the renal pelvis (8) and beginning of the ureter (10). The major vessels in the hilum (9) have been removed

1	Cortex	6	Minor calyx
2	Medulla	7	Major calyx
3	Renal column	8	Renal pelvis
4	Renal papilla	9	Hilum
5	Medullary pyramid	10	Ureter

• The renal medulla (2) is made up of the medullary pyramids (5), whose apices form the renal papillae (4) which project into the minor calyces (6).
• The renal columns (3) are the parts of the cortex that intervene between pyramids (5).
• Several minor calyces (6), which receive urine discharged into them from the collecting ducts that open on the renal papillae (4), unite to form a major calyx (7).
• The two or three major calyces (7) unite to form the renal pelvis (8) which passes out through the hilum (9) to become the ureter (10), often with a slight constriction at the junction.
• The hilum is the slit-like space on the medial surface of the kidney where the vessels and renal pelvis enter or leave.

C Cast of the aorta and kidneys, from the front   ▷

Red = arteries
Yellow = urinary tracts
On the right side the ureters (unlabelled) are double, each arising from a separate set of calyces. On the left the arteries are double (4 and 5)

1	Early branching of right renal artery
2	Coeliac trunk
3	Superior mesenteric artery
4	Accessory left renal artery
5	Left renal artery

B Cast of the right kidney, from the front

Red = renal artery
Yellow = urinary tract
The posterior division (2) of the renal artery (1) here passes behind the pelvis (10) and upper calyx (upper 8), but all other vessels are in front of the urinary tract; hence this is a right kidney seen from the front (vein, artery, ureter from front to back, and the hilum on the medial side—see page 235), not a left kidney from behind

1	Renal artery	6	Anterior inferior segment artery
2	Posterior division (forming posterior segment artery)	7	Inferior segment artery
3	Anterior division	8	Major calyx
4	Superior segment artery	9	Minor calyx
5	Anterior superior segment artery (double)	10	Pelvis of kidney
		11	Ureter

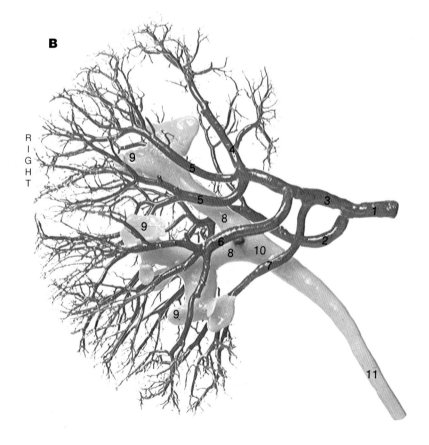

• The kidney has five arterial segments, named posterior, superior, anterior superior, anterior inferior and inferior. Typically the renal artery (1) divides into anterior (3) and posterior (2) divisions; the posterior supplies the posterior segment and the anterior supplies the remainder. However, the pattern of branching displays many variations.
• This specimen shows a fairly typical pattern, although the superior segment (4) obtains a small additional branch from the posterior division (2), and the anterior superior segment receives two major branches (5).

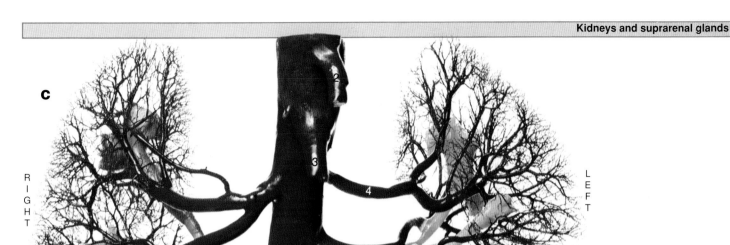

C

RIGHT

LEFT

• Accessory renal arteries represent segmental vessels that arise directly from the aorta. In this specimen, the left accessory vessel (C4) supplies the superior and anterior superior segments, leaving the 'normal' vessel to supply the posterior, anterior inferior and inferior segments.
• The left renal vein (D7) crosses the aorta *below* the origin of the superior mesenteric artery (D6). (The splenic vein crosses the aorta *above* the origin of that artery and below the coeliac trunk, D5.)

1	Right renal vein	7	Left renal vein
2	Right suprarenal vein	8	Left suprarenal veins
3	Inferior vena cava	9	Left renal artery
4	Aorta	10	Accessory renal arteries
5	Coeliac trunk	11	Right renal artery
6	Superior mesenteric artery		

D Cast of the kidneys and great vessels, from the front

Red = arteries
Blue = veins
Yellow = urinary tracts

Here both kidneys show double ureters (unlabelled), and there are accessory renal arteries (10) to the lower poles of both kidneys. The suprarenal glands (also unlabelled) are outlined by their venous patterns, and the short right suprarenal vein (2) is shown draining directly to the inferior vena cava (3). On the left there are two suprarenal veins (8), both draining to the left renal vein (7)

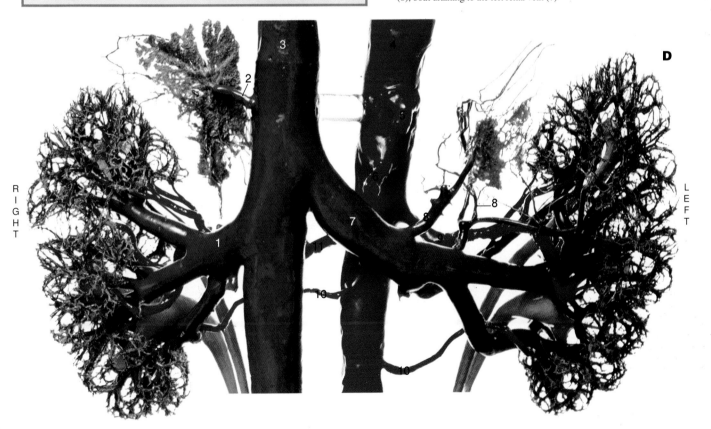

D

RIGHT

LEFT

A

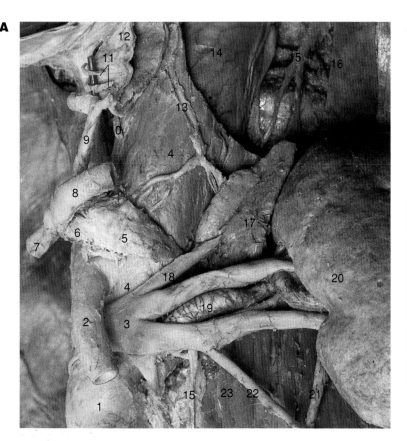

A Left kidney and suprarenal gland, from the front

The left kidney (20) and suprarenal gland (17) are seen on the posterior abdominal wall. Much of the diaphragm has been removed but the oesophageal opening remains, with the end of the oesophagus (12) opening out into the cardiac part of the stomach and a (double) anterior vagal trunk (11) overlying the red marker. The posterior vagal trunk (10) is behind and to the right of the oesophagus. Part of the pleura has been cut away (16) to show the sympathetic trunk (15) on the side of the lower thoracic vertebrae. The left coeliac ganglion and the coeliac plexus (5) are at the root of the coeliac trunk (6)

1	Abdominal aorta	12	Lower end of oesophagus
2	Superior mesenteric artery	13	Inferior phrenic vessels
3	Left renal vein	14	Thoracic aorta
4	Left crus of diaphragm	15	Sympathetic trunk
5	Left coeliac ganglion and coeliac plexus	16	Pleura (cut edge)
6	Coeliac trunk	17	Left suprarenal gland
7	Common hepatic artery	18	Left suprarenal vein
8	Splenic artery	19	Left renal artery
9	Left gastric artery	20	Left kidney
10	Posterior vagal trunk	21	Left ureter
11	Anterior vagal trunk (double, over marker)	22	Left gonadal vein
		23	Psoas major

B

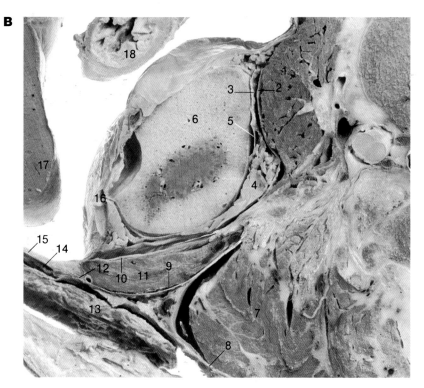

C

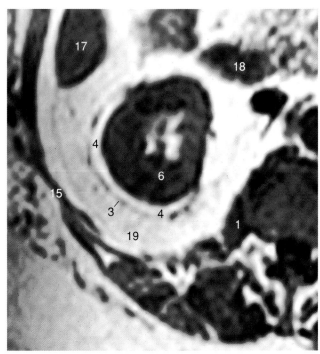

D

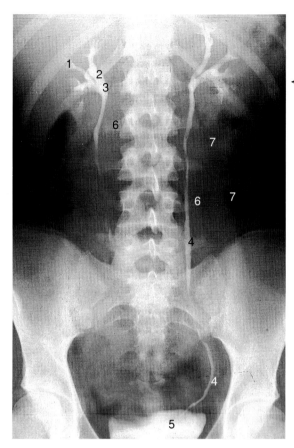

◁

D Intravenous urogram (IVU)

Contrast medium injected intravenously is excreted by the kidneys to outline the calyces (1 and 2), renal pelvis (3) and the ureters (4) which enter the bladder (5) in the pelvis

1 Minor caylx	5 Bladder
2 Major caylx	6 Transverse processes of lumbar
3 Renal pelvis	vertebrae
4 Ureter	7 Psoas shadow

• Radiologically the ureters normally lie near the tips of the transverse processes of the lumbar vertebrae.

E Upper abdomen, coronal MR image

1 Right crus	5 Kidney
2 Oesophageal opening	6 Aorta
3 Left crus	7 Psoas major
4 Second lumbar intervertebral	
disc	

▽

E

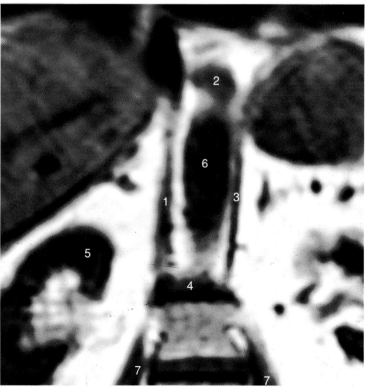

Right kidney and renal fascia, B in transverse section from below, C axial MR image

In the transverse section of the lower part of the right kidney (B), seen from below looking towards the thorax, the renal fascia (3) has been dissected out from the perirenal fat (4) and the kidney's own capsule (5). (There was a small cyst on the surface of this kidney.) The section also displays the three layers (8, 9 and 10) of the lumbar fascia (12; see the notes on page 94). Compare the features seen in the MR image with the section

◁

1 Psoas major	11 Quadratus lumborum
2 Psoas sheath	12 Lumbar fascia
3 Renal fascia	13 External oblique
4 Perirenal fat	14 Internal oblique
5 Renal capsule	15 Transversus abdominis
6 Right kidney	16 Peritoneum
7 Erector spinae	17 Right lobe of liver
8 Posterior layer ⎫ of lumbar	18 Coil of small intestine
9 Middle layer ⎬ fascia	19 Pararenal fat
10 Anterior layer ⎭	

• Outside the kidney's own capsule (renal capsule, 5), there is a variable amount of fat (perirenal fat, 4) and outside this is a condensation of connective tissue forming the renal fascia (3). Retroperitoneal fat, mainly found posteriorly and often called pararenal fat (19), lies outside this fascia, which forms a separate compartment for the suprarenal gland (too high to be seen in this section).

A Surface markings of the kidneys, from behind
The upper pole of the left kidney rises to the level of the eleventh rib, but the right kidney is slightly lower (due to the bulk of the liver on the right). The hilum of each kidney is 5 cm (2 in) from the midline. The lower edge of the costodiaphragmatic recess of the pleura crosses the twelfth rib; compare with the dissection below (B6)

1 Eleventh rib
2 Twelfth rib
3 Right kidney
4 Spinous process of first lumbar vertebra
5 Spinous process of fourth lumbar vertebra
6 Left kidney
7 Lower edge of pleura

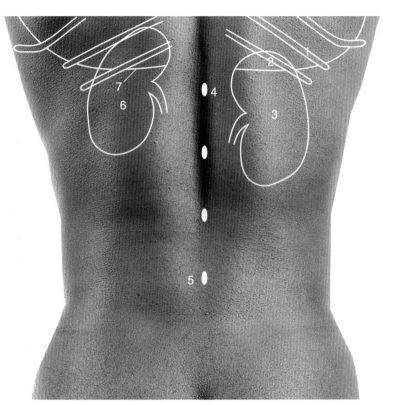

A

B Right kidney, from behind
Most thoracic and abdominal muscles have been removed to show the three nerves (5, 8 and 9) that lie behind the kidney (7). Much more important is the relationship of the upper part of the kidney to the pleura. A window has been cut in the parietal pleura above the twelfth rib (1) to open into the costodiaphragmatic recess (2), whose lower limit (6) runs transversely behind the kidney and in front of the obliquely placed twelfth rib

1 Twelfth rib
2 Costodiaphragmatic recess of pleura
3 Subcostal vein
4 Subcostal artery
5 Subcostal nerve
6 Lower edge of pleura
7 Kidney
8 Iliohypogastric nerve
9 Ilio-inguinal nerve
10 Extraperitoneal tissue
11 Psoas major
12 Transverse process of second lumbar vertebra

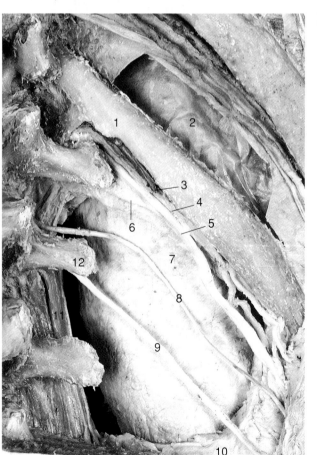

B

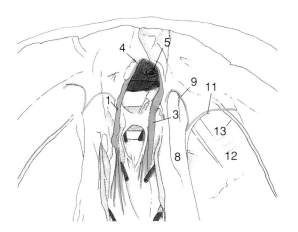

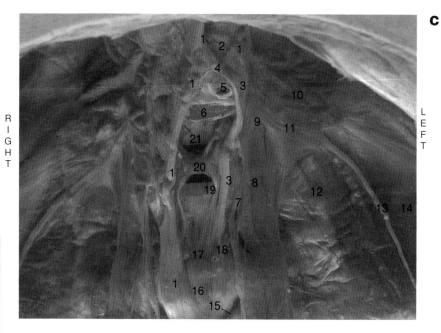

C

1 Right crus	14 Lumbar part of
2 Oesophageal opening	thoracolumbar fascia
3 Left crus	15 Third lumbar artery
4 Median arcuate ligament	16 Second lumbar
5 Coeliac trunk	intervertebral disc
6 Aorta	17 Second lumbar vertebra
7 Sympathetic trunk	18 Second lumbar artery
8 Psoas major	19 First lumbar artery
9 Medial arcuate ligament	20 Abnormal communication
10 Diaphragm	between crura
11 Lateral arcuate ligament	(superficial to marker)
12 Quadratus lumborum	21 Subcostal artery
13 Subcostal nerve	

C Posterior abdominal wall. Crura of the diaphragm

Abdominal contents have been removed and the aorta (6) has been transected immediately below the origin of the coeliac trunk (5), which is just below the median arcuate ligament (4) where the two crura (1 and 3) unite (see page 239, E1 and 3)

- The right crus of the diaphragm (C1) has a more extensive origin (from the upper three lumbar vertebrae and intervening discs) than the left (C3) (from the upper two) because of the greater bulk of the liver on the right; the crura help to pull the liver downwards when the diaphragm contracts.
- Fibres of the *right* crus (C1) form the *right and left* boundaries of the oesophageal opening (C2).

D Posterior abdominal wall, left side

The ureter (5) passes down on psoas major (17) deep to the testicular artery (16) and vein (15); in this specimen the artery has arisen from the renal artery under cover of the renal vein (3) and not from the aorta (20) which is its normal origin. The subcostal, iliohypogastric and ilio-inguinal nerves (11, 9 and 7) emerge from behind the kidney (6). The fourth lumbar artery (14) runs laterally superficial to the lower part of quadratus lumborum (8) above the iliolumbar ligament (13)

1 Suprarenal vein	12 Transversus abdominis
2 Suprarenal gland	13 Iliac crest and iliolumbar
3 Renal vein	ligament
4 Renal artery	14 Fourth lumbar artery
5 Ureter	15 Testicular vein
6 Lower pole of kidney	16 Testicular artery
7 Ilio-inguinal nerve	17 Psoas major
8 Quadratus lumborum	18 Genitofemoral nerve
9 Iliohypogastric nerve	19 Inferior mesenteric artery
10 Lumbar part of	20 Aorta and aortic plexus
thoracolumbar fascia	21 Sympathetic trunk and
11 Subcostal nerve	ganglion

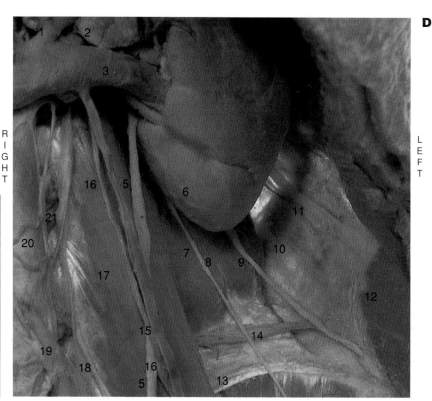

D

A

RIGHT

LEFT

A Posterior abdominal and pelvic walls

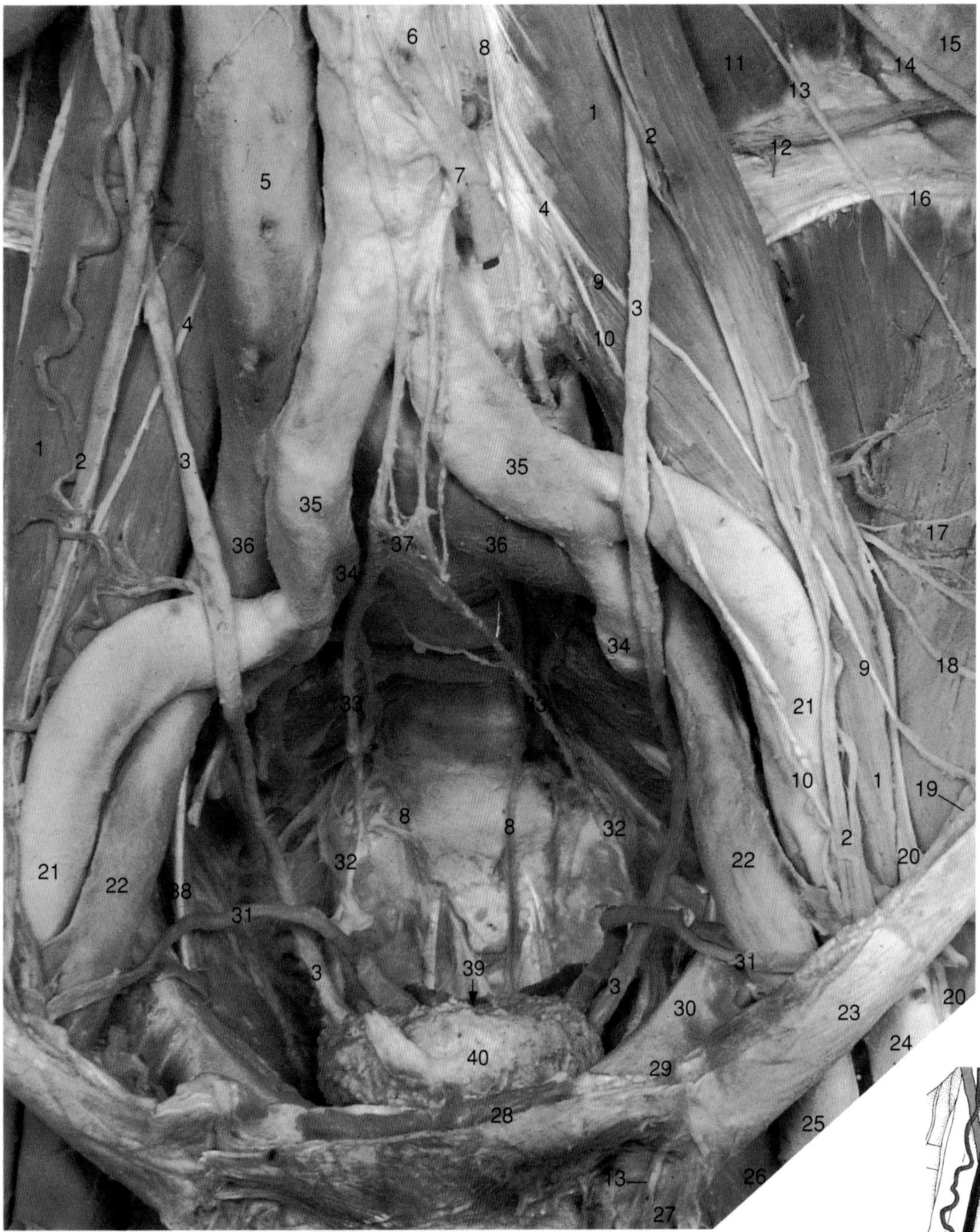

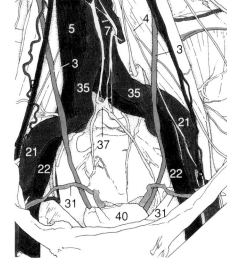

All peritoneum and viscera (except for the bladder, 40, ureter, 3, and ductus deferens or vas deferens, 31) have been removed, to display vessels and nerves

1 Psoas major
2 Testicular vessels
3 Ureter
4 Genitofemoral nerve
5 Inferior vena cava
6 Aorta and aortic plexus
7 Inferior mesenteric artery and plexus
8 Sympathetic trunk and ganglia
9 Femoral } branch of genito-
10 Genital } femoral nerve
11 Quadratus lumborum
12 Fourth lumbar artery
13 Ilio-inguinal nerve
14 Iliohypogastric nerve
15 Lumbar part of thoracolumbar fascia
16 Iliolumbar ligament
17 Iliacus and branches from femoral nerve and iliolumbar artery
18 Lateral femoral cutaneous nerve arising from femoral nerve
19 Deep circumflex iliac artery
20 Femoral nerve
21 External iliac artery
22 External iliac vein
23 Inguinal ligament
24 Femoral artery

25 Femoral vein
26 Position of femoral canal
27 Spermatic cord
28 Rectus abdominis
29 Lacunar ligament
30 Pectineal ligament
31 Ductus deferens
32 Inferior hypogastric (pelvic) plexus and pelvic splanchnic nerves
33 Hypogastric nerve
34 Internal iliac artery
35 Common iliac artery
36 Common iliac vein
37 Superior hypogastric plexus
38 Obturator nerve and vessels
39 Rectum (cut edge)
40 Bladder

• The aorta (A6) bifurcates into the common iliac arteries (A35) at the level of the fourth lumbar vertebra.

• The common iliac veins (A36) unite at the level of the fifth lumbar vertebra to form the inferior vena cava (A5), which lies on the right of the aorta (A6).

• On psoas major (A1) the ureter (A3) lies with the genitofemoral nerve (A4) behind it and the testicular vessels (A2) in front of it. A normal genitofemoral nerve is seen on the right side of this specimen, but on the left it has divided unusually early (above the level of the aortic bifurcation) into its femoral and genital branches (A9 and 10).

• The ureter (A3) enters the pelvis at the bifurcation of the common iliac artery (A35) crossing the external iliac artery (A21) and running down in front of the internal iliac artery (A34).

• In the pelvis the ureter (A3) is crossed superficially by the ductus deferens (A31).

• The single midline superior hypogastric plexus (A37) divides to form the right and left hypogastric nerves (A33) which enter the pelvis to contribute to the right and left inferior hypogastric plexuses (A32), collectively known as the pelvic plexus.

• The external iliac vessels (A21 and 22) pass beneath the inguinal ligament (A23) to become the femoral vessels, the vein (A25) lying medial to the artery (A24). The femoral nerve (A20) is lateral to the artery.

B Left lumbar plexus, from the front

Psoas major has been removed to show the constituent nerves of the plexus which are embedded within the muscle. Because of the removal of most of the anterolateral abdominal wall (except for the lowest parts of the external oblique, 11, internal oblique, 10, and transversus, 15), the iliohypogastric (8) and ilio-inguinal (7) nerves have fallen too far medially; they should not overlie iliacus (9)

1	Third lumbar vertebra and anterior longitudinal ligament
2	Sympathetic trunk and ganglia
3	Rami communicantes
4	Ventral ramus of fourth lumbar nerve
5	Iliolumbar ligament
6	Quadratus lumborum
7	Ilio-inguinal nerve
8	Iliohypogastric nerve
9	Iliacus
10	Internal oblique
11	External oblique
12	External oblique aponeurosis
13	Upper surface of inguinal ligament
14	Superficial inguinal ring
15	Transversus abdominis
16	Obturator nerve
17	Femoral nerve
18	Genitofemoral nerve
19	Lateral femoral cutaneous nerve
20	Ventral ramus of fifth lumbar nerve
21	Lumbosacral trunk
22	Ventral ramus of first sacral nerve

• The lumbosacral trunk (21), formed by part of the ventral ramus of the fourth lumbar nerve (4) and the whole of the ventral ramus of the fifth lumbar nerve (20), is the contribution which the lumbar plexus makes to the sacral plexus.

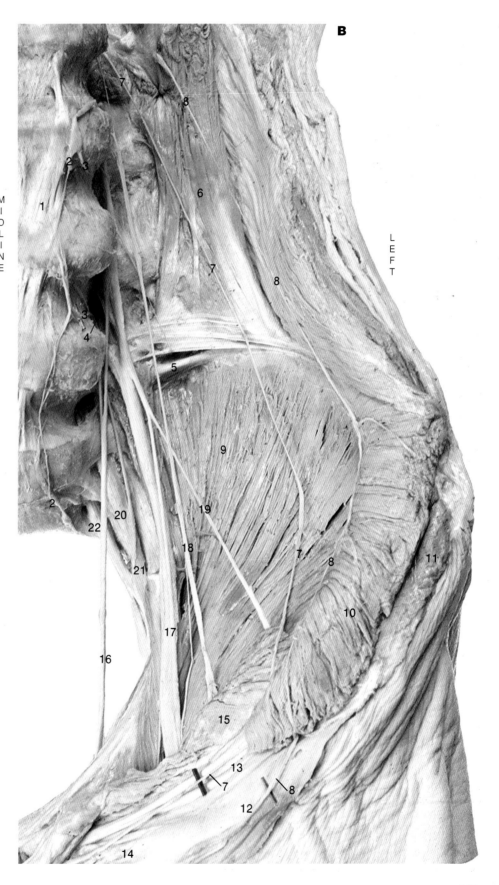

A

A Muscles of the left half of the pelvis and upper thigh, from the front

All fasciae have been removed but the inguinal ligament (16), formed from part of the external oblique aponeurosis, has been preserved. Psoas major (3) and iliacus (4) are seen entering the thigh deep to the inguinal ligament. On the front of the thigh there is an unusually large gap between the adjacent borders of pectineus (14) and adductor longus (11), revealing part of the adductor brevis (13)

1	Promontory of sacrum
2	Fifth lumbar intervertebral disc
3	Psoas major
4	Iliacus
5	Iliac crest
6	Anterior superior iliac spine
7	Tensor fasciae latae
8	Vastus lateralis
9	Rectus femoris
10	Sartorius
11	Adductor longus
12	Gracilis
13	Adductor brevis
14	Pectineus
15	Pubic tubercle
16	Inguinal ligament
17	Coccygeus
18	Obturator internus
19	Piriformis

• The medial border of psoas major (A3) overlaps the side of the pelvic brim.
• Above the inguinal ligament (A16) iliacus (A4) forms the floor of the iliac fossa. On the right side, this is where the caecum and appendix lie (page 231, E).
• Piriformis (A19) and obturator internus (A18) are muscles of the posterior and lateral walls of the pelvis; they are also classified as muscles of the lower limb.
• Coccygeus (A17, B and C2) and levator ani (C18 and 21) are the muscles of the pelvic floor, otherwise known as the pelvic diaphragm.
• Below the inguinal ligament (A16), iliacus (A4), psoas major (A3), pectineus (A14), adductor brevis (A13) and adductor longus (A11) form the floor of the femoral triangle (page 292), whose lateral boundary is the medial border of sartorius (A10) and medial boundary is the medial border of adductor longus (A11). Adductor longus is usually adjacent to pectineus (A14), so excluding adductor brevis (A13) from the floor of the triangle.
• Gracilis (A12, B13) is the most medial muscle of the thigh.
• The anterior superior iliac spine (A6) and the pubic tubercle (A15), which give attachment to the ends of the inguinal ligament (A16), are important palpable landmarks in the inguinal region (see page 204).

• The part of obturator internus (B17) *above* the attachment of levator ani (interrupted line in B) is part of the lateral wall of the pelvic cavity, while the part *below* the attachment is in the perineum and forms part of the lateral wall of the ischio-anal (ischiorectal) fossa (page 258).
• Piriformis (B3) passes out of the pelvis into the gluteal region through the *greater* sciatic foramen *above* the ischial spine (B19), while obturator internus (B17) passes out through the *lesser* sciatic foramen *below* the ischial spine (B19).
• The posterior part of the *ilio*coccygeus part of the levator ani (C21) arises from the *ischial* spine (B19, C19), not from any part of the ileum; the name is derived from animals in which the muscle has a higher origin.

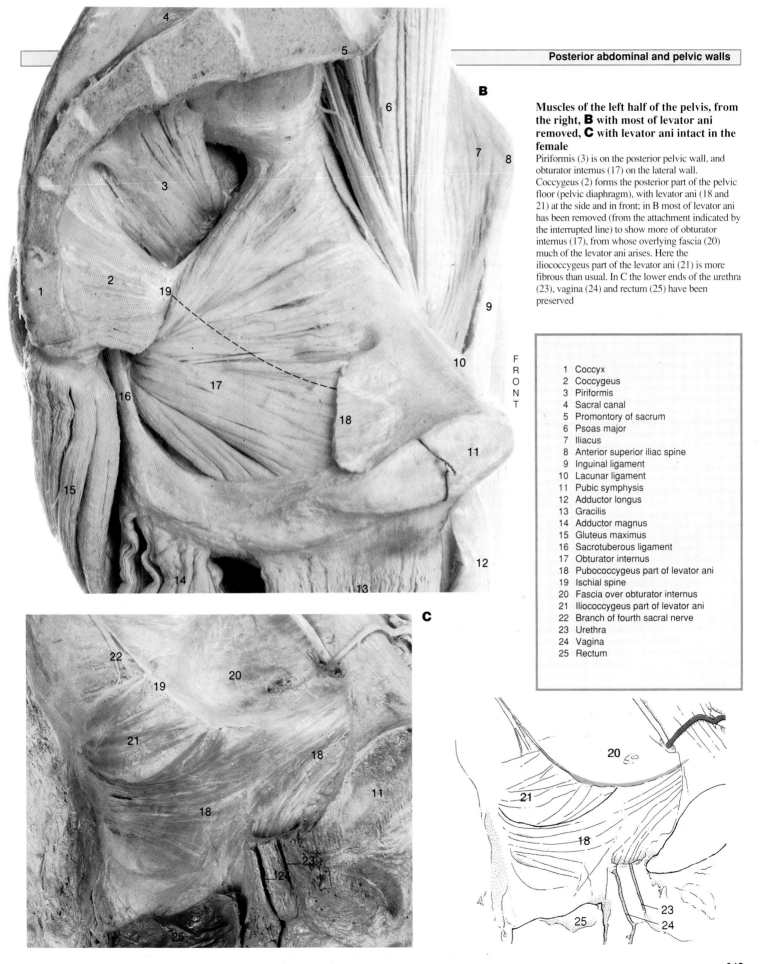

B

C

Muscles of the left half of the pelvis, from the right, B with most of levator ani removed, C with levator ani intact in the female

Piriformis (3) is on the posterior pelvic wall, and obturator internus (17) on the lateral wall. Coccygeus (2) forms the posterior part of the pelvic floor (pelvic diaphragm), with levator ani (18 and 21) at the side and in front; in B most of levator ani has been removed (from the attachment indicated by the interrupted line) to show more of obturator internus (17), from whose overlying fascia (20) much of the levator ani arises. Here the iliococcygeus part of the levator ani (21) is more fibrous than usual. In C the lower ends of the urethra (23), vagina (24) and rectum (25) have been preserved

FRONT

1	Coccyx
2	Coccygeus
3	Piriformis
4	Sacral canal
5	Promontory of sacrum
6	Psoas major
7	Iliacus
8	Anterior superior iliac spine
9	Inguinal ligament
10	Lacunar ligament
11	Pubic symphysis
12	Adductor longus
13	Gracilis
14	Adductor magnus
15	Gluteus maximus
16	Sacrotuberous ligament
17	Obturator internus
18	Pubococcygeus part of levator ani
19	Ischial spine
20	Fascia over obturator internus
21	Iliococcygeus part of levator ani
22	Branch of fourth sacral nerve
23	Urethra
24	Vagina
25	Rectum

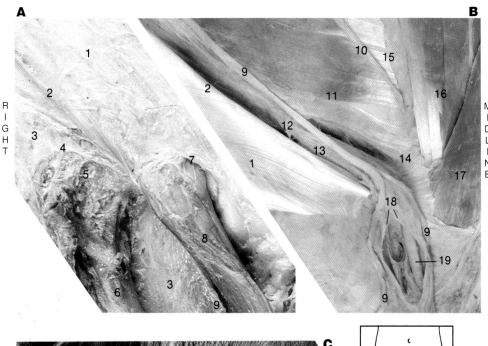

A

B

R I G H T

M I D L I N E

Right inguinal region in the male, A superficial dissection, B with the external oblique aponeurosis and spermatic cord incised

In A the spermatic cord (8) is seen emerging from the superficial inguinal ring (7) and covered by the external spermatic fascia. In B, with the external oblique aponeurosis reflected and the anterior wall of the rectus sheath removed, the cord is emerging from the deep inguinal ring (12) with the cremasteric fascia (13) now the most superficial covering. All three coverings of the cord have been incised (18) to show the ductus deferens (19)

1	External oblique aponeurosis
2	Inguinal ligament
3	Fascia lata
4	Upper margin of saphenous opening
5	Cribriform fascia
6	Great saphenous vein
7	Upper margin of superficial inguinal ring
8	Spermatic cord
9	Ilio-inguinal nerve
10	Iliohypogastric nerve
11	Internal oblique
12	Deep inguinal ring
13	Cremasteric fascia and cremaster muscle over spermatic cord
14	Conjoint tendon
15	Edge of rectus sheath
16	Rectus abdominis
17	Pyramidalis
18	Incised margin of coverings of cord
19	Ductus deferens

C Right testis and epididymis, and the penis, from the right

The scrotum, spermatic cord (2) and the tunica vaginalis (1) of the testis (5) have been opened up. The testis has been rotated to show that the ductus deferens (7) is the upward continuation of the tail of the epididymis (6); in its normal position the testis (5) hangs with the epididymis (3 and 6) on its posterolateral side, not anteromedial as here

1	Tunica vaginalis
2	Spermatic cord
3	Head of epididymis
4	Appendix of testis
5	Testis
6	Tail of epididymis
7	Ductus deferens
8	Body of penis
9	Foreskin (retracted)
10	Corona of glans
11	Glans penis
12	External urethral orifice

• The spermatic cord (A8) consists of the ductus deferens, the obliterated remains of the processus vaginalis of peritoneum, three arteries (testicular, cremasteric and deferential), the pampiniform plexus of veins, the genital branch of the genitofemoral nerve, sympathetic nerve fibres (accompanying the arteries) from the testicular and pelvic plexuses, and lymph vessels from the testis.

• The *coverings* of the cord consist of the internal spermatic fascia (derived from the transversalis fascia at the deep inguinal ring), the cremasteric fascia and cremaster muscle (B13, from the transversus and internal oblique muscles), and the external spermatic fascia (from the external oblique aponeurosis at the superficial inguinal ring, A7).

• The external oblique aponeurosis (A1) and the external spermatic fascia (which is the outermost covering of the spermatic cord, as at A8) are in continuity at the superficial inguinal ring (A7). The 'ring' only becomes a gap with a free margin if the fascia is cut away from the aponeurosis—as has been done for a short distance exactly at the label A7 on the medial side of the cord.

• The lowest fibres of the internal oblique (B11), together with the underlying transversus fibres, arch over the cord (as at B11) to form the conjoint tendon (B14).

• The inguinal canal is the oblique gap in the anterior abdominal wall above the inguinal ligament and between the deep inguinal ring (B12) laterally and the superficial inguinal ring (A7) medially.

• In the male the inguinal canal contains the spermatic cord and the ilio-inguinal nerve; the cord enters the canal through the deep inguinal ring (B12), but the ilio-inguinal nerve (B9) enters from the side by running deep to the external oblique aponeurosis (in A it can be seen shining through the aponeurosis just below and to the right of the label 2). Both the cord and the nerve leave the canal through the superficial inguinal ring (A7).

D Right inguinal region, in the female

The external oblique aponeurosis (1) has been incised and reflected to show the position of the deep inguinal ring (5) which marks the lateral end of the inguinal canal. The round ligament of the uterus (8) emerges from the superficial inguinal ring (7), which marks the medial end of the canal, and becomes lost in the fat of the labium majus (9). The ilio-inguinal nerve (2) also passes through the canal and out of the superficial ring

1	External oblique aponeurosis
2	Ilio-inguinal nerve
3	Upper surface of inguinal ligament
4	Internal oblique
5	Position of deep inguinal ring
6	Conjoint tendon
7	Position of superficial inguinal ring
8	Round ligament of uterus
9	Fat of labium majus
10	Great saphenous vein

• In the female the inguinal canal contains the round ligament of the uterus and the ilio-inguinal nerve.
• The processus vaginalis is normally obliterated, but if it remains patent within the female inguinal canal it is sometimes known as the canal of Nuck.

E Right inguinal and femoral regions, in the female

Part of the fascia lata of the thigh has been removed to show the femoral nerve (21), artery (20) and vein (18) beneath the inguinal ligament (19), and also the position of the femoral canal (17), medial to the vein (18). The femoral structures have been included here because of the importance of the femoral canal as a site for hernia in the female (see page 249)

1	Anterior superior iliac spine
2	External oblique aponeurosis
3	Cut edge of rectus sheath
4	Rectus abdominis
5	Superficial epigastric vein
6	Superficial inguinal ring
7	Round ligament of uterus
8	Mons pubis
9	Gracilis
10	Adductor longus
11	Pectineus
12	Great saphenous vein
13	Superficial external pudendal vessels
14	Fascia lata
15	Accessory saphenous vein
16	Lower edge of saphenous opening
17	Position of femoral canal
18	Femoral vein
19	Inguinal ligament
20	Femoral artery
21	Femoral nerve
22	Medial ⎫ femoral cutaneous nerve
23	Intermediate ⎭
24	Sartorius
25	Superficial circumflex iliac vessels
26	Fascia lata overlying tensor fasciae latae

• The round ligament of the uterus (D8, E7) is a very much smaller structure than the spermatic cord of the male but it pursues a similar course through the inguinal canal. Theoretically it has similar coverings to those of the cord but they are usually too small to be defined. The round ligament disappears into the labium majus (D9).

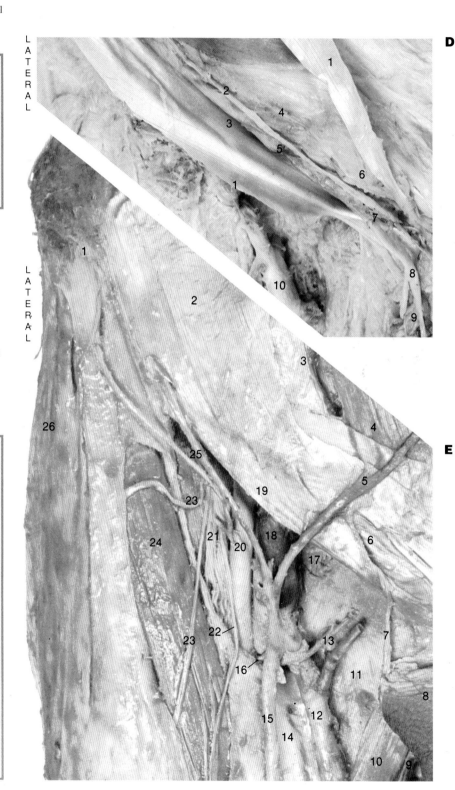

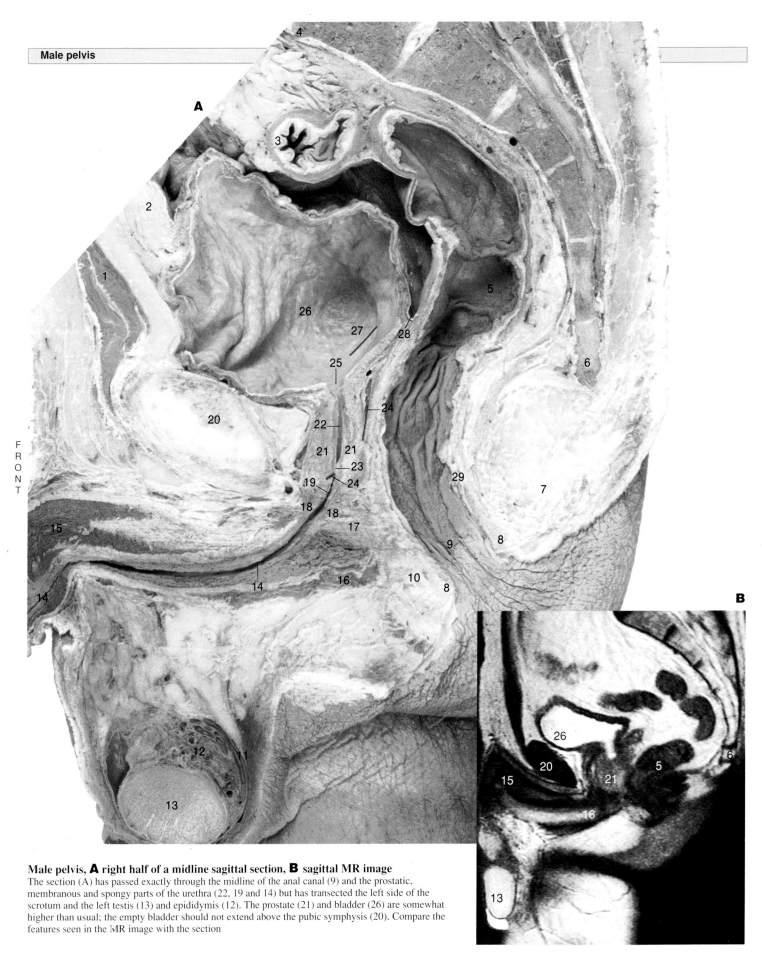

Male pelvis, A right half of a midline sagittal section, B sagittal MR image

The section (A) has passed exactly through the midline of the anal canal (9) and the prostatic, membranous and spongy parts of the urethra (22, 19 and 14) but has transected the left side of the scrotum and the left testis (13) and epididymis (12). The prostate (21) and bladder (26) are somewhat higher than usual; the empty bladder should not extend above the pubic symphysis (20). Compare the features seen in the MR image with the section

C

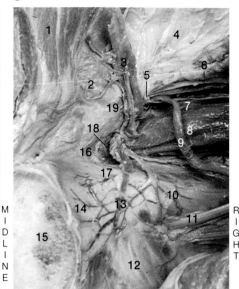

D

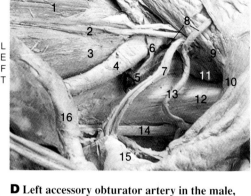

1 Rectus abdominis
2 Extraperitoneal fat
3 Sigmoid colon
4 Promontory of sacrum
5 Rectum
6 Coccyx
7 Anococcygeal body
8 External anal sphincter
9 Anal canal with anal columns of mucous
  membrane
10 Perineal body
11 Ductus deferens
12 Epididymis
13 Testis
14 Spongy part of urethra and corpus
   spongiosum
15 Corpus cavernosum
16 Bulbospongiosus
17 Perineal membrane
18 Sphincter urethrae
19 Membranous part of urethra
20 Pubic symphysis
21 Prostate
22 Prostatic part of urethra
23 Seminal collicus
24 Bristle in ejaculatory duct
25 Internal urethral orifice
26 Bladder
27 Bristle passing up into right ureteral orifice
28 Rectovesical pouch
29 Puborectalis fibres of levator ani

D Left accessory obturator artery in the male, from the right

This is a similar view to that in C but on the left side, showing an accessory obturator artery (13) passing from the inferior epigastric (8) over the superior pubic ramus (12) to enter the obturator foramen with the obturator nerve (14)

• The lowest part of the peritoneal cavity is the rectovesical pouch (A28), between the front of the rectum (A5) and the posterior surface (base) of the bladder (A26).
• The lower end of the rectum (A5) and the anal canal (A9) are maintained at right angles to one another by a sling formed by the puborectalis fibres of both levator ani muscles (A29), which become continuous with the upper end of the external anal sphincter (A8).
• The various constituents of the spermatic cord come together at the deep inguinal ring (C5), which is in the transversalis fascia (C4) *lateral* to the inferior epigastric vessels (C3). The ductus deferens (C9) therefore appears to emerge from the ring by hooking round the lateral side of the vessels.
• The inguinal triangle (Hesselbach's triangle) is the area bounded laterally by the inferior epigastric vessels (C3), medially by the lateral border of rectus abdominis (C1) and below by the inguinal ligament (C19). A *direct* inguinal hernia passes forwards through this triangle, *medial* to the inferior epigastric vessels.
• An *indirect* inguinal hernia passes through the deep inguinal ring (C5) *lateral* to the inferior epigastric vessels (C3).
• A femoral hernia passes into the femoral canal through the femoral ring (C18), bounded medially by the lacunar ligament (C16) and laterally by the femoral vein (which becomes the external iliac vein, C8, as it passes beneath the inguinal ligament).

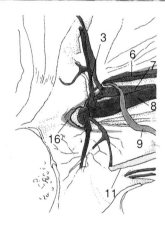

C Right deep inguinal ring and inguinal triangle, in the male

This is a view looking into the right half of the pelvis from the left, showing the posterior surface of the lower part of the anterior abdominal wall, above the pubic symphysis. The femoral ring (18), the entrance to the femoral canal, is below the medial end of the inguinal ligament (19). The inferior epigastric vessels (3) lie medial to the deep inguinal ring (5)

1 Iliacus
2 Testicular vessels
3 Psoas major
4 External iliac artery
5 External iliac vein (cut end)
6 Deep circumflex iliac vein
7 Ductus deferens
8 Inferior epigastric artery
9 Inguinal ligament
10 Lacunar ligament
11 Femoral ring
12 Superior ramus of pubis and pectineal
   ligament
13 Accessory obturator artery
14 Obturator nerve
15 Bladder
16 Right common iliac artery and vein

• The anastomosis between the pubic branches of the inferior epigastric and obturator arteries may be unusually large, forming the vessel known as the accessory or abnormal obturator artery (D13), in which case the normal obturator branch from the internal iliac may be absent.
• The accessory obturator artery *usually* lies at the *lateral* margin of the femoral ring (D11) but may lie at the medial edge of the ring, i.e. at the lateral margin of the lacunar ligament (D10), where it may be at risk if the ligament has to be incised to enlarge the femoral ring in operations to reduce a femoral hernia.

1 Rectus abdominis	11 Obturator nerve
2 Conjoint tendon	12 Origin of levator ani from fascia overlying
3 Inferior epigastric vessels	obturator internus
4 Transversalis fascia overlying transversus	13 Pubic branches of inferior epigastric vessels
abdominis	14 Body of pubis
5 Deep inguinal ring	15 Pubic symphysis
6 Testicular vessels	16 Lacunar ligament
7 External iliac artery	17 Pectineal ligament
8 External iliac vein	18 Femoral ring
9 Ductus deferens	19 Inguinal ligament
10 Superior ramus of pubis	

A

A Pelvis, right inguinal region and penis, from above

In the pelvis, most of the bladder (18) has been removed to show part of the base (upper surface) of the prostate (17), and the left seminal vesicle (16) lying lateral to the ductus deferens (15). The ductus in the pelvis crosses superficial to the ureter (9). The external iliac artery (8) passes under the inguinal ligament (1) to become the femoral artery (36). On the dorsum of the penis the fascia has been removed, showing the single midline deep dorsal vein (27) with a dorsal artery (28) and dorsal nerve (29) on each side

1	External oblique aponeurosis and inguinal ligament
2	Internal oblique
3	Iliacus
4	Femoral nerve
5	Psoas major
6	Femoral } branch of
7	Genital } genitofemoral nerve
8	External iliac artery
9	Ureter
10	Common iliac artery
11	Internal iliac artery
12	Fifth lumbar intervertebral disc
13	Sigmoid colon (cut lower end)
14	Rectum
15	Ductus deferens
16	Seminal vesicle
17	Base of prostate
18	Trigone of bladder
19	Internal urethral orifice
20	Ureteral orifice
21	Superior vesical artery
22	Inferior vesical artery
23	Obturator artery
24	Obturator nerve
25	Spermatic cord
26	Inferior epigastric artery
27	Deep dorsal vein }
28	Dorsal artery } of penis
29	Dorsal nerve }
30	Adductor longus
31	Pectineus
32	Deep external pudendal artery
33	Femoral vein
34	Great saphenous vein
35	Superficial circumflex iliac vein
36	Femoral artery

• The obturator artery (A23, C19) runs below the obturator nerve (A24, C10), with the vein below the artery, but in C there is an accessory obturator vein (C8) draining to the inferior epigastric vein (C40).

• Each ductus deferens (A15, B3, C6) lies on the medial side of its own seminal vesicle (A16, B2, C21), and crosses superficial to the ureter (A9, C11).

• The neck of the bladder is the part containing the internal urethral orifice (A19, C37), at the lower angle of the trigone (A18, C38).

• The base of the bladder is its posterior surface (B5).

• The base of the prostate is not its posterior surface (B6) but its upper surface (A17), in contact with the neck of the bladder and pierced by the urethra (A19, C37).

• The trigone of the bladder (A18, C38), at the lower part of the base or posterior surface, is the relatively fixed area with smooth mucous membrane between the internal urethral orifice (A19, C37) and the two ureteral openings (A20 on the right side, C39 on the left).

• In the male pelvis the ureter (A9, C11) is crossed superficially by the ductus deferens (A15, C6). (In the female pelvis it is crossed superficially by the uterine artery—page 256, A4 and 5).

• The ureter (A9, C11) enters the pelvis at the bifurcation of the common iliac artery (A10), crossing the external iliac artery and vein (C4 and 5) and running down the side wall of the pelvis in front of the internal iliac artery (A11, C12).

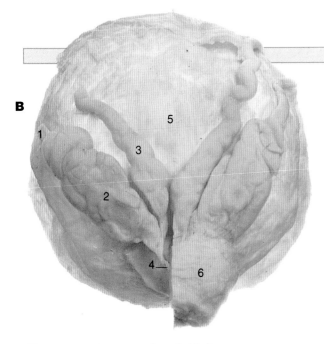

B Bladder and prostate, from behind

The bladder (5) has been distended and the left half of the prostate removed to show the ductus deferens (3) and the seminal vesicle (2) uniting to form the ejaculatory duct (4)

1	Ureter	5	Base of bladder
2	Seminal vesicle	6	Posterior surface of
3	Ductus deferens		prostate
4	Left ejaculatory duct		

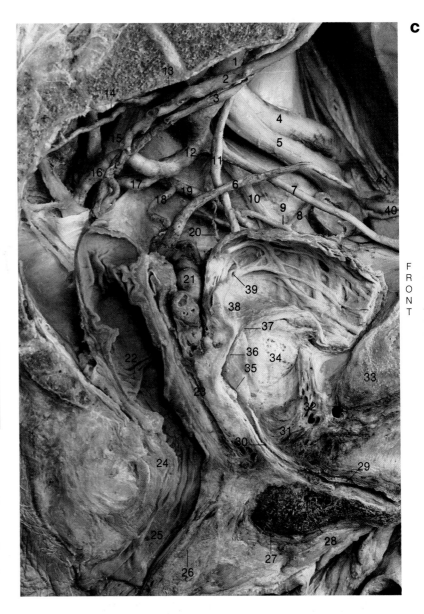

C Left side of the male pelvis, from the right

In this midline sagittal section, the prostate (34) is enlarged, lengthening the prostatic urethra (36) and accentuating the trabeculae of the bladder. The mucous membrane of the bladder (whose trigone is labelled at 38) has been removed to show muscular trabeculae in the wall. Variations in the branches of the internal iliac artery (12) are common, and here the obturator artery (19) gives origin to the superior vesical (9) and inferior vesical (20) as well as the middle rectal (18). The largest branch of the internal iliac, the superior gluteal (13), is largely hidden behind the superior rectal vessels (2 and 3). The ureter (11) is crossed superficially by the ductus deferens (6)

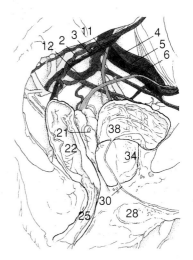

1	Common iliac artery	16	Inferior gluteal artery	32	Vesicoprostatic venous plexus
2	Superior rectal artery	17	Internal pudendal artery	33	Pubic symphysis
3	Superior rectal vein	18	Middle rectal artery	34	Prostate (enlarged)
4	External iliac artery	19	Obturator artery	35	Seminal colliculus
5	External iliac vein	20	Inferior vesical artery	36	Prostatic part of urethra
6	Ductus deferens	21	Seminal vesicle	37	Internal urethral orifice
7	Obliterated umbilical artery	22	Lower end of rectum	38	Trigone of bladder
8	Accessory obturator vein	23	Rectovesical fascia	39	Ureteral orifice
9	Superior vesical artery	24	Puborectalis part of levator ani	40	Inferior epigastric vessels
10	Obturator nerve	25	Anal canal	41	Testicular vessels and deep
11	Ureter	26	External anal sphincter		inguinal ring
12	Internal iliac artery	27	Bulbospongiosus		
13	Superior gluteal artery	28	Bulb of penis		
14	Lateral sacral artery	29	Bulbar part of spongy urethra		
15	Ventral ramus of first sacral	30	Membranous part of urethra		
	nerve	31	Urogenital diaphragm		

A Arteries and nerves of the pelvis, left side

In this left half section of the pelvis, all peritoneum, fascia, veins and visceral arteries have been removed together with the left levator ani, so displaying the whole of the internal surface of obturator internus (20). On the posterior pelvic wall the vessels in general lie superficial to the nerves. In this specimen the external iliac artery (15) is unusually tortuous, and the anterior trunk of the internal iliac artery (12) has divided unusually high up into its terminal branches, the internal pudendal (13) and the inferior gluteal (5). The superior gluteal artery (8) has perforated the lumbosacral trunk

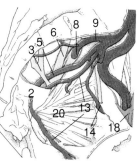

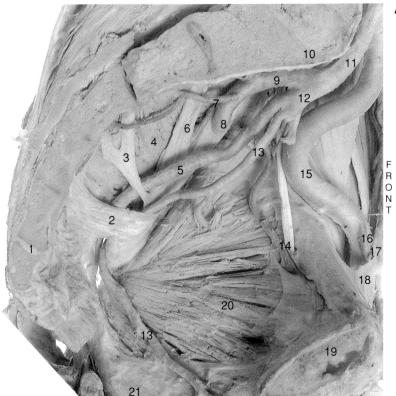

1 Sacrococcygeal joint	10 Sacral promontory
2 Coccygeus and sacrospinous ligament	11 Internal iliac artery
3 Union of ventral rami of second and third sacral nerves	12 Anterior trunk of internal iliac artery
4 Piriformis	13 Internal pudendal artery
5 Inferior gluteal artery	14 Obturator nerve and artery
6 Ventral ramus of first sacral nerve	15 External iliac artery
7 Lateral sacral artery	16 Inferior epigastric artery
8 Superior gluteal artery piercing lumbosacral trunk	17 Inguinal ligament
9 Posterior trunk of internal iliac artery	18 Lacunar ligament
	19 Pubic symphysis
	20 Obturator internus
	21 Ischial tuberosity

B

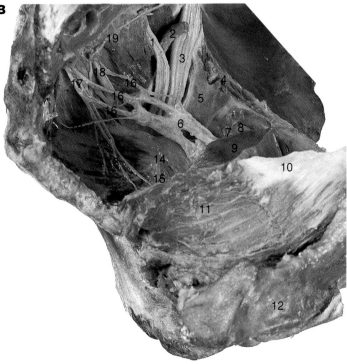

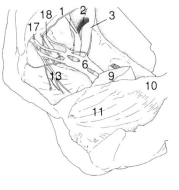

B Left inferior hypogastric plexus, from the right

In this view of the left side of the pelvis from the right, the right pelvic wall has been removed but the right levator ani (11) forming part of the pelvic floor (pelvic diaphragm) has been preserved and is seen from its right (perineal) side. Pelvic splanchnic nerves (16) arise from the ventral rami of the second and third sacral nerves (18 and 17) and contribute to the inferior hypogastric plexus (6)

1 Ventral ramus of first sacral nerve
2 Superior gluteal artery
3 Lumbosacral trunk
4 Arcuate line of ilium
5 Fascia overlying obturator internus
6 Left inferior hypogastric plexus
7 Left seminal vesicle
8 Left ductus deferens
9 Rectum
10 Lateral surface of fascia overlying right obturator internus
11 Right levator ani and ischio-anal (ischiorectal) fossa
12 Right ischiopubic ramus
13 Left coccygeus and nerves to levator ani
14 Ischial spine
15 Left levator ani
16 Pelvic splanchnic nerves (nervi erigentes)
17 Ventral ramus of third sacral nerve
18 Ventral ramus of second sacral nerve
19 Part of left sympathetic trunk

◁ • Before they leave the pelvis, the internal pudendal artery (A13) lies in front of the inferior gluteal (A5). The perineal part of the internal pudendal is seen here overlying the lower part of the obturator internus (A20) because the fascia forming the pudendal canal (in which it lies, page 257, D20) has been removed.

• The superior gluteal artery (A8) usually passes backwards above piriformis (A4) between the lumbosacral trunk and the ventral ramus of the first sacral nerve (A6) (but sometimes between the first and second ventral rami). Here it has passed between fibres of the lumbosacral trunk.

• The inferior gluteal artery (A5) passes backwards below piriformis (A4) between the ventral rami of the first (A6) and second (A3) (or second and third) sacral nerves.

• The left and right inferior hypogastric plexuses (B6) together form the pelvic plexus. Their parasympathetic fibres are from the pelvic splanchnic nerves (B16), and the sympathetic contributions are from the hypogastric nerves (page 242, A33) and ganglia of the sacral part of the sympathetic trunk (B19).

C Pelvic ligaments, left side, from the right

In this median sagittal section of the pelvis all soft tissues have been removed except the ligaments

Interrupted line = position of origin of levator ani

1	Sacral promontory
2	Iliac fossa
3	Anterior superior iliac spine
4	Anterior inferior iliac spine and origin of straight head of rectus femoris
5	Inguinal ligament
6	Lacunar ligament
7	Pectineal ligament
8	Pubic symphysis
9	Obturator foramen
10	Obturator membrane
11	Falciform process of sacrotuberous ligament
12	Ischial tuberosity
13	Sacrotuberous ligament
14	Lesser sciatic foramen
15	Ischial spine
16	Sacrospinous ligament
17	Greater sciatic foramen
18	Ventral sacro-iliac ligament

• The ligaments classified as 'the ligaments of the pelvis' (vertebropelvic ligaments) are the sacrotuberous (C13), sacrospinous (C16) and iliolumbar (seen in the posterior view on page 297, C2).

• The sacrotuberous and sacrospinous ligaments convert the greater and lesser sciatic *notches* of the hip bone (page 261, 18 and 15) into *foramina* (C17 and C14).

• The lacunar ligament (C6) passes backwards from the medial end of the inguinal ligament (C5) to the medial end of the pectineal line of the pubis, to which the pectineal ligament (C7) is attached.

• The lower attachment of the sacrotuberous ligament is to the medial side of the ischial tuberosity, but it gives off two slips. One is the falciform process (C11), which passes towards the ischial ramus to form the lower boundary of the pudendal canal (page 257, D20). The other runs into the ischial attachment of the long head of biceps (page 291, C5).

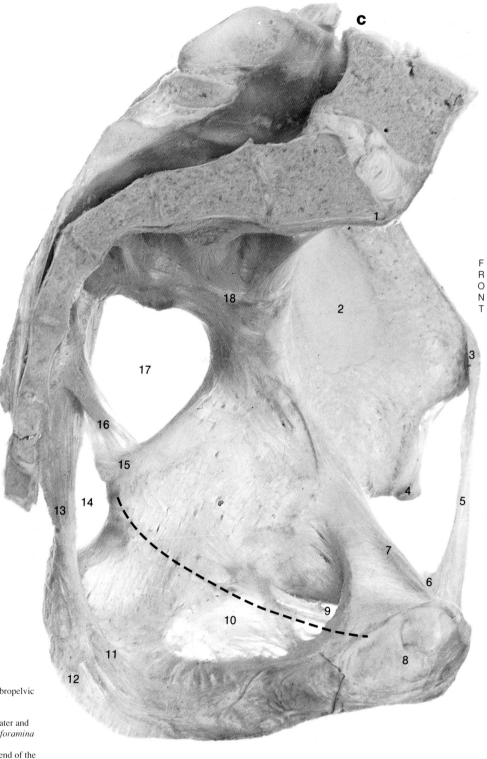

C

FRONT

A

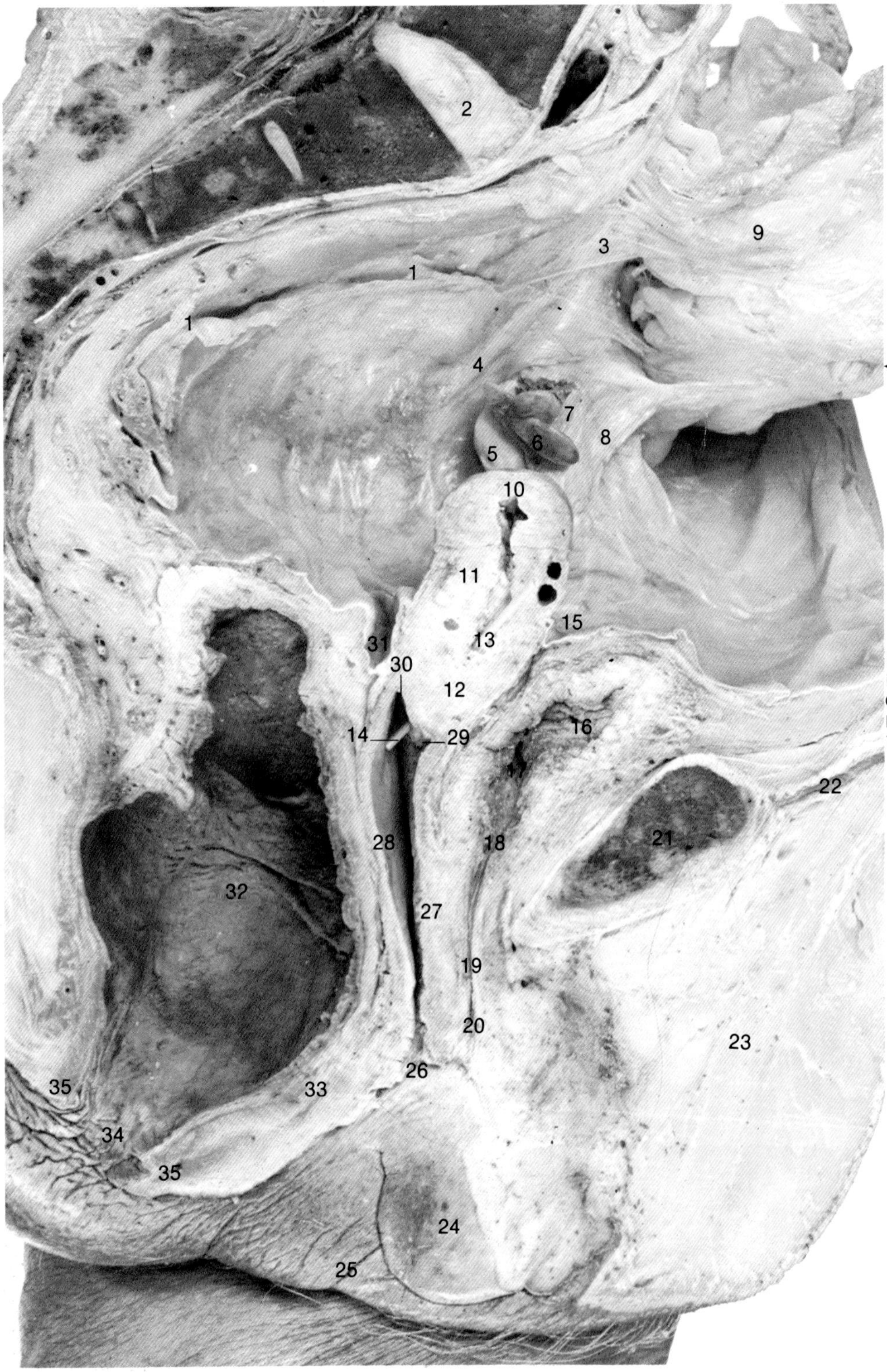

Female pelvis, A left half of a midline sagittal section, B sagittal MR image

In A the lower end of the rectum (32) is dilated, and the bladder (16), uterus (11) and vagina (27 and 28) are contracted. The section has opened up the whole length of the urethra (19), but the cervix of the uterus (12) is rarely exactly in the midline and the line of the cervical canal is indicated by the marker in the internal and external os (13 and 14). Compare features in the MR image in B with the section

FRONT

1 Line of attachment of right limb of sigmoid mesocolon
2 Fifth lumbar intervertebral disc
3 Apex of sigmoid mesocolon
4 Ureter underlying peritoneum
5 Ovary
6 Uterine tube
7 Suspensory ligament of ovary containing ovarian vessels
8 Left limb of sigmoid mesocolon overlying external iliac vessels
9 Sigmoid colon (reflected to left and upwards)
10 Fundus ⎫
11 Body ⎬ of uterus
12 Cervix ⎭
13 Marker in internal os
14 Marker in external os
15 Vesico-uterine pouch
16 Bladder
17 Marker in left ureteral orifice
18 Internal urethral orifice
19 Urethra
20 External urethral orifice
21 Pubic symphysis
22 Rectus abdominis (turned forwards)
23 Fat of mons pubis
24 Labium minus
25 Labium majus
26 Vestibule
27 Anterior wall ⎫
28 Posterior wall ⎬ of vagina
29 Anterior fornix ⎪
30 Posterior fornix ⎭
31 Recto-uterine pouch (of Douglas)
32 Rectum
33 Perineal body
34 Anal canal
35 External anal sphincter

• The apex of the sigmoid mesocolon (A3) is a guide to the left ureter (A4) which enters the pelvis under the peritoneum at this point (in both sexes).
• The recto-uterine pouch (A31, pouch of Douglas) overlies the posterior fornix of the vagina (A30), but the vesico-uterine pouch (A15) does not reach the anterior fornix (A29).

B

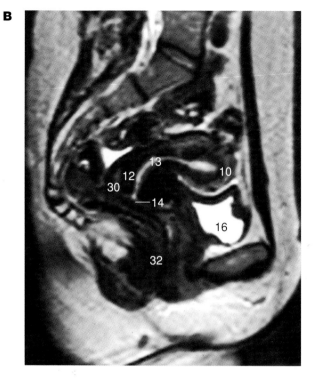

D

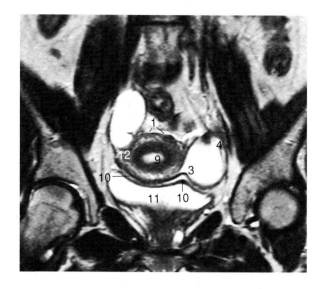

1 Recto-uterine pouch
2 Ligament of ovary
3 Uterine ⎫
4 Tubal ⎬ extremity of ovary
5 Infundibulum ⎫
6 Ampulla ⎬ of uterine tube
7 Isthmus ⎭
8 Round ligament of uterus
9 Fundus of uterus
10 Vesico-uterine pouch
11 Bladder
12 Mesosalpinx
13 Posterior surface of broad ligament
14 Mesovarium
15 Suspensory ligament of ovary with ovarian vessels
16 Overspill of contrast into recto-uterine pouch

Female pelvis, C uterus and ovaries, from above and in front, D coronal MR image, E hysterosalpingogram

Looking down into the pelvis from the front in C, the fundus of the uterus (9) overlies the bladder (11) with the peritoneum of the vesico-uterine pouch (10) intervening. These relationships are seen in the MR image. In E contrast medium has filled the uterus and tubes (9, 7, 6 and 5) and spilled out into the peritoneal cavity (16)

C

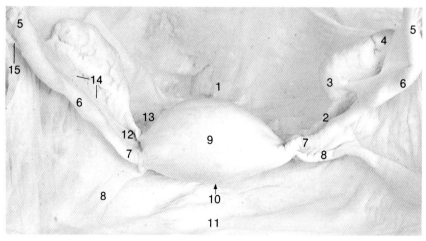

FRONT

E

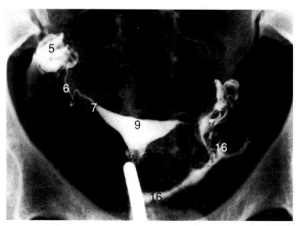

FRONT

A

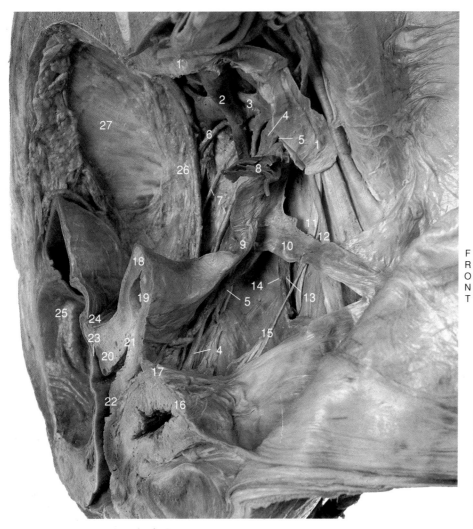

Female pelvis, **A** left half, obliquely from above and behind

Looking obliquely into the left half of the pelvis from the front, with the anterior abdominal wall turned forwards, the peritoneum of the vesico-uterine pouch (17) has been incised and the uterus (19) displaced backwards to show the ureter (4) running towards the bladder and being crossed by the uterine artery (5). The uterosacral ligament (26) passes backwards at the side of the rectum (25) towards the pelvic surface of the sacrum. The root of the sigmoid mesocolon (1) has been left in place to emphasize that the left ureter (4) passes from the abdomen into the pelvis beneath it

F
R
O
N
T

1	Sigmoid mesocolon
2	Internal iliac vein
3	Internal iliac artery
4	Ureter
5	Uterine artery
6	Middle rectal artery
7	Vaginal artery (double)
8	Fimbriated end of uterine tube
9	Ampulla of uterine tube
10	Round ligament of uterus
11	Obturator nerve
12	Obliterated umbilical artery
13	Obturator artery
14	Obturator vein
15	Superior vesical artery
16	Peritoneum overlying bladder
17	Vesico-uterine pouch
18	Fundus ⎫
19	Body ⎬ of uterus
20	Cervix ⎭
21	Anterior fornix ⎫
22	Cavity ⎬ of vagina
23	Posterior fornix ⎭
24	Recto-uterine pouch (of Douglas)
25	Rectum
26	Uterosacral ligament
27	Peritoneum overlying piriformis

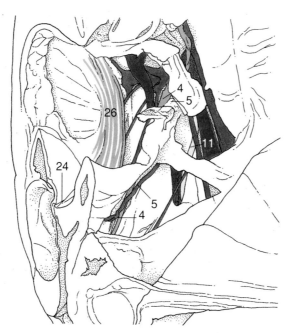

• Because the body and cervix of the uterus (A19 and 20) are rarely exactly in the midline, the section in A has not passed through the cervical canal, so the continuity between the cavity of the uterus and the vagina (A22) cannot be seen. The projection of the cervix into the vagina gives rise to the anterior and posterior fornices (A21 and 23).

• In the pelvis the ureter (A4) is crossed superficially by the uterine artery (A5). In the male pelvis it is crossed by the ductus deferens (pages 250 and 251).

• The uterosacral ligaments (A26), passing backwards on either side of the rectum to the sacrum and internal iliac vessels, and the lateral cervical ligaments (tissue underlying the ureter and uterine artery, A4 and 5, often called the cardinal or Mackenrodt's ligaments and passing to the lateral pelvic wall) are condensations of retroperitoneal tissue of great importance in supporting the uterine cervix (A20) in its normal position.

B FRONT

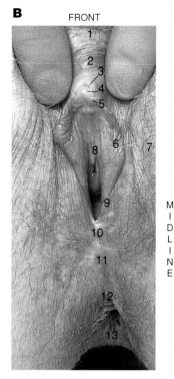

C FRONT

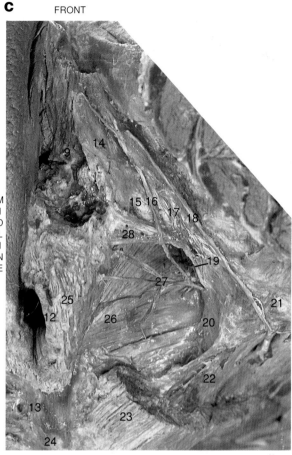

1	Mons pubis
2	Anterior commissure
3	Prepuce of clitoris
4	Clitoris
5	Frenulum of clitoris
6	Labium minus
7	Labium majus
8	External urethral orifice
9	Vagina
10	Posterior commissure
11	Perineal body
12	Margin of anus
13	Anococcygeal body
14	Bulbospongiosus overlying bulb of vestibule
15	Perineal membrane
16	Posterior labial nerve
17	Ischiocavernosus overlying crus of clitoris
18	Perineal branch of posterior femoral cutaneous nerve
19	Pudendal nerve
20	Pudendal canal
21	Ischial tuberosity
22	Sacrotuberous ligament
23	Gluteus maximus
24	Coccyx
25	External anal sphincter
26	Levator ani
27	Inferior rectal nerve
28	Superficial transverse perineal muscle overlying posterior border of perineal membrane
29	Obturator internus and fascia

Female perineum, B surface features, C left ischio-anal fossa, from below, D left ischio-anal fossa, from behind

In B the labia minora (6) have been separated to show the orifice of the vagina (9) with the urethra (8) opening into it anteriorly, 2.5 cm (1 in) behind the clitoris (4). In C and D fat and vessels have been removed from the ischio-anal fossa to show the pudendal canal (20) in the lateral wall, with levator ani (26) sloping downwards and medially to the external anal sphincter (25). The inferior rectal nerve (27) leaves the pudendal nerve (19) by piercing the wall of the pudendal canal (20) and crosses the fossa to reach the external anal sphincter (25)

D

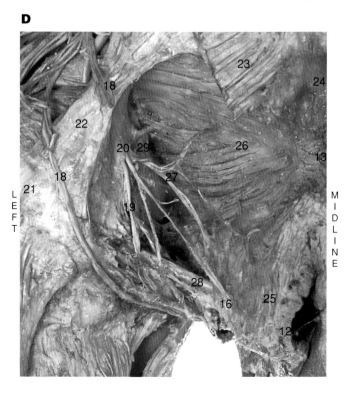

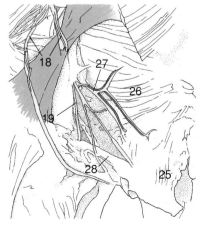

• The ischiorectal fossa is now properly and more correctly called the ischio-anal fossa; the anal canal (C and D12), not the rectum, is its lower medial boundary. The walls and contents are similar in both sexes.

• The vulva is the anterior part of the female perineum containing the external genitalia.

• The external genitalia consist of the mons pubis (B1), labia majora (B7), labia minora (B6), clitoris (B4), vestibule of the vagina (the lower end with the vaginal orifice, B9), the bulb of the vestibule (C14), the greater vestibular (Bartholin's) glands (under the posterior end of the bulb of the vestibule), and the lesser vestibular glands (small mucous glands in the labia minora).

• The vestibule of the vagina is bounded by the labia minora (B6), and contains the external urethral orifice (B8), the vaginal orifice (B9, with the hymen at its margin in the virgin) and the ducts of the greater and lesser vestibular glands.

• The pudendal cleft is the region between the two labia majora (B7).

A Male perineum

The central area is shown, with the scrotum (1) pulled upwards and forwards

1 Scrotum overlying left testis
2 Raphe overlying bulb of penis
3 Perineal body
4 Margin of anus
5 Anococcygeal body

• In both sexes the ischio-anal (ischiorectal) fossa has the pudendal canal in its lateral wall. In B the canal has been opened up to display its contents: the internal pudendal artery (B18) and the terminal branches of the pudendal nerve—the perineal nerve (B17) and the dorsal nerve of the penis (B21) or clitoris.

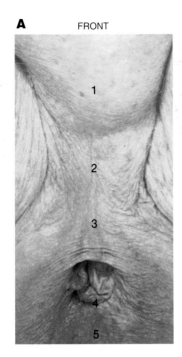

A FRONT

B Male perineum and ischio-anal (ischiorectal) fossae

All the fat has been removed from the ischio-anal fossae so that a clear view is obtained of the perineal surface of levator ani (22) and of the vessels and nerves within the fossae. On the left side (right of the picture) the perineal membrane (10) is intact but on the right side it and the underlying muscle (urogenital diaphragm) have been removed

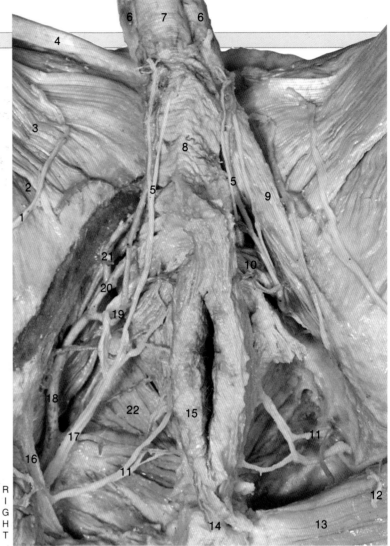

1 Perineal branch of posterior femoral cutaneous nerve
2 Adductor magnus
3 Gracilis
4 Adductor longus
5 Posterior scrotal vessels and nerves
6 Corpus cavernosum of penis
7 Corpus spongiosum of penis
8 Bulbospongiosus overlying bulb of penis
9 Ischiocavernosus overlying crus of penis
10 Superficial transverse perineal muscle overlying posterior border of perineal membrane
11 Inferior rectal vessels and nerve in ischio-anal fossa
12 Perforating cutaneous nerve
13 Gluteus maximus
14 Anococcygeal body
15 Margin of anus
16 Sacrotuberous ligament
17 Perineal nerve
18 Internal pudendal artery
19 Perineal artery
20 Artery to bulb
21 Dorsal nerve and artery of penis
22 Levator ani

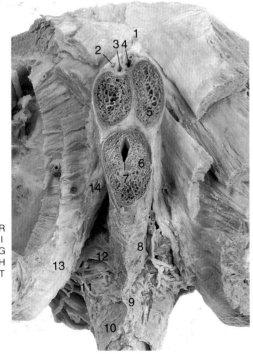

C

1 Pubic symphysis
2 Dorsal nerve of penis
3 Dorsal artery of penis
4 Deep dorsal vein of penis
5 Corpus cavernosum
6 Corpus spongiosum
7 Urethra
8 Bulbospongiosus
9 Perineal body
10 External anal sphincter
11 Inferior rectal vessels and nerve crossing ischio-anal fossa
12 Superficial transverse perineal muscle overlying perineal membrane
13 Ischiopubic ramus
14 Ischiocavernosus

C Root of penis, from below and in front

The front part of the penis has been removed to show the root, formed by the two corpora cavernosa dorsally (5) and the single corpus spongiosum ventrally (6) containing the urethra (7)

Lower limb

Left hip bone, lateral surface

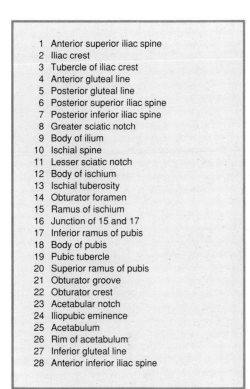

1 Anterior superior iliac spine
2 Iliac crest
3 Tubercle of iliac crest
4 Anterior gluteal line
5 Posterior gluteal line
6 Posterior superior iliac spine
7 Posterior inferior iliac spine
8 Greater sciatic notch
9 Body of ilium
10 Ischial spine
11 Lesser sciatic notch
12 Body of ischium
13 Ischial tuberosity
14 Obturator foramen
15 Ramus of ischium
16 Junction of 15 and 17
17 Inferior ramus of pubis
18 Body of pubis
19 Pubic tubercle
20 Superior ramus of pubis
21 Obturator groove
22 Obturator crest
23 Acetabular notch
24 Iliopubic eminence
25 Acetabulum
26 Rim of acetabulum
27 Inferior gluteal line
28 Anterior inferior iliac spine

• The hip (innominate) bone is formed by the union of the ilium (9), ischium (12) and pubis (18).
• It bears on its lateral surface the cup-shaped acetabulum (25), to which the ilium, ischium and pubis each contribute a part (see page 286).
• The two hip bones articulate in the midline anteriorly at the pubic symphysis; posteriorly they are separated by the sacrum, forming the sacro-iliac joints. The two hip bones with the sacrum and coccyx constitute the pelvis.
• The ischiopubic ramus is formed by the union (16) of the ramus of the ischium (15) with the inferior ramus of the pubis (17).

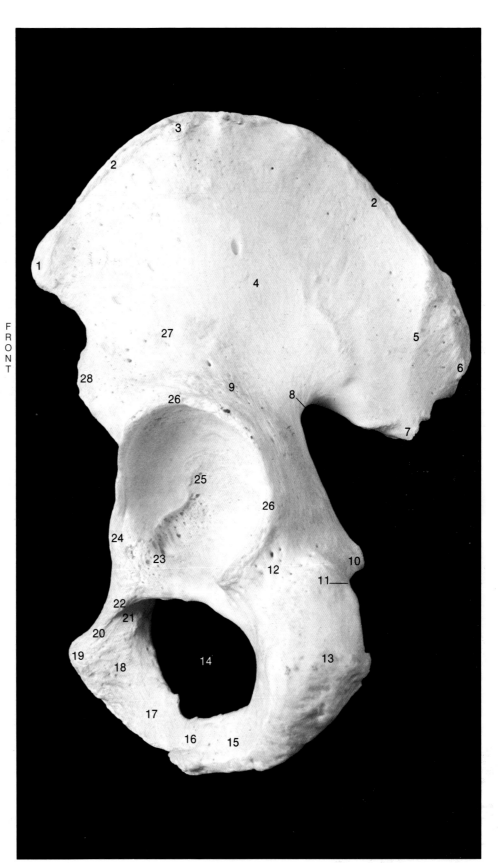

FRONT

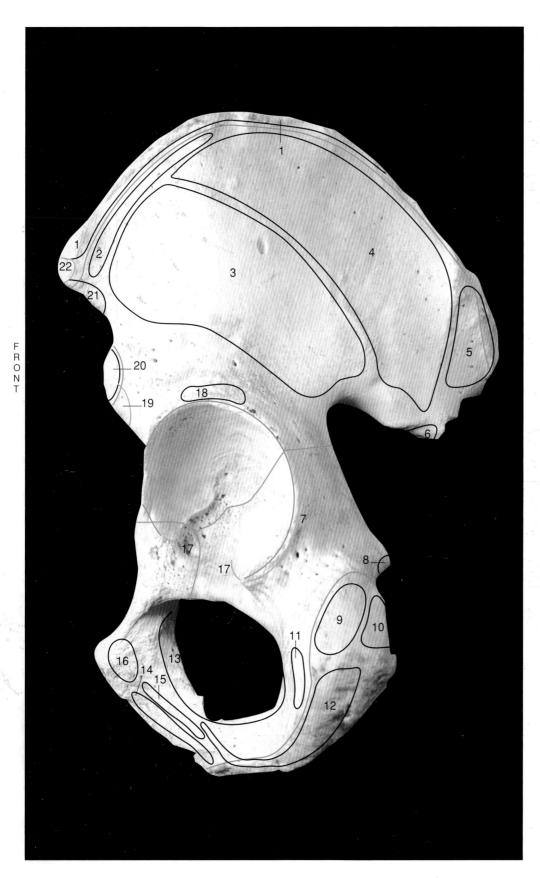

**Left hip bone, lateral surface.
Attachments**

Blue lines = epiphysial lines; green lines =
capsule attachment of hip joint; pale green lines =
ligament attachments

1 External oblique
2 Tensor fasciae latae
3 Gluteus minimus
4 Gluteus medius
5 Gluteus maximus
6 Piriformis
7 Ischiofemoral ligament
8 Superior gemellus
9 Semimembranosus
10 Semitendinosus and long head
    of biceps
11 Quadratus femoris
12 Adductor magnus
13 Obturator externus
14 Gracilis
15 Adductor brevis
16 Adductor longus
17 Transverse ligament
18 Reflected head of rectus femoris
19 Iliofemoral ligament
20 Straight head of rectus femoris
21 Sartorius
22 Inguinal ligament

FRONT

Left hip bone, medial surface

1 Iliac fossa
2 Anterior superior iliac spine
3 Anterior inferior iliac spine
4 Arcuate line
5 Iliopubic eminence
6 Obturator groove
7 Superior ramus of pubis
8 Pecten of pubis (pectineal line)
9 Body of pubis
10 Pubic tubercle
11 Pubic crest
12 Obturator foramen
13 Ischiopubic ramus
14 Ischial tuberosity
15 Lesser sciatic notch
16 Ischial spine
17 Body of ischium
18 Greater sciatic notch
19 Auricular surface
20 Posterior inferior iliac spine
21 Posterior superior iliac spine
22 Iliac tuberosity
23 Iliac crest

• The auricular surface of the ilium (19) is the articular surface for the sacro-iliac joint.

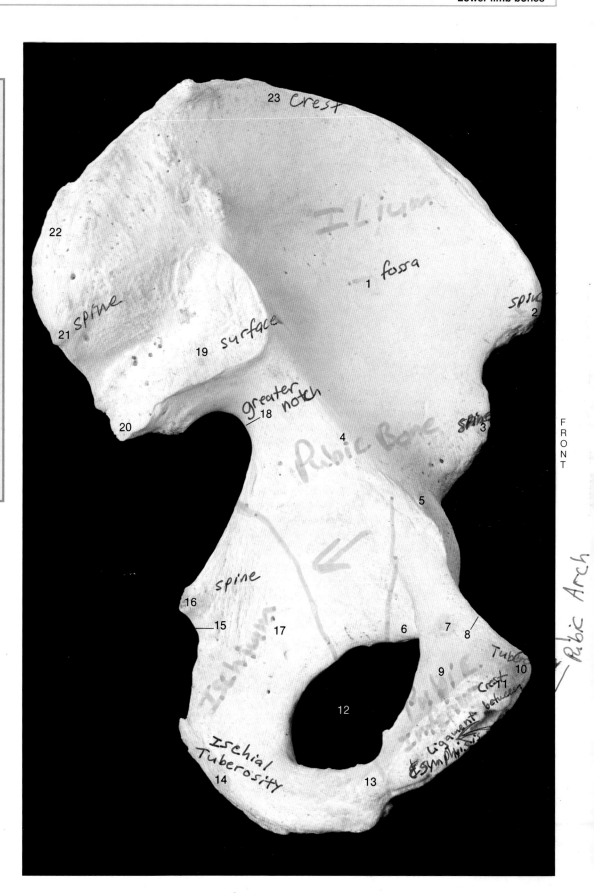

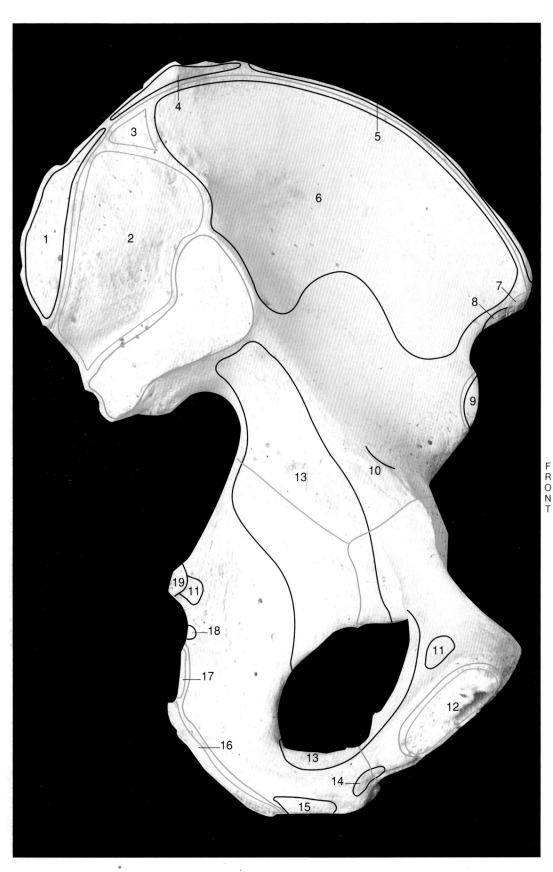

Left hip bone, medial surface. Attachments
Blue lines = epiphysial lines; green line = capsule attachment of sacro-iliac joint; pale green lines = ligament attachments

1 Erector spinae
2 Interosseous sacro-iliac ligament
3 Iliolumbar ligament
4 Quadratus lumborum
5 Transversus abdominis
6 Iliacus
7 Inguinal ligament
8 Sartorius
9 Straight head of rectus femoris
10 Psoas minor
11 Levator ani
12 Pubic symphysis
13 Obturator internus
14 Sphincter urethrae
15 Superficial transverse perineal and ischiocavernosus
16 Falciform process of sacrotuberous ligament
17 Sacrotuberous ligament
18 Inferior gemellus
19 Coccygeus and sacrospinous ligament

FRONT

Left hip bone, from above

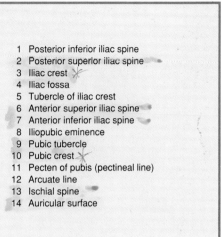

1 Posterior inferior iliac spine
2 Posterior superior iliac spine
3 Iliac crest
4 Iliac fossa
5 Tubercle of iliac crest
6 Anterior superior iliac spine
7 Anterior inferior iliac spine
8 Iliopubic eminence
9 Pubic tubercle
10 Pubic crest
11 Pecten of pubis (pectineal line)
12 Arcuate line
13 Ischial spine
14 Auricular surface

● The arcuate line on the ilium (12) and the pecten and crest of the pubis (11 and 10) form part of the brim of the pelvis (the rest of the brim being formed by the promontory and upper surface of the lateral part of the sacrum—see page 84).
● The pecten of the pubis (11) is more commonly called the pectineal line.

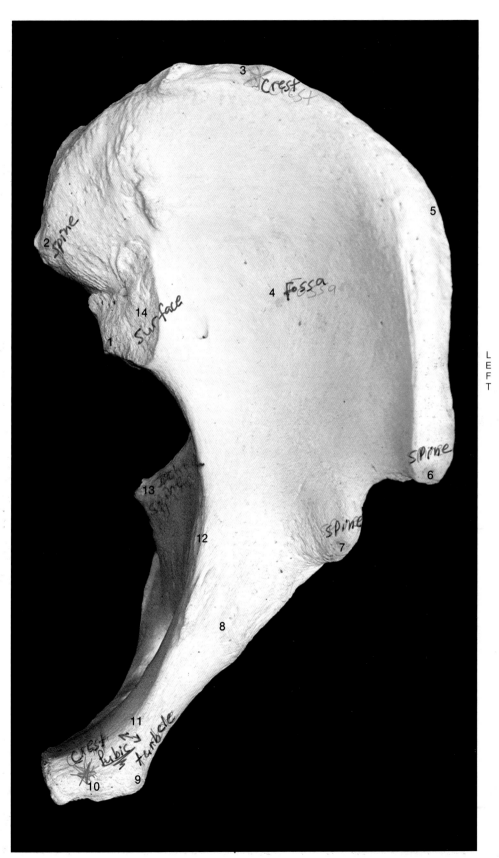

FRONT

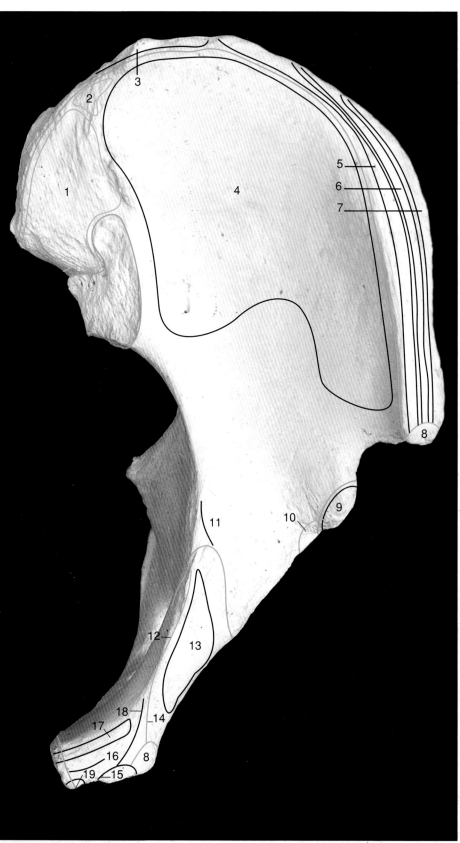

Left hip bone from above. Attachments
Blue lines = epiphysial lines; green line = capsule attachment of sacro-iliac joint; pale green lines = ligament attachments

1 Interosseous sacro-iliac ligament
2 Iliolumbar ligament
3 Quadratus lumborum
4 Iliacus
5 Transversus abdominis
6 Internal oblique
7 External oblique
8 Inguinal ligament
9 Straight head of rectus femoris
10 Iliofemoral ligament
11 Psoas minor
12 Pectineal ligament
13 Pectineus
14 Lacunar ligament
15 Anterior wall of rectus sheath
16 Pyramidalis
17 Lateral head of rectus abdominis
18 Conjoint tendon
19 Medial head of rectus abdominis

• The inguinal ligament (8) is formed by the lower border of the aponeurosis of the external oblique muscle, and extends from the anterior superior iliac spine to the pubic tubercle.
• The lacunar ligament (14, sometimes called the pectineal part of the inguinal ligament) is the part of the inguinal ligament that extends backwards from the medial end of the inguinal ligament to the pecten of the pubis.
• The pectineal ligament (12) is the lateral extension of the lacunar ligament along the pecten. It is not classified as a part of the inguinal ligament, and must not be confused with the alternative name for the lacunar ligament, i.e. with the pectineal part of the inguinal ligament.
• The conjoint tendon (18) is formed by the aponeuroses of the internal oblique and transversus muscles, and is attached to the pubic crest and the adjoining part of the pecten, blending medially with the anterior wall of the rectus sheath.

A Left hip bone. Ischial tuberosity, from behind and below

1 Ischial spine
2 Lesser sciatic notch
3 Upper part of tuberosity
4 Transverse ridge
5 Lower part of tuberosity
6 Longitudinal ridge
7 Ischiopubic ramus
8 Obturator groove
9 Acetabular notch
10 Rim of acetabulum
11 Acetabulum

B Left hip bone, from the front

1 Tubercle of iliac crest
2 Anterior superior iliac spine
3 Anterior inferior iliac spine
4 Rim of acetabulum
5 Acetabular notch
6 Ischial tuberosity
7 Ischiopubic ramus
8 Obturator foramen
9 Body of pubis
10 Pubic crest
11 Pubic tubercle
12 Obturator groove
13 Obturator crest
14 Pecten of pubis (pectineal line)
15 Iliopubic eminence
16 Iliac fossa

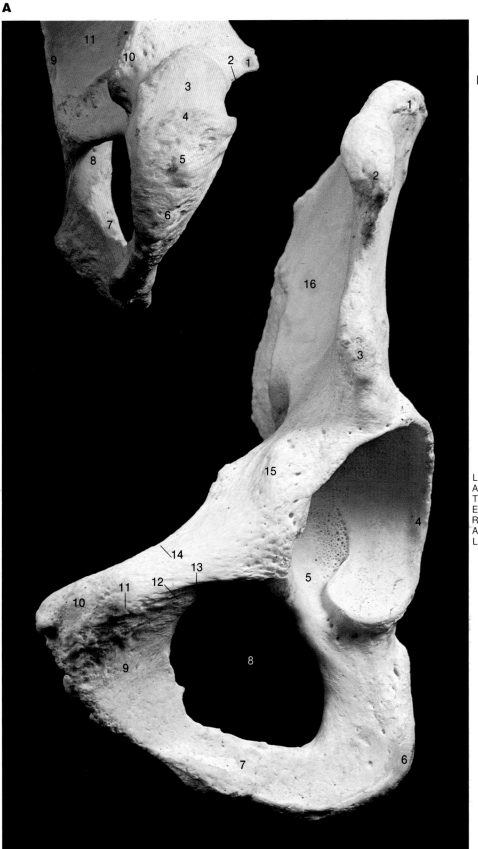

A

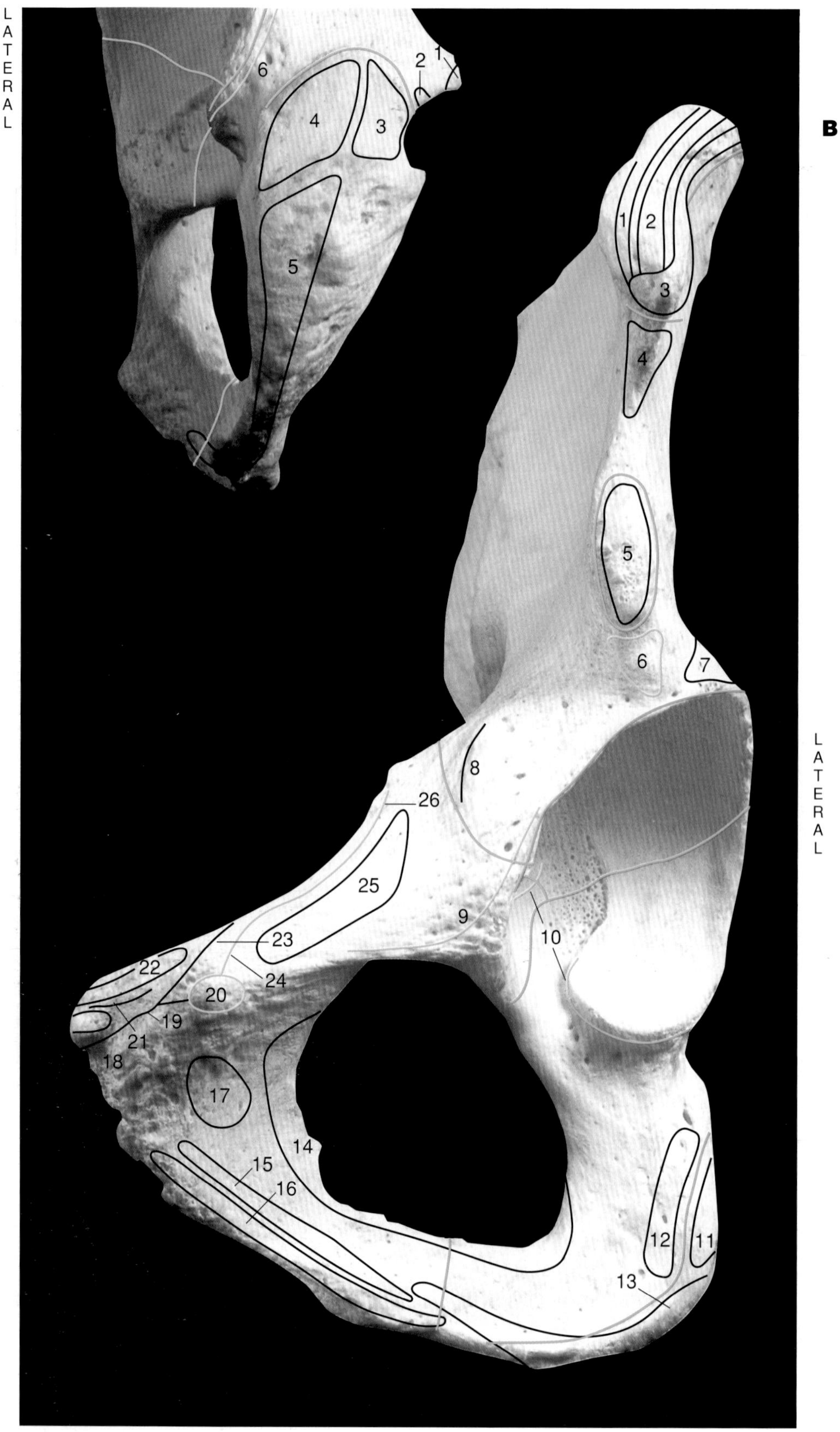

LATERAL

A Left hip bone. Ischial tuberosity, from behind and below. Attachments
Blue lines = epiphysial lines; green line = capsular attachment of hip joint; pale green lines = ligament attachments

1	Superior gemellus
2	Inferior gemellus
3	Semitendinosus and long head of biceps
4	Semimembranosus
5	Adductor magnus
6	Ischiofemoral ligament

• The area on the ischial tuberosity medial to the adductor magnus attachment (5) is covered by fibrofatty tissue and the ischial bursa underlying gluteus maximus.

B Left hip bone, from the front. Attachments
Blue lines = epiphysial lines; green line = capsular attachment of hip joint; pale green lines = ligament attachments

LATERAL

1	Transversus abdominis
2	Internal oblique
3	External oblique and inguinal ligament
4	Sartorius
5	Straight head of rectus femoris
6	Iliofemoral ligament
7	Reflected head of rectus femoris
8	Psoas minor
9	Pubofemoral ligament
10	Transverse ligament
11	Semimembranosus
12	Quadratus femoris
13	Adductor magnus
14	Obturator externus
15	Adductor brevis
16	Gracilis
17	Adductor longus
18	Medial head of rectus abdominis
19	Rectus sheath
20	Inguinal ligament
21	Pyramidalis
22	Lateral head of rectus abdominis
23	Conjoint tendon
24	Lacunar ligament
25	Pectineus
26	Pectineal ligament

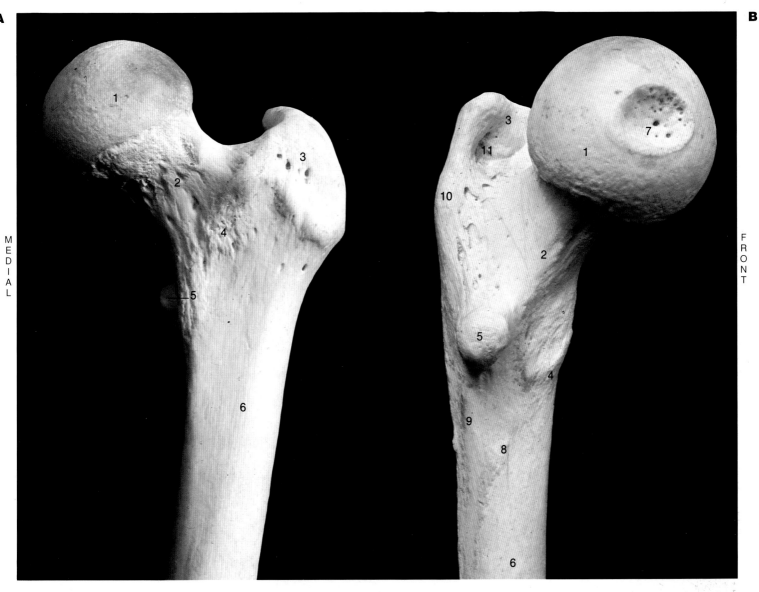

Left femur, upper end, A from the front, B from the medial side

1 Head
2 Neck
3 Greater trochanter
4 Intertrochanteric line
5 Lesser trochanter
6 Shaft
7 Fovea of head
8 Spiral line
9 Pectineal line
10 Quadrate tubercle on intertrochanteric crest
11 Trochanteric fossa

• The intertrochanteric *line* (4) is at the junction of the neck (2) and shaft (6) on the anterior surface; the intertrochanteric *crest* is in a similar position on the posterior surface (10, and page 268, A9).
• The neck makes an angle with the shaft of about 125°.
• The pectineal line of the femur (9) must not be confused with the pectineal line (pecten) of the pubis (page 263), nor with the spiral line of the femur (8) which is usually more prominent than the pectineal line.

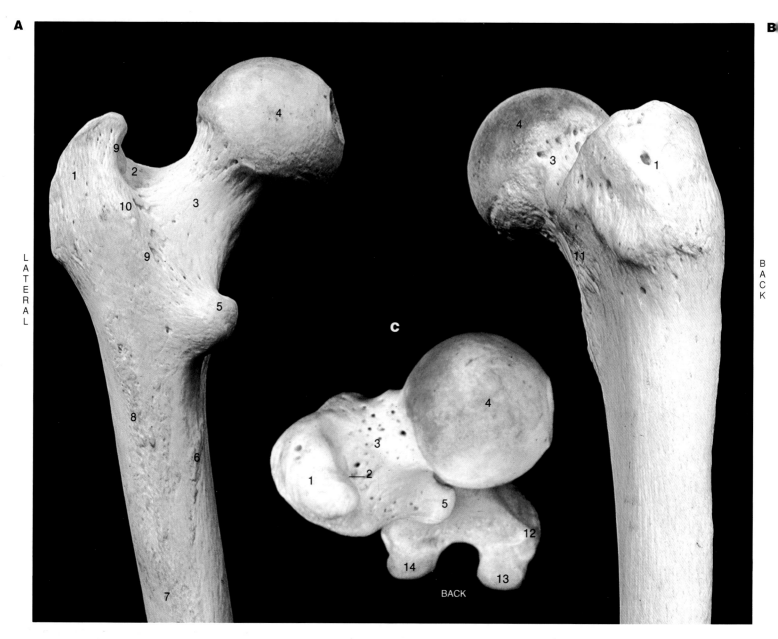

Left femur, upper end, A from behind, B from the lateral side, C from above

• The neck of the femur passes forwards as well as upwards and medially (C3), making an angle of about 15° with the transverse axis of the lower end (the angle of femoral torsion).
• The lesser trochanter (5) projects backwards and medially.

1	Greater trochanter
2	Trochanteric fossa
3	Neck
4	Head
5	Lesser trochanter
6	Spiral line
7	Linea aspera
8	Gluteal tuberosity
9	Intertrochanteric crest
10	Quadrate tubercle
11	Inter trochanteric line
12	Adductor tubercle
13	Medial condyle
14	Lateral condyle

12, 13, 14 at lower end

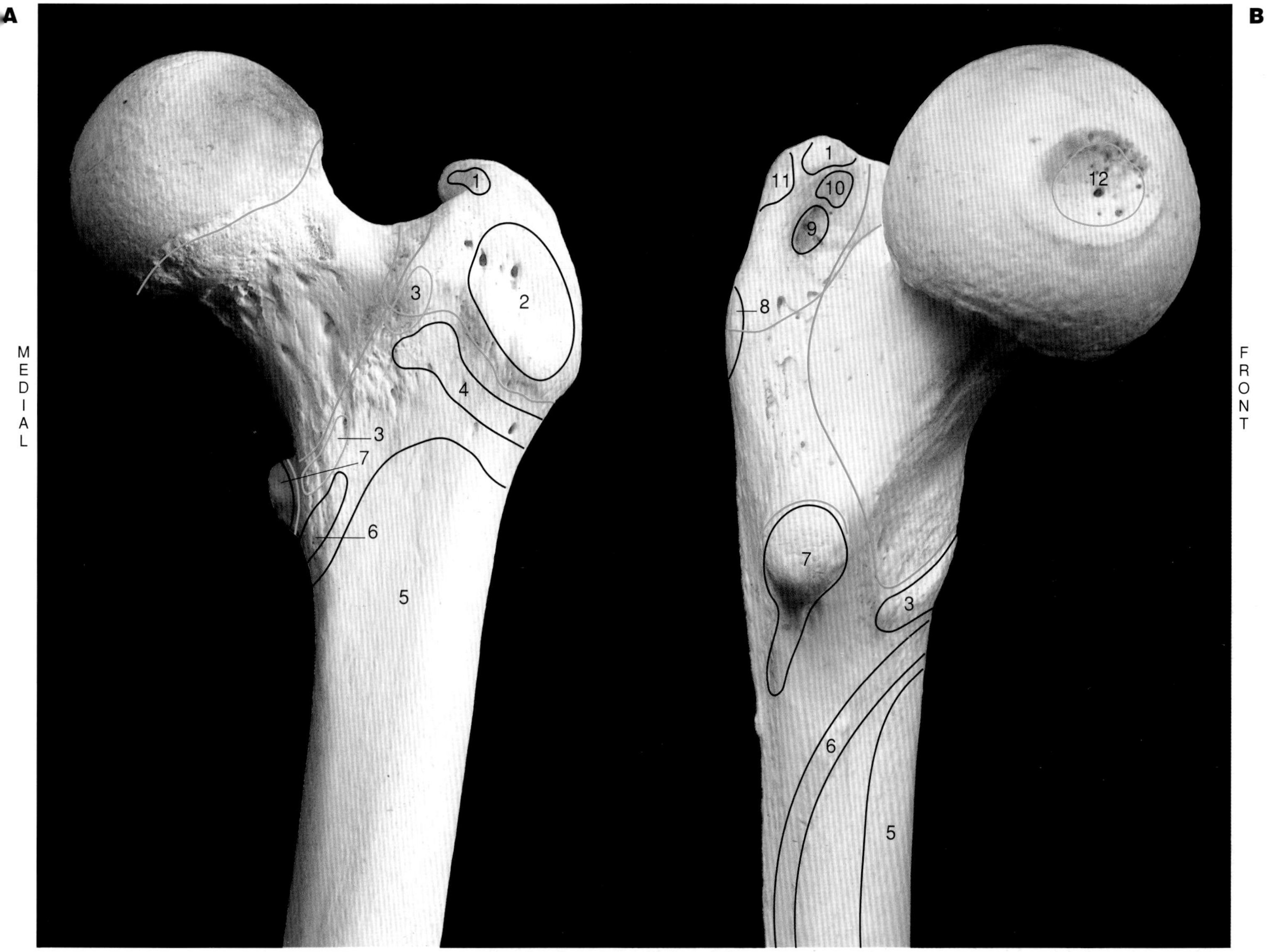

Left femur, upper end, A from the front, B from the medial side. Attachments

Blue lines = epiphysial lines; green line = capsular attachment of hip joint; pale green lines = ligament attachments

1	Piriformis
2	Gluteus minimus
3	Iliofemoral ligament
4	Vastus lateralis
5	Vastus intermedius
6	Vastus medialis
7	Psoas major and iliacus
8	Quadratus femoris
9	Obturator externus
10	Obturator internus and gemelli
11	Gluteus medius
12	Ligament of head of femur

• The iliofemoral ligament has the shape of an inverted V, with the stem attached to the anterior inferior iliac spine of the hip bone (page 266, B6), and the lateral and medial bands attached to the upper (lateral) and lower (medial) ends of the intertrochanteric line (3), blending with the capsule of the hip joint.

• The tendon of psoas major is attached to the lesser trochanter (7); many of the muscle fibres of iliacus are inserted into the psoas tendon but some reach the femur below the trochanter.

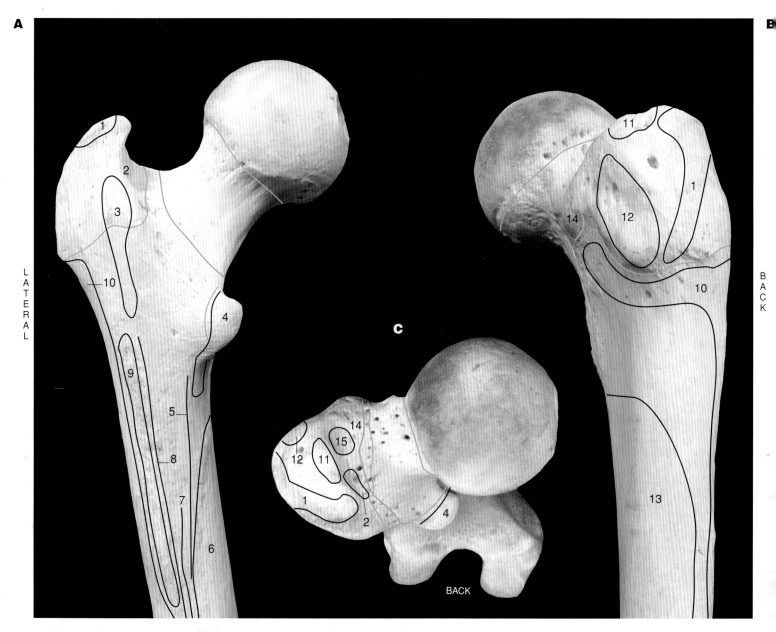

Left femur, upper end, A from behind, B from the lateral side, C from above.
Attachments
Blue lines = epiphysial lines; green line = capsule attachment of hip joint; pale green lines = ligament attachments

• On the front of the femur (page 269) the capsule of the hip joint is attached to the intertrochanteric line, but at the back the capsule is attached to the neck of the femur and does not extend as far laterally as the intertrochanteric crest (page 268, A9).

1	Gluteus medius
2	Obturator externus
3	Quadratus femoris
4	Psoas major and iliacus
5	Pectineus
6	Vastus medialis
7	Adductor brevis
8	Adductor magnus
9	Gluteus maximus
10	Vastus lateralis
11	Piriformis
12	Gluteus minimus
13	Vastus intermedius
14	Iliofemoral ligament (lateral band)
15	Obturator internus and gemelli

D Left femur, upper end, from the front ▷
This is the posterior half of a cleared and bisected specimen, to show the major groups of bone trabeculae

1	From medial ⎫ surface of shaft to head
2	From lateral ⎭
3	From medial ⎫ surface of shaft
4	From lateral ⎭ to greater trochanter
5	Calcar femorale
6	Triangular area of few trabeculae

• The calcar femorale (5) is a dense concentration of trabeculae passing from the region of the lesser trochanter to the under-surface of the neck.

E Left femur, shaft, from behind

1	Gluteal tuberosity	4	Linea aspera
2	Lesser trochanter	5	Medial supracondylar line
3	Pectineal line	6	Lateral supracondylar line

• The rough linea aspera (4) often shows distinct medial and lateral lips; the lateral lip continues upwards as the gluteal tuberosity (1).

F Left femur, shaft, from behind. Attachments

1	Vastus lateralis	7	Adductor brevis
2	Quadratus femoris	8	Vastus medialis
3	Gluteus maximus	9	Adductor longus
4	Adductor magnus	10	Short head of biceps
5	Psoas and iliacus	11	Vastus intermedius
6	Pectineus		

• For diagrammatic clarity the muscle attachments to the linea aspera have been slightly separated.

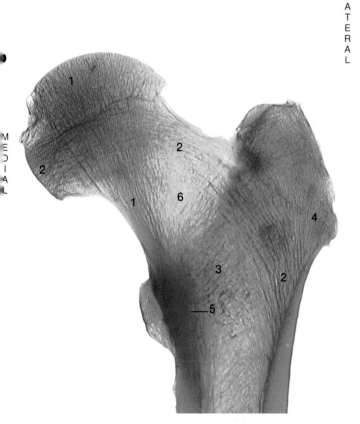

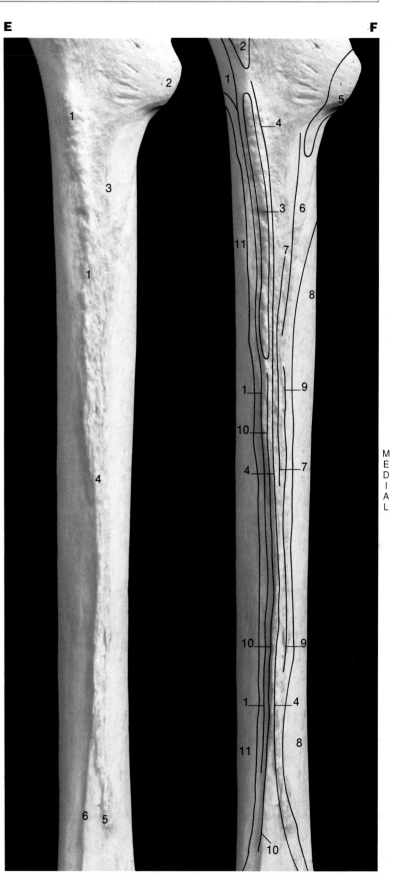

271

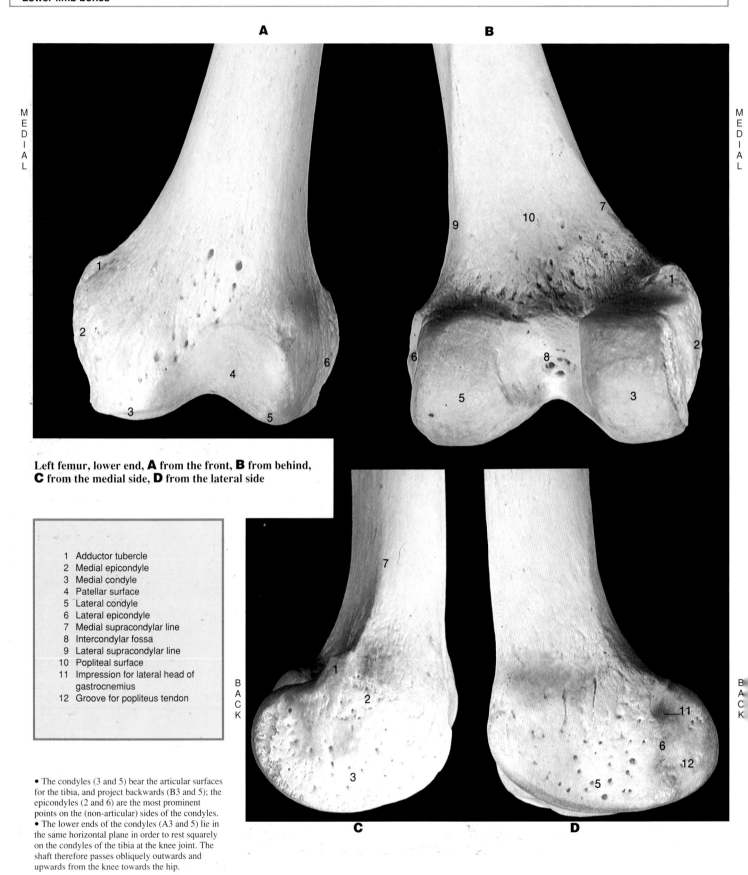

Left femur, lower end, A from the front, B from behind, C from the medial side, D from the lateral side

1 Adductor tubercle
2 Medial epicondyle
3 Medial condyle
4 Patellar surface
5 Lateral condyle
6 Lateral epicondyle
7 Medial supracondylar line
8 Intercondylar fossa
9 Lateral supracondylar line
10 Popliteal surface
11 Impression for lateral head of gastrocnemius
12 Groove for popliteus tendon

• The condyles (3 and 5) bear the articular surfaces for the tibia, and project backwards (B3 and 5); the epicondyles (2 and 6) are the most prominent points on the (non-articular) sides of the condyles.
• The lower ends of the condyles (A3 and 5) lie in the same horizontal plane in order to rest squarely on the condyles of the tibia at the knee joint. The shaft therefore passes obliquely outwards and upwards from the knee towards the hip.

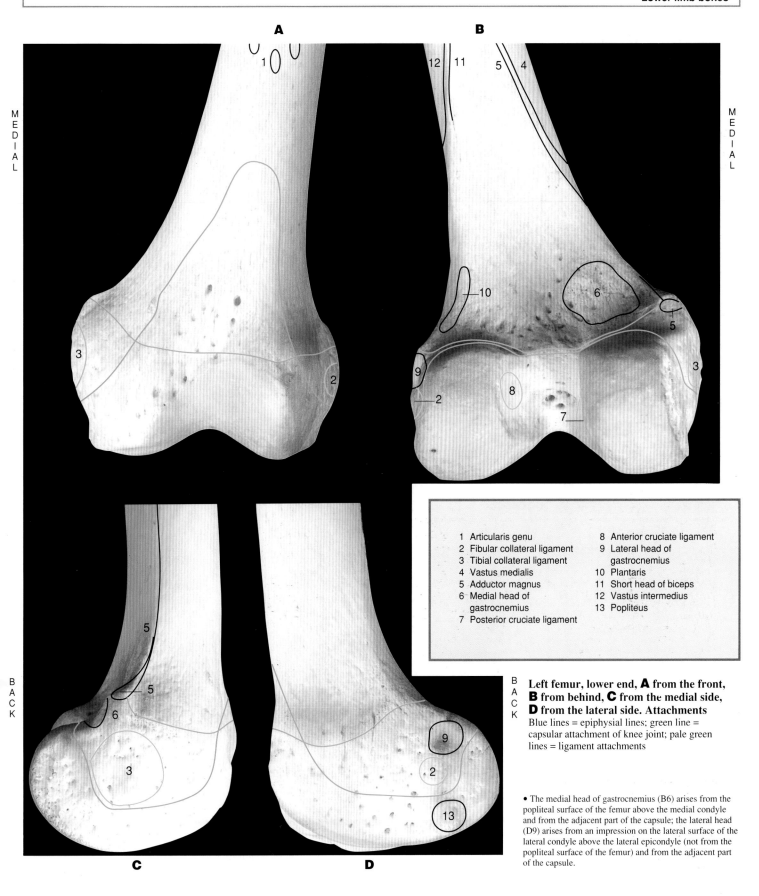

MEDIAL

MEDIAL

BACK

BACK

A

B

C

D

1 Articularis genu	8 Anterior cruciate ligament
2 Fibular collateral ligament	9 Lateral head of
3 Tibial collateral ligament	gastrocnemius
4 Vastus medialis	10 Plantaris
5 Adductor magnus	11 Short head of biceps
6 Medial head of	12 Vastus intermedius
gastrocnemius	13 Popliteus
7 Posterior cruciate ligament	

**Left femur, lower end, A from the front,
B from behind, C from the medial side,
D from the lateral side. Attachments**
Blue lines = epiphysial lines; green line =
capsular attachment of knee joint; pale green
lines = ligament attachments

• The medial head of gastrocnemius (B6) arises from the
popliteal surface of the femur above the medial condyle
and from the adjacent part of the capsule; the lateral head
(D9) arises from an impression on the lateral surface of the
lateral condyle above the lateral epicondyle (not from the
popliteal surface of the femur) and from the adjacent part
of the capsule.

273

A

B

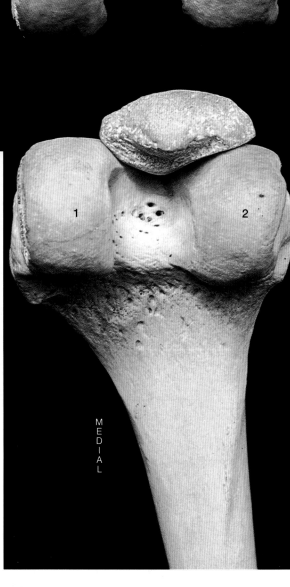

C

D

MEDIAL

MEDIAL

MEDIAL

MEDIAL

LATERAL

Left patella, A anterior surface, B articular (posterior) surface

Left patella, C anterior surface, D articular (posterior) surface. Attachments
Pale green line = ligament attachment

1	Base
2	Apex
3	Facet for lateral condyle of femur
4	Vertical ridge
5	Facet for medial condyle of femur

• The lateral part of the articular surface (B3) is larger than the medial (B5).
• The articular surface does not extend on to the apex (B2).

1	Vastus intermedius	parts of quadriceps tendon
2	Rectus femoris	
3	Vastus medialis	
4	Vastus lateralis	
5	Facets for femur in flexion	
6	Facets for femur in extension	
7	Area for medial condyle in extreme flexion	
8	Area for infrapatellar fat pad	
9	Patellar ligament	

Left femur and patella articulated, E from below with knee extended, F from below and behind with knee flexed
In flexion note the increased area of contact between the medial condyle of the femur (1) and the patella

1	Medial condyle
2	Lateral condyle

• The most medial facet of the patella (D7) only comes into contact with the medial condyle in extreme flexion as in F.

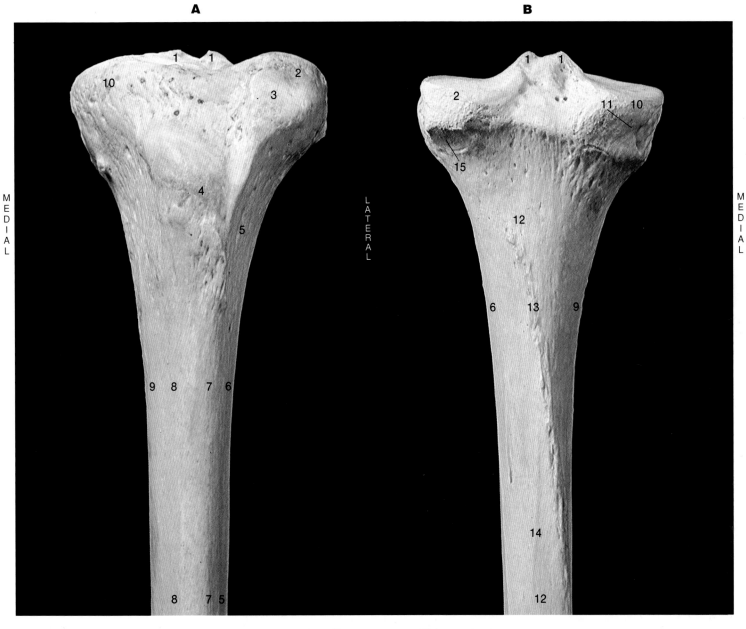

Left tibia, upper end, A from the front, B from behind

1	Tubercles of intercondylar eminence
2	Lateral condyle
3	Impression for iliotibial tract
4	Tuberosity
5	Lateral surface
6	Interosseous border
7	Anterior border
8	Medial surface
9	Medial border
10	Medial condyle
11	Groove for semimembranosus
12	Posterior surface
13	Soleal line
14	Vertical line
15	Articular facet for fibula

• The shaft of the tibia has three borders—anterior (7), medial (9) and interosseous (6)—and three surfaces—medial (8), lateral (5) and posterior (12).

• Much of the anterior border (7) forms a slightly curved crest commonly known as the shin. Most of the smooth medial surface (8) is subcutaneous. The posterior surface contains the soleal and vertical lines (13 and 14).

• The tuberosity (4) is at the upper end of the anterior border.

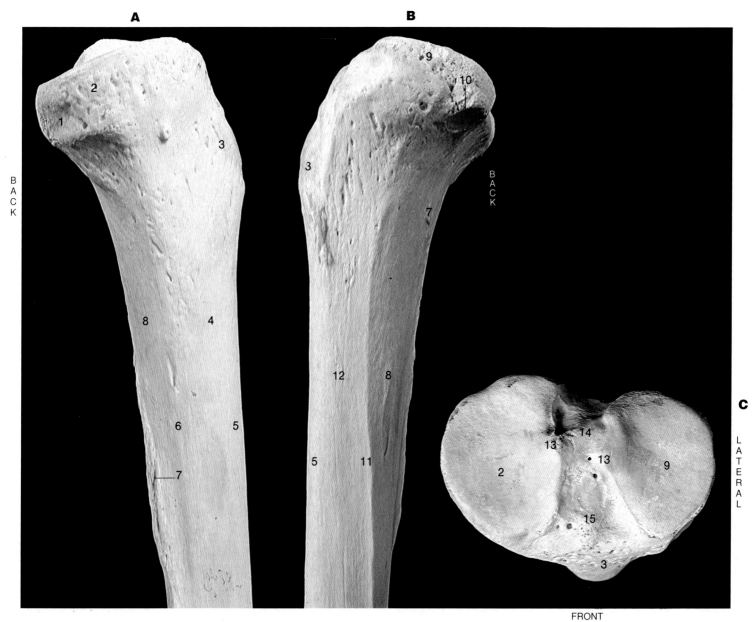

Left tibia, upper end, **A** from the medial side, **B** from the lateral side, **C** from above

1	Groove for semimembranosus	9	Lateral condyle
2	Medial condyle	10	Articular facet for fibula
3	Tuberosity	11	Interosseous border
4	Medial surface	12	Lateral surface
5	Anterior border	13	Tubercles of intercondylar eminence
6	Medial border	14	Posterior intercondylar area
7	Soleal line	15	Anterior intercondylar area
8	Posterior surface		

• The medial condyle (C2) is larger than the lateral condyle (C9).
• The articular facet for the fibula is on the postero-inferior aspect of the lateral condyle (B10).

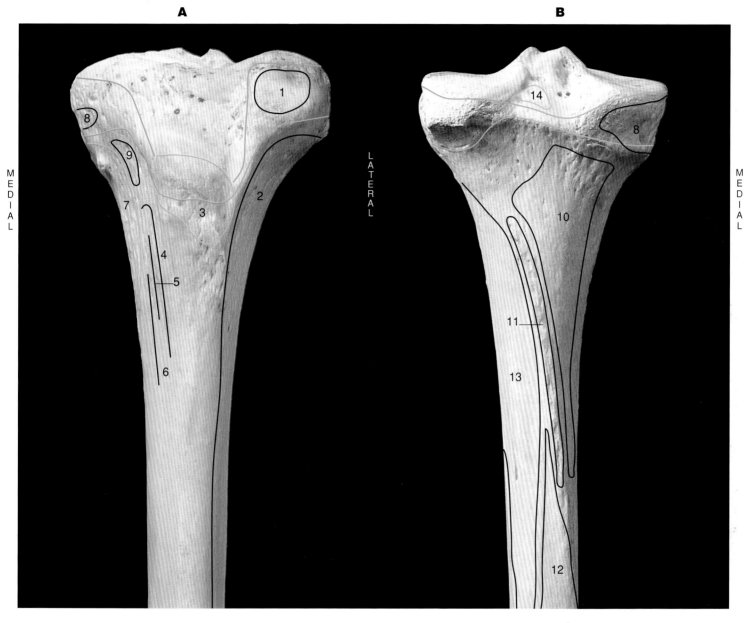

Left tibia, upper end, A from the front, B from behind. Attachments
Blue lines = epiphysial lines; green line = capsular attachment of knee joint; pale green lines = ligament attachments

1	Iliotibial tract	8	Semimembranosus
2	Tibialis anterior	9	Vastus medialis
3	Patellar ligament	10	Popliteus
4	Sartorius	11	Soleus
5	Gracilis	12	Flexor digitorum longus
6	Semitendinosus	13	Tibialis posterior
7	Tibial collateral ligament	14	Posterior cruciate ligament

A   **B**   **C**

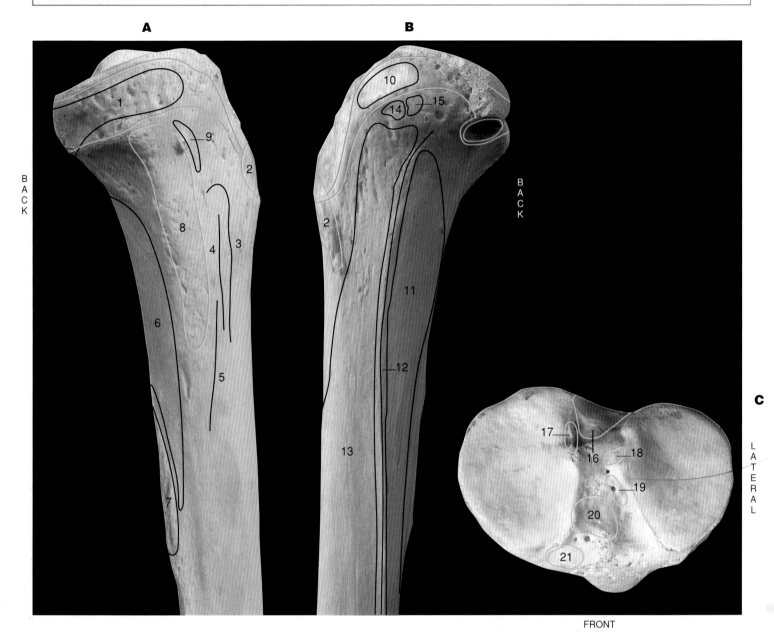

Left tibia, upper end, A from the medial side, B from the lateral side, C from above.
Attachments

Blue lines = epiphysial lines; green lines = capsular attachments of knee joint and superior tibiofibular joint; pale green lines = ligament attachments

1	Semimembranosus	12	Interosseous membrane
2	Patellar ligament	13	Tibialis anterior
3	Sartorius	14	Extensor digitorum longus
4	Gracilis	15	Peroneus longus
5	Semitendinosus	16	Posterior cruciate ligament
6	Popliteus	17	Posterior horn of medial meniscus
7	Soleus	18	Posterior horn of lateral meniscus
8	Tibial collateral ligament	19	Anterior horn of lateral meniscus
9	Vastus medialis	20	Anterior cruciate ligament
10	Iliotibial tract	21	Anterior horn of medial meniscus
11	Tibialis posterior		

• Although arising mainly from the fibula (see page 281), extensor digitorum longus (B14) and peroneus longus (B15) have a small attachment to the tibia above tibialis anterior (B13).
• The horns of the lateral meniscus (C18 and 19) are attached close to one another on either side of the intercondylar eminence, but the horns of the medial meniscus (C17 and 21) are widely separated (see page 305).
• The tibial attachment of the anterior cruciate ligament (C20) is to the top of the intercondylar area, but the attachment of the posterior cruciate ligament (C16) extends 'over the top' on to the posterior surface.

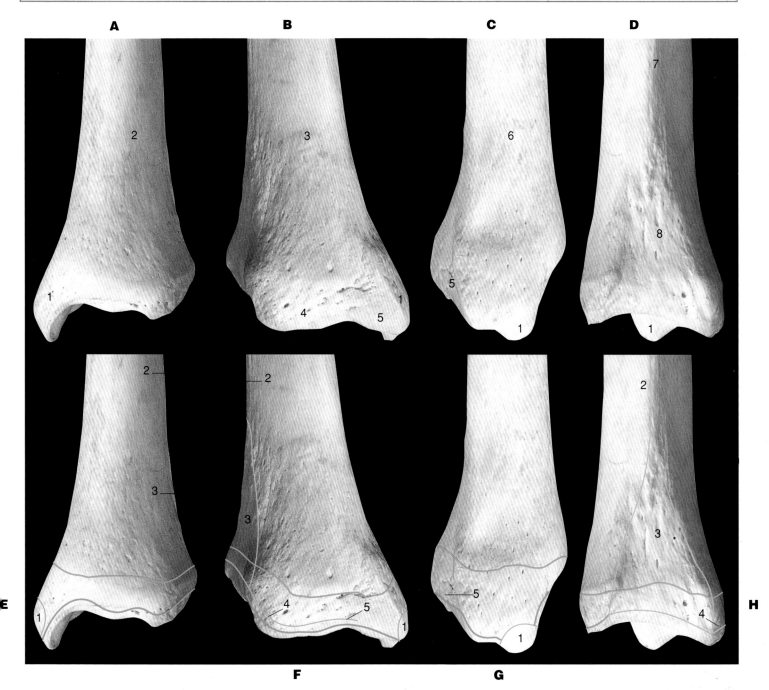

A   B   C   D

E   F   G   H

Left tibia, lower end, A from the front, B from behind, C from the medial side, D from the lateral side

1	Medial malleolus
2	Anterior surface
3	Posterior surface
4	Groove for flexor hallucis longus
5	Groove for tibialis posterior
6	Medial surface
7	Interosseous border
8	Fibular notch

• The lower end of the tibia has five surfaces—anterior, posterior, medial, lateral and inferior (for the inferior surface see page 282).
• The medial surface (C6) is continuous below with the medial surface of the medial malleolus (C1) (the lateral malleolus is the lower end of the fibula, see page 280).
• The fibular notch (D8) is triangular and constitutes the lateral surface of the lower end.

• The medial collateral ligament (G1) is commonly known as the deltoid ligament.
• The lowest fibres of the posterior tibiofibular ligament (attached most medially to the tibia) are known as the inferior transverse ligament (F4 and 5).

Left tibia, lower end, E from the front, F from behind, G from the medial side, H from the lateral side. Attachments
Blue line = epiphysial line; green line = capsular attachment of ankle joint; pale green lines= ligament attachments

1	Medial collateral ligament
2	Interosseous membrane
3	Interosseous ligament
4	Posterior tibiofibular ligament
5	Inferior transverse ligament

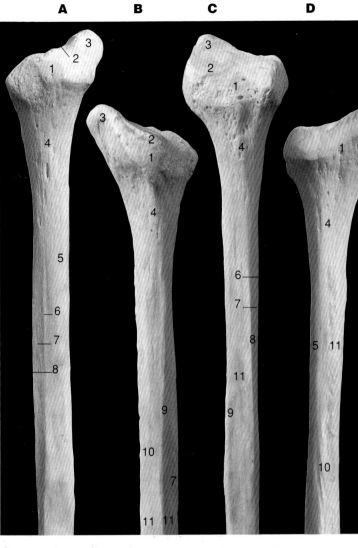

A   B   C   D

Left fibula, upper end, A from the front, B from behind, C from the medial side, D from the lateral side

1 Head	6 Anterior border
2 Articular facet on upper surface	7 Medial surface
	8 Interosseous border
3 Apex (styloid process)	9 Medial crest
4 Neck	10 Posterior border
5 Lateral surface	11 Posterior surface

● The fibula has three borders—anterior (A6), interosseous (A8) and posterior (B10)—and three surfaces—medial (A7), lateral (A5) and posterior (B11).

● At first sight much of the shaft appears to have four borders and four surfaces, but this is because the posterior surface (B11) is divided into two parts (medial and lateral) by the medial crest (B9).

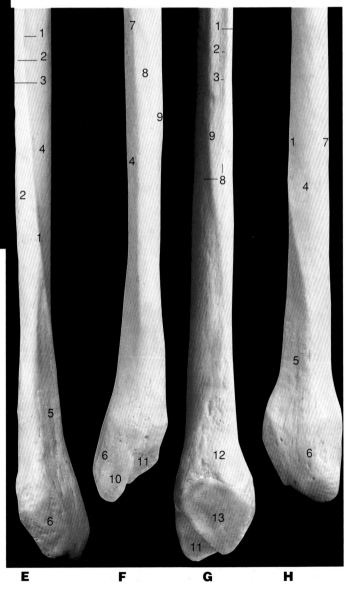

E   F   G   H

Left fibula, lower end, E from the front, F from behind, G from the medial side, H from the lateral side

1 Anterior border	9 Medial crest
2 Medial surface	10 Groove for peroneus brevis
3 Interosseous border	11 Malleolar fossa
4 Lateral surface	12 Surface for interosseous ligament
5 Triangular subcutaneous area	
6 Lateral malleolus	13 Articular surface of lateral malleolus
7 Posterior border	
8 Posterior surface	

● At the lower end the lateral surface (H4) comes to face posteriorly, so leaving the triangular subcutaneous area (H5) above the lateral malleolus (H6).

● The anterior border (E1) is easily identified by following it upwards from the apex of the triangular subcutaneous area (E5); the interosseous border (E3) is usually 2–3 mm behind the anterior border (although in the upper part of the shaft these two borders may fuse into one).

● The malleolar fossa (G11) is posterior to the articular surface (G13).

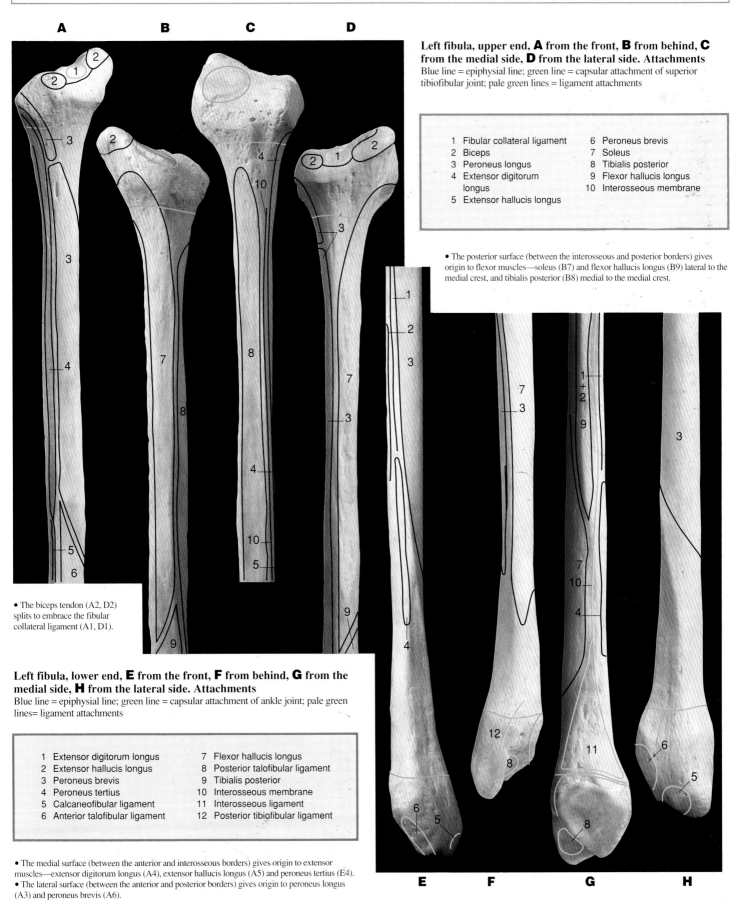

A B C D

Left fibula, upper end, A from the front, B from behind, C from the medial side, D from the lateral side. Attachments
Blue line = epiphysial line; green line = capsular attachment of superior tibiofibular joint; pale green lines = ligament attachments

1	Fibular collateral ligament	6	Peroneus brevis
2	Biceps	7	Soleus
3	Peroneus longus	8	Tibialis posterior
4	Extensor digitorum longus	9	Flexor hallucis longus
5	Extensor hallucis longus	10	Interosseous membrane

• The posterior surface (between the interosseous and posterior borders) gives origin to flexor muscles—soleus (B7) and flexor hallucis longus (B9) lateral to the medial crest, and tibialis posterior (B8) medial to the medial crest.

• The biceps tendon (A2, D2) splits to embrace the fibular collateral ligament (A1, D1).

Left fibula, lower end, E from the front, F from behind, G from the medial side, H from the lateral side. Attachments
Blue line = epiphysial line; green line = capsular attachment of ankle joint; pale green lines= ligament attachments

1	Extensor digitorum longus	7	Flexor hallucis longus
2	Extensor hallucis longus	8	Posterior talofibular ligament
3	Peroneus brevis	9	Tibialis posterior
4	Peroneus tertius	10	Interosseous membrane
5	Calcaneofibular ligament	11	Interosseous ligament
6	Anterior talofibular ligament	12	Posterior tibiofibular ligament

• The medial surface (between the anterior and interosseous borders) gives origin to extensor muscles—extensor digitorum longus (A4), extensor hallucis longus (A5) and peroneus tertius (E4).
• The lateral surface (between the anterior and posterior borders) gives origin to peroneus longus (A3) and peroneus brevis (A6).

E F G H

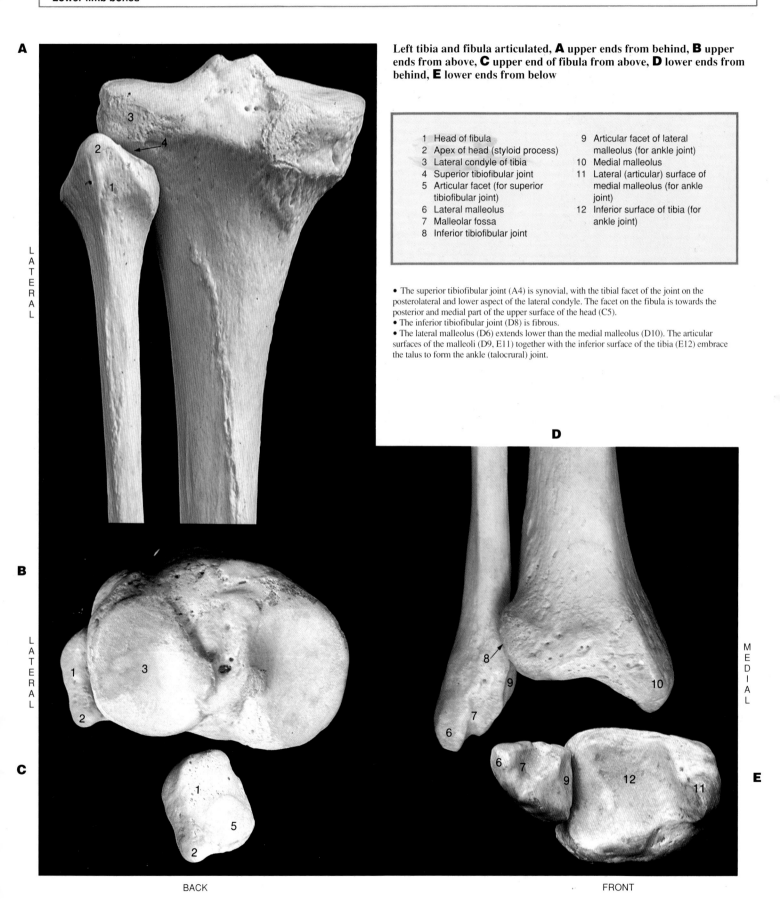

A

LATERAL

Left tibia and fibula articulated, **A** upper ends from behind, **B** upper ends from above, **C** upper end of fibula from above, **D** lower ends from behind, **E** lower ends from below

1 Head of fibula
2 Apex of head (styloid process)
3 Lateral condyle of tibia
4 Superior tibiofibular joint
5 Articular facet (for superior tibiofibular joint)
6 Lateral malleolus
7 Malleolar fossa
8 Inferior tibiofibular joint

9 Articular facet of lateral malleolus (for ankle joint)
10 Medial malleolus
11 Lateral (articular) surface of medial malleolus (for ankle joint)
12 Inferior surface of tibia (for ankle joint)

• The superior tibiofibular joint (A4) is synovial, with the tibial facet of the joint on the posterolateral and lower aspect of the lateral condyle. The facet on the fibula is towards the posterior and medial part of the upper surface of the head (C5).
• The inferior tibiofibular joint (D8) is fibrous.
• The lateral malleolus (D6) extends lower than the medial malleolus (D10). The articular surfaces of the malleoli (D9, E11) together with the inferior surface of the tibia (E12) embrace the talus to form the ankle (talocrural) joint.

D

B

LATERAL

C

MEDIAL

E

BACK

FRONT

A

B

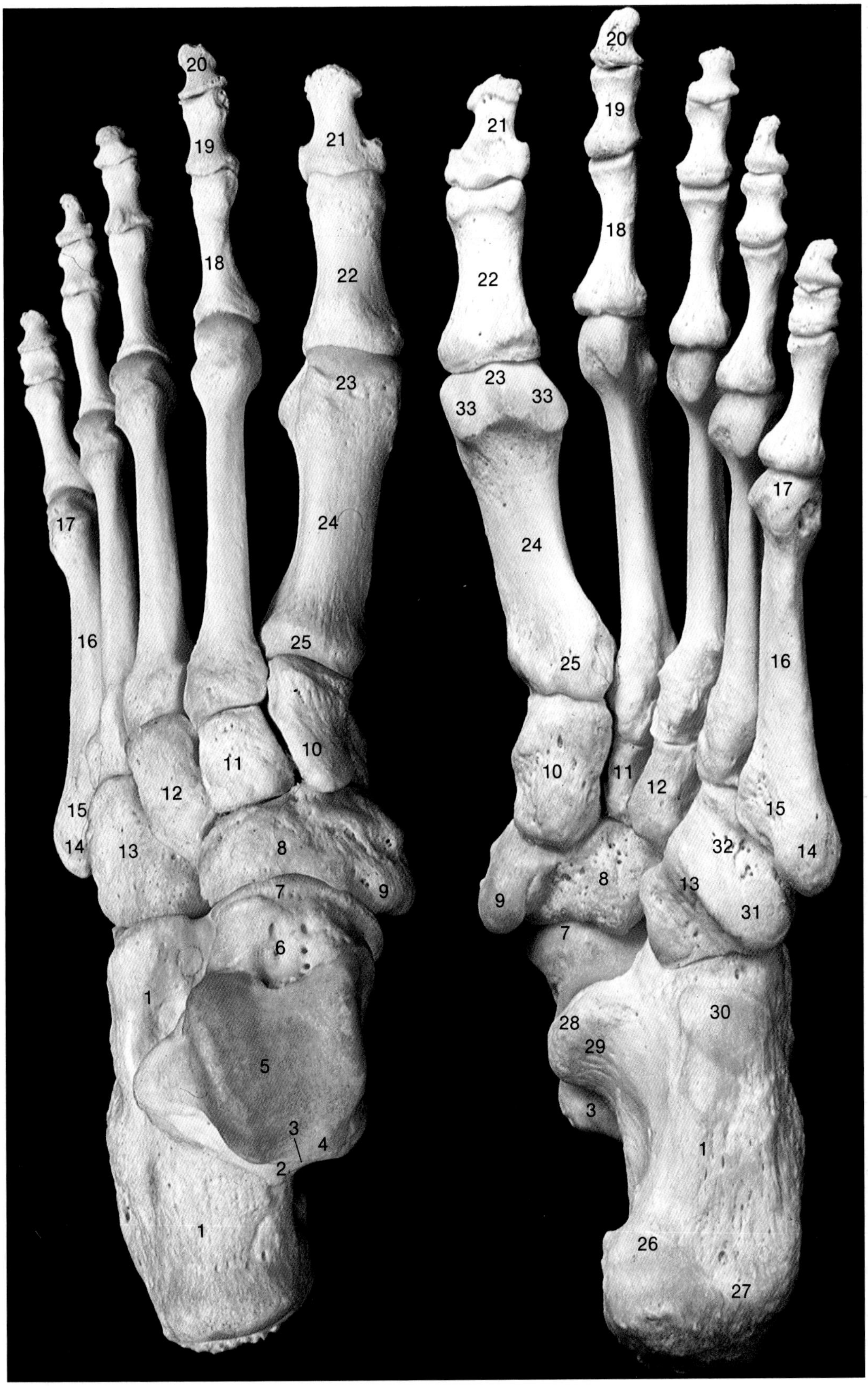

Bones of the left foot, A from above (dorsum), B from below (plantar surface)

1   Calcaneus
2   Lateral tubercle of talus
3   Groove on talus for flexor hallucis longus
4   Medial tubercle of talus
5   Trochlear surface of body of talus
6   Neck of talus
7   Head of talus
8   Navicular
9   Tuberosity of navicular
10 Medial cuneiform
11 Intermediate cuneiform
12 Lateral cuneiform
13 Cuboid
14 Tuberosity of base of fifth metatarsal
15 Base of fifth metatarsal
16 Shaft of fifth metatarsal
17 Head of fifth metatarsal
18 Proximal phalanx of second toe
19 Middle phalanx of second toe
20 Distal phalanx of second toe
21 Distal phalanx of great toe
22 Proximal phalanx of great toe
23 Head of first metatarsal
24 Shaft of first metatarsal
25 Base of first metatarsal
26 Medial process of calcaneus
27 Lateral process of calcaneus
28 Sustentaculum tali of calcaneus
29 Groove on calcaneus for flexor hallucis longus
30 Anterior tubercle of calcaneus
31 Tuberosity of cuboid
32 Groove on cuboid for peroneus longus
33 Grooves for sesamoid bones in flexor hallucis brevis

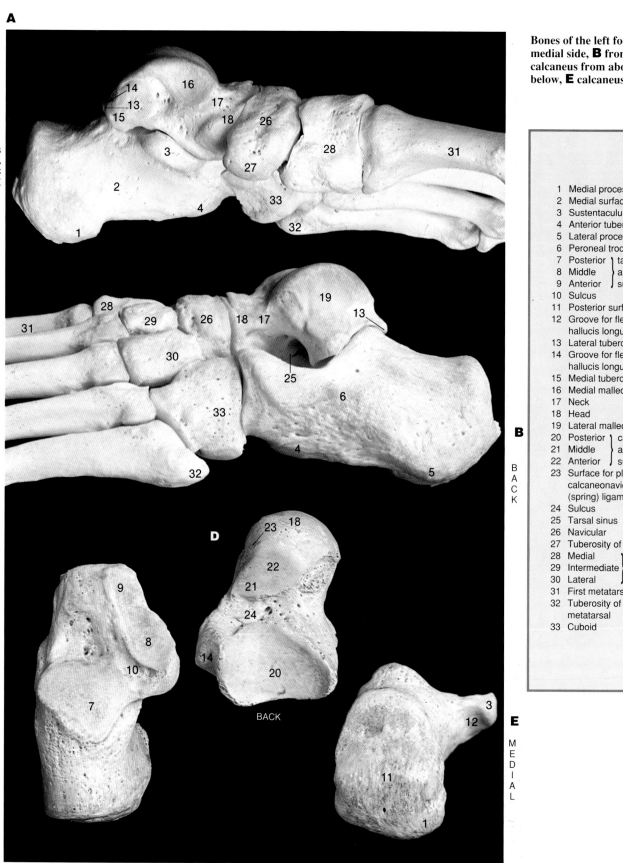

Bones of the left foot, **A** from the medial side, **B** from the lateral side, **C** calcaneus from above, **D** talus from below, **E** calcaneus from behind

1	Medial process
2	Medial surface
3	Sustentaculum tali
4	Anterior tubercle
5	Lateral process
6	Peroneal trochlea
7	Posterior } talal articular — of calcaneus
8	Middle } articular
9	Anterior } surface
10	Sulcus
11	Posterior surface
12	Groove for flexor hallucis longus
13	Lateral tubercle
14	Groove for flexor hallucis longus
15	Medial tubercle
16	Medial malleolar surface
17	Neck
18	Head
19	Lateral malleolar surface — of talus
20	Posterior } calcanean articular
21	Middle } articular
22	Anterior } surface
23	Surface for plantar calcaneonavicular (spring) ligament
24	Sulcus
25	Tarsal sinus
26	Navicular
27	Tuberosity of navicular
28	Medial
29	Intermediate } cuneiform
30	Lateral
31	First metatarsal
32	Tuberosity of base of fifth metatarsal
33	Cuboid

A   **B**

Bones of the left foot, A from above, B from below. Attachments
Joint capsules and minor ligaments have been omitted. Pale green lines = ligament attachments

1   Tendo calcaneus (Achilles' tendon)
2   Plantaris
3   Extensor digitorum brevis
4   Calcaneocuboid part of bifurcate ligament
5   Calcaneonavicular part of bifurcate ligament
6   Peroneus brevis
7   Peroneus tertius
8   Fourth ⎫
9   Third ⎬ dorsal
10   Second ⎬ interosseous
11   First ⎭
12   Abductor hallucis
13   Extensor hallucis brevis
14   Extensor hallucis longus
15   Extensor digitorum longus and brevis
16   Extensor digitorum longus
17   First ⎫
18   Second ⎬ plantar
19   Third ⎬ interosseous
20   Abductor digiti minimi
21   Flexor digitorum brevis
22   Flexor accessorius
23   Long plantar ligament
24   Plantar calcaneocuboid (short plantar) ligament
25   Plantar calcaneonavicular (spring) ligament
26   Tibialis posterior
27   Tibialis anterior
28   Flexor hallucis brevis
29   Flexor digiti minimi brevis
30   Adductor hallucis
31   Flexor hallucis longus
32   Flexor digitorum longus
33   Opponens digiti minimi (part of 29)
34   Peroneus longus

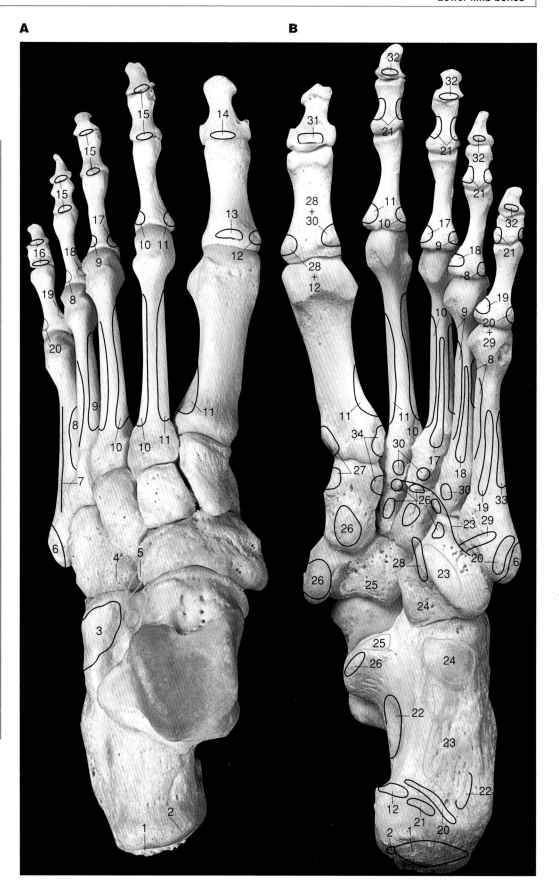

Left calcaneus, A from above, C from behind. B Left talus, from below

Curved lines indicate corresponding articular surfaces; green = capsular attachment of talocalcanean (subtalar), and talocalcaneonavicular joints; pale green lines = ligament attachments

1	Calcaneofibular ligament
2	Lateral ⎫ talocalcanean ligament
3	Medial ⎭
4	Tibiocalcanean part of deltoid ligament
5	Interosseous talocalcanean ligament
6	Inferior extensor retinaculum
7	Cervical ligament
8	Extensor digitorum brevis
9	Calcaneocuboid ⎫ parts of
10	Calcaneonavicular ⎭ bifurcate ligament
11	Area for bursa
12	Tendo calcaneus (Achilles' tendon)
13	Plantaris
14	Area for fibrofatty tissue

• The interosseous talocalcanean ligament (5) is formed by thickening of the adjacent capsules of the talocalcanean and talocalcaneonavicular joints.
• For different interpretations of the term 'subtalar joint' see the notes on page 320.

Secondary centres of ossification of left lower limb bones
D Hip bone, lower lateral part
E and **F** Femur, upper and lower ends
G and **H** Tibia, upper and lower ends
J and **K** Fibula, upper and lower ends
L Calcaneus
M Metatarsal and phalanges of second toe
N Metatarsal and phalanges of great toe

Figures in years, commencement of ossification → fusion.
P = puberty, B = ninth intra-uterine month. See introduction on page 114
• In the hip bone (D) one or more secondary centres appear in the Y-shaped cartilage between ilium, ischium and pubis. Other centres (not illustrated) are usually present for the iliac crest, anterior inferior iliac spine, and (possibly) the pubic tubercle and pubic crest (all P → 25).
• The patella (not illustrated) begins to ossify from one or more centres between the third and sixth year.
• All the phalanges, and the first metatarsal, have a secondary centre at their proximal ends; the other metatarsals have one at their distal ends.
• Of the tarsal bones, the largest, the calcaneus, begins to ossify in the third intra-uterine month and the talus about three months later. The cuboid may begin to ossify either just before or just after birth, with the lateral cuneiform in the first year, medial cuneiform at two years and the intermediate cuneiform and navicular at three years.
• The calcaneus (L) is the only tarsal bone to have a secondary centre.

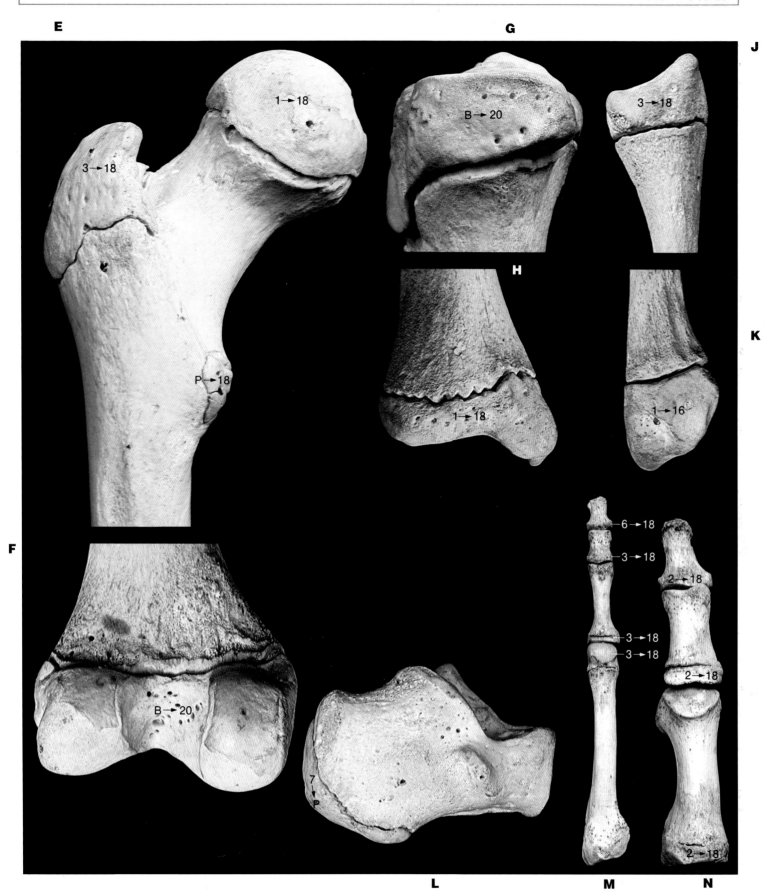

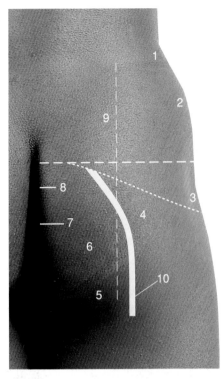

A Right gluteal region. Surface features
The interrupted lines divide the gluteal region into quadrants (see the note below). The iliac crest (1) with the posterior superior iliac spine (9), the tip of the coccyx (7), the ischial tuberosity (6) and the tip of the greater trochanter of the femur (3) are palpable landmarks. A line drawn from a point midway between the posterior superior iliac spine (9) and the tip of the coccyx (7) to the tip of the greater trochanter (3) marks the lower border of piriformis (dotted white line) which is a key feature of the gluteal region, where the most important structure is the sciatic nerve (indicated here in yellow, 10; see dissections and notes opposite).

1	Iliac crest
2	Gluteus medius
3	Tip of greater trochanter of femur
4	Gluteus maxinus
5	Fold of buttock
6	Ischial tuberosity
7	Tip of coccyx
8	Natal cleft
9	Posterior superior iliac spine
10	Sciatic nerve

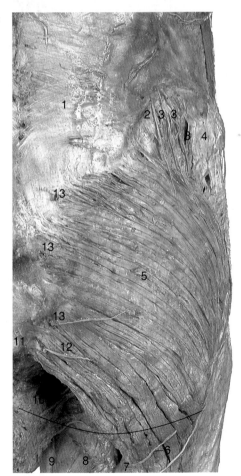

B Right gluteal region. Superficial nerves
Skin and subcutaneous tissue have been removed, preserving cutaneous branches from the first three lumbar (3) and first three sacral (13) nerves, the cutaneous branches of the posterior femoral cutaneous nerve (6) and the perforating cutaneous nerve (12). The curved line near the bottom of the picture indicates the position of the gluteal fold (fold of the buttock). The muscle fibres of gluteus maximus (5) run downwards and laterally, and its lower border does not correspond to the gluteal fold

1	Posterior layer of lumbar fascia overlying erector spinae
2	Iliac crest
3	Cutaneous branches of dorsal rami of first three lumbar nerves
4	Gluteal fascia overlying gluteus medius
5	Gluteus maximus
6	Gluteal branches of the posterior femoral cutaneous nerve
7	Semitendinosus
8	Adductor magnus
9	Gracilis
10	Ischio-anal fossa and levator ani
11	Coccyx
12	Perforating cutaneous nerve
13	Gluteal branches of dorsal rami of first three sacral nerves

• The first three lumbar nerves and the first three sacral nerves supply skin over the gluteal region (by the lateral branches of their dorsal rami, 3 and 13) but the intervening fourth and fifth lumbar nerves do not have a cutaneous distribution in this region.
• The gluteal region or buttock is sometimes used as a site for intramuscular injections. The correct site is in the upper outer quadrant of the buttock, and for delimiting this quadrant it is essential to remember that the upper boundary of the buttock is the uppermost part of the iliac crest. The lower boundary is the fold of the buttock. Dividing the area between these two boundaries by a vertical line midway between the midline and the lateral side of the body indicates that the upper outer quadrant is well above and to the right of the label 5 in B, and this is the safe site for injection—well above and to the right of the sciatic nerve which is displayed in the dissections opposite.

Right gluteal region, C with most of gluteus maximus removed, D with the sciatic nerve displaced

The removal of the central part of gluteus maximus (1) displays piriformis (2) which is the guide to the surrounding structures. The superior gluteal artery (3) and nerve (4) are above it, running between gluteus medius (5) and minimus (7). The inferior gluteal nerve (6) and vessels (22) are below piriformis (2), and part of the nerve is seen entering gluteus maximus (1), the rest having been removed with the muscle. Also emerging below piriformis are the sciatic nerve (14 and 15) with the nerve to quadratus femoris (D23) under cover of it, the posterior femoral cutaneous nerve (16) superficially, and more medially the nerve to obturator internus (19), the internal pudendal artery (20) and the pudendal nerve (21). Obturator internus (10) with a gemellus on either side (9 and 11) and quadratus femoris (13) lie in that order below piriformis. In D the sciatic nerve has been displaced slightly laterally to show the underlying nerve to quadratus femoris (23, in front of the upper white marker; the lower marker is behind the nerve to obturator internus, 19)

M
I
D
L
I
N
E

1 Gluteus maximus
2 Piriformis
3 Superior gluteal artery
4 Superior gluteal nerve
5 Gluteus medius
6 Inferior gluteal nerve
7 Gluteus minimus
8 Greater trochanter of femur
9 Superior gemellus
10 Obturator internus
11 Inferior gemellus
12 Obturator externus
13 Quadratus femoris
14 Common peroneal } part of
15 Tibial } sciatic nerve
16 Posterior femoral cutaneous nerve
17 Ischial tuberosity
18 Sacrotuberous ligament
19 Nerve to obturator internus
20 Internal pudendal artery
21 Pudendal nerve
22 Inferior gluteal artery
23 Nerve to quadratus femoris

C

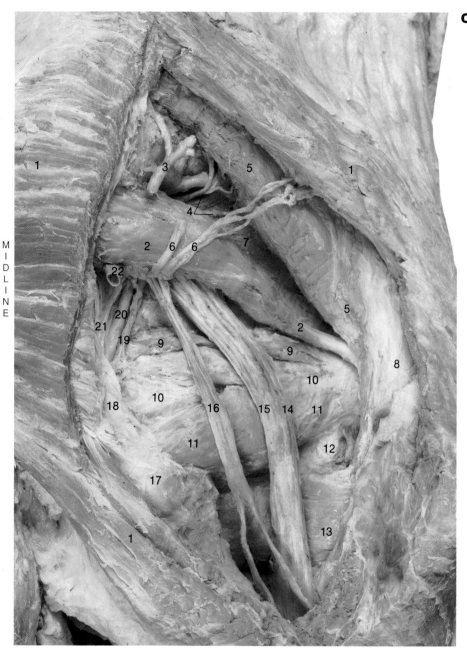

D

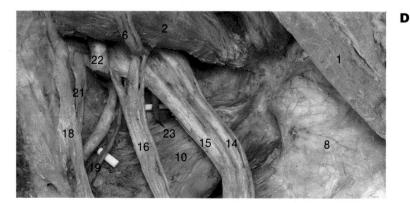

• Emerging from the pelvis into the gluteal region above piriformis (2) are the superior gluteal nerve and vessels (4 and 3).
• Emerging from the pelvis into the gluteal region below piriformis are the inferior gluteal nerve and vessels (6 and 22), the sciatic nerve (14 and 15), the posterior femoral cutaneous nerve (16) and the nerve to quadratus femoris (23).
• Emerging from the pelvis below piriformis to enter the perineum are the pudendal nerve (21), the internal pudendal vessels (20) and the nerve to obturator internus (19), in that order from medial to lateral.
• The two parts of the sciatic nerve (common peroneal and tibial, 14 and 15) usually divide from one another at the top of the popliteal fossa (page 302) but are sometimes separate as they emerge beneath piriformis, and the common peroneal may even perforate piriformis.
• After curving laterally beneath piriformis the sciatic nerve lies midway between the ischial tuberosity (17) and the greater trochanter of the femur (8); these two bony points are surface markings for the upper part of the nerve as it passes centrally down the back of the thigh.

A

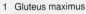

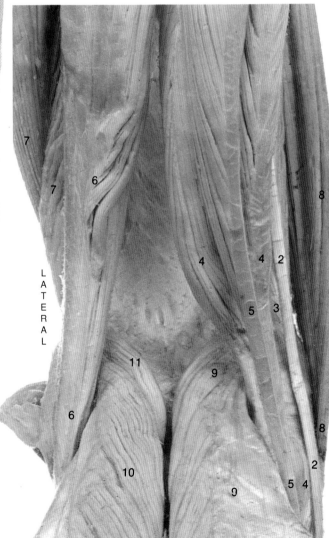

Back of the left thigh. Muscles, **A** in the upper part, **B** in the lower part bordering the popliteal fossa

All fascia, vessels and nerves have been removed. Biceps (6) passes downwards and laterally, forming in B the upper lateral boundary of the popliteal fossa. Semimembranosus (4) and semitendinosus (5) pass down on the medial side, forming in B the upper medial boundary of the popliteal fossa, where the tendon of semitendinosus (B5) overlies semimembranosus (B4)

1	Gluteus maximus
2	Gracilis
3	Adductor magnus
4	Semimembranosus
5	Semitendinosus
6	Biceps
7	Vastus lateralis
8	Sartorius
9	Medial } head of gastrocnemius
10	Lateral
11	Plantaris

• The long head of biceps (the part seen in A, 6), semimembranosus (4) and semitendinosus (5) are commonly called the hamstrings. The short head of biceps, which is under cover of the long head and arises from the back of the shaft of the femur and not from the ischial tuberosity (as the other muscles do), is not classified as a hamstring. The true hamstrings span both the hip and knee joint; they extend the hip and flex the knee.

• The origins of the hamstrings from the ischial tuberosity are under cover of the lower border of gluteus maximus (1), but are seen in C opposite, where gluteus maximus has been partly removed.

C

C Back of the right upper thigh

Gluteus maximus (10) has been reflected laterally and the gap between semitendinosus (4) and biceps (5) has been opened up to show the sciatic nerve (7) and its muscular branches

1 Ischial tuberosity
2 Gracilis
3 Semimembranosus
4 Semitendinosus
5 Long head of biceps
6 Anastomotic branch of inferior gluteal artery
7 Sciatic nerve
8 Quadratus femoris
9 Upper part of adductor magnus ('adductor minimus')
10 Gluteus maximus
11 First perforating artery
12 Nerve to short head of biceps
13 Iliotibial tract overlying vastus lateralis
14 Short head of biceps
15 Popliteal vein
16 Popliteal artery
17 Opening in adductor magnus
18 Fourth perforating artery
19 Adductor magnus
20 Nerve to semimembranosus
21 Third perforating artery
22 Nerve to semitendinosus
23 Nerve to semimembranosus and adductor magnus
24 Nerve to long head of biceps
25 Second perforating artery

L A T E R A L

• The only muscular branch to arise from the lateral side of the sciatic nerve (i.e. from the common peroneal part of the nerve—7, uppermost label near the top of the picture) is the nerve to the short head of biceps (12). All the other muscular branches—to the long head of biceps (24), semimembranosus (20), semimembranosus and adductor magnus (23) and semitendinosus (22)—arise from the medial side of the sciatic nerve (7, near the centre of the picture) (i.e. from the tibial part of the nerve).

D

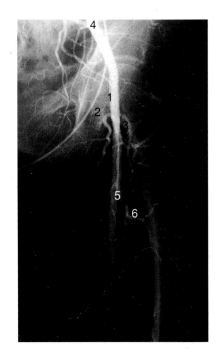

D Femoral arteriogram

1 Femoral artery
2 Medial circumflex femoral artery
3 Lateral circumflex femoral artery
4 External iliac artery
5 Profunda femoris artery
6 Perforating artery

A

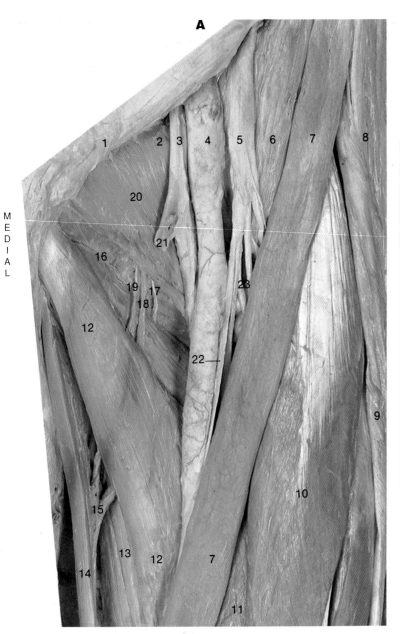

Left femoral region, **A** femoral vessels and nerve, **B** profunda femoris artery

The superficial vessels and nerves and the fascia lata have been removed to display in A the femoral vein (3), artery (4) and nerve (5) and the surrounding muscles. In B the femoral artery (4) has been displaced laterally to show the profunda femoris branch (24)

1	Inguinal ligament
2	Position of femoral canal
3	Femoral vein
4	Femoral artery
5	Femoral nerve
6	Iliacus
7	Sartorius
8	Fascia lata overlying tensor fasciae latae
9	Iliotibial tract overlying vastus lateralis
10	Rectus femoris
11	Vastus medialis
12	Adductor longus
13	Adductor magnus
14	Gracilis
15	Nerve and vessels to gracilis
16	Adductor brevis
17	Nerve to adductor brevis ⎫ from anterior
18	Nerve to adductor longus ⎬ branch of
19	Nerve to gracilis ⎭ obturator nerve
20	Pectineus
21	Great saphenous vein
22	Saphenous nerve
23	Muscular branches of femoral nerve overlying lateral circumflex femoral vessels
24	Profunda femoris artery
25	Medial circumflex femoral artery

B

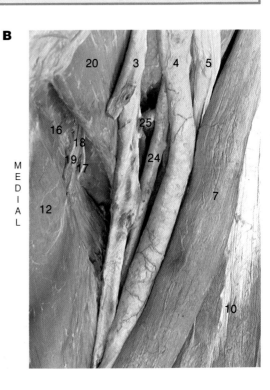

• The boundaries of the femoral triangle are the inguinal ligament (1), the *medial* border of sartorius (7) and the *medial* border of adductor longus (12).
• The adjacent borders of pectineus (20) and adductor longus (12) are usually in contact with one another, but if they are not (as in this specimen) the anterior branch of the obturator nerve and its muscular branches (17 to 19) are visible in the floor of the triangle lying in front of adductor brevis (16).
• The femoral canal (2) is the medial compartment of the femoral sheath (removed) which contains in its middle compartment the femoral vein (3), and in the lateral compartment the femoral artery (4). The femoral nerve (5) is *lateral* to the sheath, not within it.
• The profunda femoris artery (24) arises from the posterolateral surface of the femoral artery (4) and so is under cover of it in A, but is shown in B when the parent vessel is displaced laterally.
• In the lower part of the femoral triangle the femoral vein (3) lies behind the artery (4) and both pass in front of adductor longus (12).
• The profunda femoris artery (24) passes behind adductor longus (as shown on page 294).

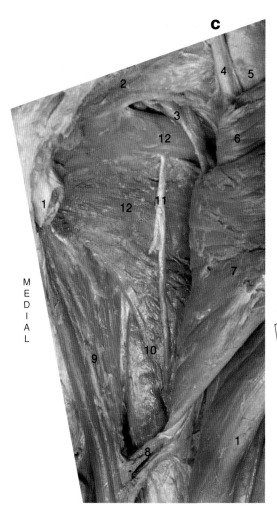

C

C Left obturator nerve

In this left femoral region, pectineus (6), adductor longus (1, lower label) and adductor brevis (7) have been detached from their origins and reflected laterally to display obturator externus (12) and the anterior (3) and posterior (11) branches of the obturator nerve

- The obturator nerve divides into its anterior and posterior branches when in the obturator foramen. The anterior branch emerges anterior to obturator externus, while the posterior branch pierces the muscle.
- The anterior branch of the obturator nerve (C3, A17 to 19) supplies adductor longus (A12 and 18), adductor brevis (A16 and 17) and gracilis (A14, 15 and 19).
- The posterior branch of the obturator nerve (C11) supplies obturator externus (C12) and part of adductor magnus (C10). (The rest ot adductor magnus is supplied by the sciatic nerve—page 291, C23.)

1	Adductor longus
2	Superior ramus of pubis
3	Anterior branch of obturator nerve
4	Femoral vein
5	Femoral artery
6	Pectineus
7	Adductor brevis
8	Nerve and vessels to gracilis
9	Gracilis
10	Adductor magnus
11	Posterior branch of obturator nerve
12	Obturator externus

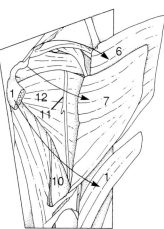

D

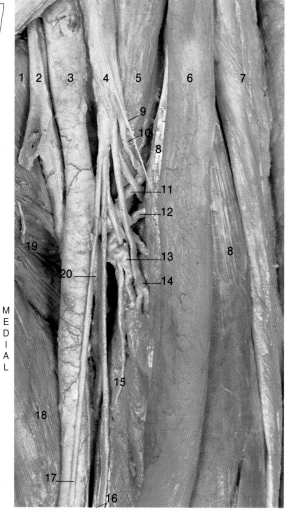

D Left femoral nerve

This is the same specimen as in A, but here sartorius (6) and rectus femoris (8) have been displaced laterally to open up the upper part of the adductor canal and show the lateral circumflex femoral vessels (11 to 13) between branches of the femoral nerve (4)

1	Pectineus	11	Ascending ⎫ branch of
2	Femoral vein	12	Transverse ⎬ lateral circumflex
3	Femoral artery	13	Descending ⎭ femoral artery
4	Femoral nerve	14	Nerve to vastus lateralis
5	Iliacus	15	Vastus intermedius and nerve
6	Sartorius	16	Vastus medialis and nerves
7	Tensor fasciae latae	17	Saphenous nerve
8	Rectus femoris	18	Adductor longus
9	Nerve to sartorius	19	Adductor brevis and nerve
10	Nerve to rectus femoris	20	Profunda femoris artery

- The adductor canal extends from the apex of the femoral triangle to the opening in adductor magnus for the femoral vessels (page 295, B6).
- The canal, which is triangular in section, is bounded laterally by vastus medialis (D16), behind by adductor longus (D18) (and lower down by adductor magnus), and in front by sartorius (D6) which forms the roof of the canal.
- The contents of the canal are the femoral artery and vein (D3 and 2, with the vein lying deep to the artery), the saphenous nerve (D17) and the nerve to vastus medialis (D16, double in this specimen).

A

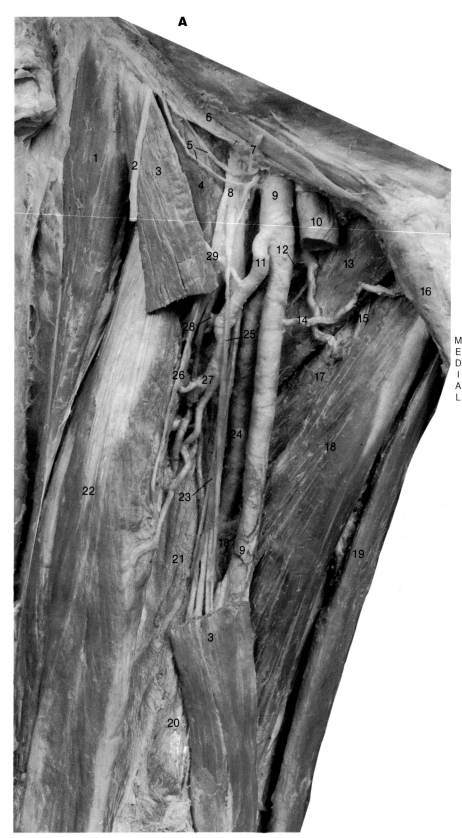

A Right femoral artery

In the upper part of the right thigh, all veins have been removed except for the uppermost part of the femoral vein (10), which is on the medial side of the femoral artery (9). The femoral nerve (8), whose femoral cutaneous branches have been removed, is lateral to the artery. Part of sartorius (3) has been resected to show the lateral circumflex femoral artery (11, here arising from the femoral artery) and the uppermost part of the adductor canal, which is the gutter behind the lower part of sartorius with vastus medialis (20) on the lateral side and adductor longus (18) medially. The profunda femoris artery (24) arises from the posterolateral side of the femoral artery (9) about 3 cm below the inguinal ligament. In the upper part of the adductor canal the saphenous nerve (25) lies in front of the nerve to vastus medialis (23)

MEDIAL

1	Tensor fasciae latae
2	Lateral femoral cutaneous nerve
3	Sartorius
4	Iliacus
5	Superficial circumflex iliac artery (double)
6	Inguinal ligament
7	Superficial epigastric artery
8	Femoral nerve
9	Femoral artery
10	Femoral vein
11	Lateral circumflex femoral artery
12	Medial circumflex femoral artery
13	Pectineus
14	Superficial external pudendal artery (low origin)
15	Anterior branch of obturator nerve
16	Spermatic cord
17	Adductor brevis
18	Adductor longus
19	Gracilis
20	Vastus medialis
21	Vastus intermedius
22	Rectus femoris
23	Nerve to vastus medialis
24	Profunda femoris artery
25	Saphenous nerve
26	Nerve to rectus femoris
27	Descending ⎫ branch of
28	Transverse ⎬ lateral circumflex
29	Ascending ⎭ femoral artery

• The lateral circumflex femoral artery (11) is usually a branch of the profunda femoris (24), but frequently, as in this specimen, it arises directly from the femoral artery (9). It divides into ascending, transverse and descending branches (29, 28 and 27).
• The medial circumflex femoral artery (12) leaves the femoral triangle by passing backwards between pectineus (13) and the tendon of psoas (hidden behind the femoral artery, 9). It emerges in the gluteal region between the lower border of quadratus femoris and the upper border of adductor magnus (page 289).
• The femoral artery (9) with the femoral vein behind it (here removed) passes down the thigh *in front* of adductor longus (18).
• The profunda femoris artery (24) with the profunda femoris vein in front of it (here removed) passes down the thigh *behind* adductor longus (18). Above adductor longus the two veins lie between the two arteries. The upper border of adductor longus is seen separating the two arteries about 2 cm above the lower cut end of sartorius (3).

B Right lower thigh, from the front and medial side

The lower part of sartorius (3) has been displaced medially to open up the lower part of the adductor canal and expose the femoral artery (4) passing through the opening in adductor magnus (6) to enter the popliteal fossa behind the knee and become the popliteal artery (page 302)

B

1 Gracilis	9 Iliotibial tract
2 Adductor magnus	10 Quadriceps tendon
3 Sartorius	11 Patella
4 Femoral artery	12 Medial patellar retinaculum
5 Saphenous nerve	13 Lowest (horizontal) fibres of vastus medialis
6 Opening in adductor magnus	
7 Vastus medialis and nerve	14 Saphenous branch of descending genicular artery
8 Rectus femoris	

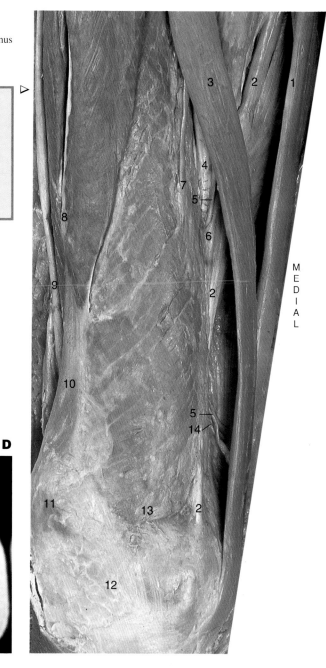

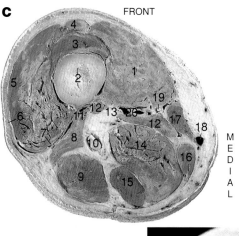

FRONT

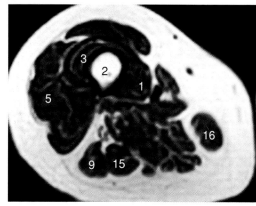

Right lower thigh, C cross section, D axial MR image

The section in C, viewed as when looking upwards from knee to hip, is at the level of the opening in adductor magnus (13) through which the femoral vessels (20) will pass to become the popliteal vessels. The vasti (1, 3 and 5) envelop the femur (2) at the sides and front, and rectus femoris (4) at this level has become narrow and tendinous. The femoral vessels (20) are between vastus medialis (1) and adductor magnus (12) and the profunda vessels (11) close to the back of the femur (2). The sciatic nerve (10) is deeply placed between biceps laterally (8 and 9) and semimembranosus medially (14). Compare features in the MR image with the section

1 Vastus medialis	11 Profunda femoris vessels
2 Femur	12 Adductor magnus
3 Vastus intermedius	13 Opening in adductor magnus
4 Rectus femoris	14 Semimembranosus
5 Vastus lateralis	15 Semitendinosus
6 Iliotibial tract of fascia lata	16 Gracilis
7 Lateral intermuscular septum	17 Sartorius
8 Short head of biceps	18 Great saphenous vein
9 Long head of biceps	19 Saphenous nerve
10 Sciatic nerve	20 Femoral vessels

A

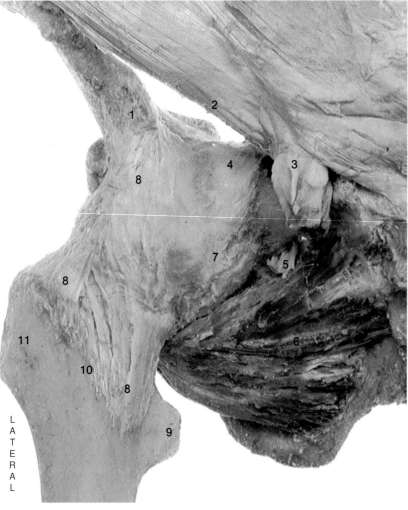

Right hip joint, A from the front, B from behind
All muscles except obturator externus (6) have been removed to display the iliofemoral (8), pubofemoral (7) and ischiofemoral (12) ligaments which reinforce the outside of the capsule of the joint

1	Anterior inferior iliac spine
2	Inguinal ligament
3	Superficial inguinal ring and spermatic cord
4	Iliopubic eminence
5	Obturator nerve
6	Obturator externus
7	Pubofemoral ligament
8	Iliofemoral ligament
9	Lesser trochanter
10	Intertrochanteric line and capsule attachment
11	Greater trochanter
12	Ischiofemoral ligament
13	Zona orbicularis
14	Intertrochanteric crest
15	Extracapsular part of neck of femur
16	Ischial tuberosity
17	Lesser sciatic notch and surface for obturator internus
18	Ischial spine

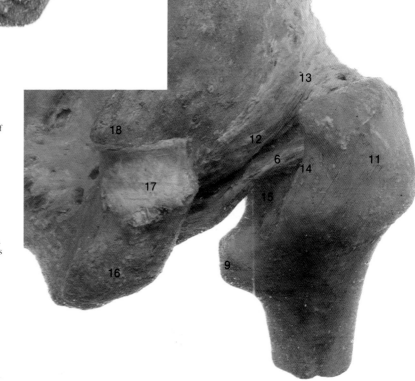

B

• The iliofemoral ligament (8) has the shape of an inverted V. It and the interosseous sacro-iliac ligament are the two strongest ligaments in the body.
• Some of the fibres of the ischiofemoral ligament (12) help to form the zona orbicularis (13)—circular fibres of the capsule that form a collar round the neck of the femur.
• Posteriorly the capsule is attached to the neck of the femur, not to the intertrochanteric crest. (Anteriorly it is attached to the intertrochanteric line.) See pages 269 and 270.
• Muscles producing movements at the hip joint:

Flexion: psoas and iliacus, with rectus femoris, sartorius, tensor fasciae latae, pectineus and adductor longus and brevis.
Extension: gluteus maximus, semimembranosus, semitendinosus, long head of biceps and the ischial part of adductor magnus.
Abduction: gluteus medius and minimus, with tensor fasciae latae and piriformis.
Adduction: adductor longus, brevis and magnus, pectineus, gracilis and quadratus femoris, with tensor fasciae latae.
Medial rotation: anterior fibres of gluteus medius and minimus.
Lateral rotation: obturator externus and internus and gemelli, piriformis, quadratus femoris, gluteus maximus and sartorius.

C

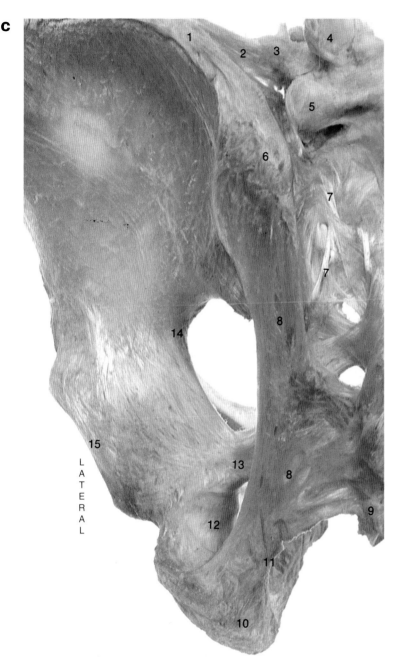

LATERAL

C **Left vertebropelvic and sacro-iliac ligaments, from behind**

All tissues except ligaments have been removed to show how the sacrotuberous and sacrospinous ligaments (8 and 13) bridge the greater and lesser sciatic notches (14 and 12), so converting them into foramina

1	Iliac crest
2	Iliolumbar ligament
3	Transverse process
4	Superior articular process ⎫ of fifth lumbar vertebra
5	Inferior articular process ⎭
6	Posterior superior iliac spine
7	Dorsal sacro-iliac ligaments
8	Sacrotuberous ligament
9	Coccyx
10	Ischial tuberosity
11	Falciform process of sacrotuberous ligament
12	Lesser sciatic notch
13	Sacrospinous ligament and ischial spine
14	Greater sciatic notch
15	Acetabular labrum

- The vertebropelvic ligaments are the iliolumbar (2), sacrotuberous (8) and sacrospinous (13) ligaments.
- The dorsal sacro-iliac ligaments (7) cover the interosseous sacro-iliac ligament.

D

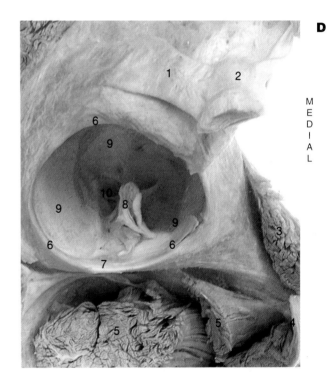

MEDIAL

D **Right hip joint with femur removed, from the right**

The femur has been disarticulated from the acetabulum and removed, leaving the acetabular labrum (6), transverse ligament (7) and the ligament of the head of the femur (8)

1	Reflected ⎫ head of rectus femoris	6	Acetabular labrum
2	Straight ⎭	7	Transverse ligament
3	Pectineus	8	Ligament of head of femur
4	Adductor longus	9	Articular surface
5	Obturator externus	10	Acetabular fossa (non-articular)

- The acetabular labrum (6) is attached to the margin of the acetabulum and is composed of fibrocartilage.
- The transverse ligament (7) fills in the acetabular notch and the gap between the two ends of the labrum (6), and is composed of fibrous tissue, not fibrocartilage.
- The ligament of the head of the femur (8) extends from the transverse ligament (7) and the margins of the acetabular notch to the fovea or pit on the medial side of the head of the femur. Like the transverse ligament it is composed of fibrous tissue.

A

Left hip joint, **A** coronal section, from the front, **B** coronal MR image

The section has almost passed through the centre of the head (18) of the femur and the centre of the greater trochanter (7). Above the neck of the femur (16), gluteus minimus (6) with gluteus medius (5) above it run down to their attachments to the greater trochanter (7), while below the neck the tendon of psoas major (2) and muscle fibres of iliacus (3) pass backwards towards the lesser trochanter. The circular fibres of the zona orbicularis (17) constrict the capsule (15) around the intracapsular part of the neck of the femur

1 External iliac artery	14 Medial circumflex
2 Psoas major	femoral vessels
3 Iliacus	15 Capsule of hip joint
4 Iliac crest	16 Neck of femur
5 Gluteus medius	17 Zona orbicularis of
6 Gluteus minimus	capsule
7 Greater trochanter	18 Head of femur
8 Vastus lateralis	19 Acetabular labrum
9 Shaft of femur	20 Rim of acetabulum
10 Vastus medialis	21 Hyaline cartilage of
11 Profunda femoris	head
vessels	22 Hyaline cartilage of
12 Adductor longus	acetabulum
13 Pectineus	

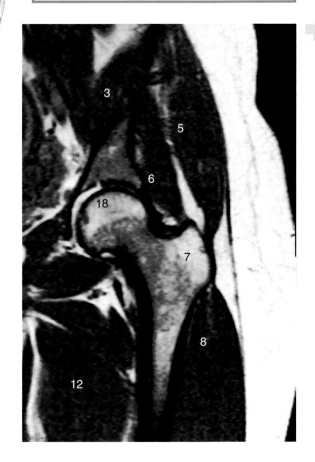

• The convergence of gluteus medius and minimus (5 and 6) on to the greater trochanter is well displayed in this section. These muscles are classified as abductors of the femur at the hip joint, but their more important action is in walking, where they act to prevent adduction—preventing the pelvis from tilting to the opposite side when the opposite limb is off the ground.

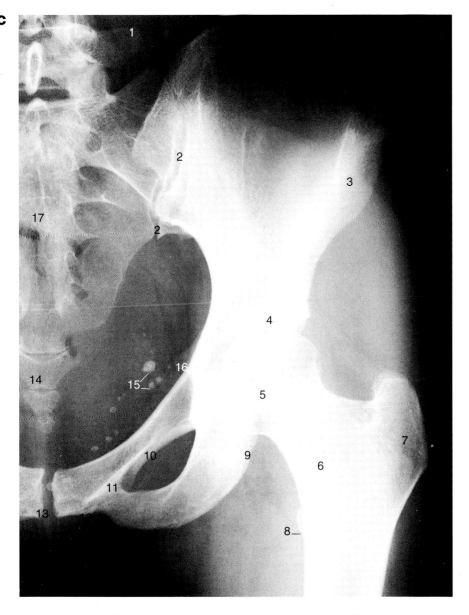

C Left hip and sacro-iliac joint radiograph
In this standard anteroposterior view of the hip joint (4 and 5), much of the joint line of the sacro-iliac joint can also be seen (2)

1	Transverse process of fifth lumbar vertebra
2	Sacro-iliac joint
3	Anterior superior iliac spine
4	Rim of acetabulum
5	Head
6	Neck
7	Greater trochanter
8	Lesser trochanter
9	Ischial tuberosity
10	Superior pubic ramus
11	Pectineal line
12	Pubic tubercle
13	Pubic symphysis
14	First coccygeal vertebra
15	Phleboliths in pelvic veins
16	Ischial spine
17	Sacrum

(4, 5, 6, 7, 8 labelled "of femur")

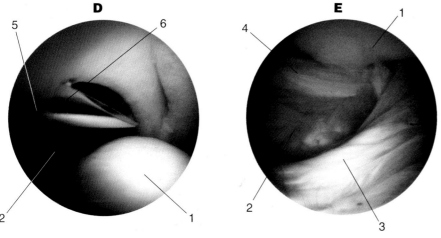

D and **E** Endoscopic views of the hip joint
Reproduced with kind permission of Richard N. Villar from *Hip Arthroscopy* (Butterworth Heinemann).

1	Femoral head
2	Synovium
3	Ligamentum teres
4	Transverse ligament
5	Zona orbicularis
6	Irrigation needle

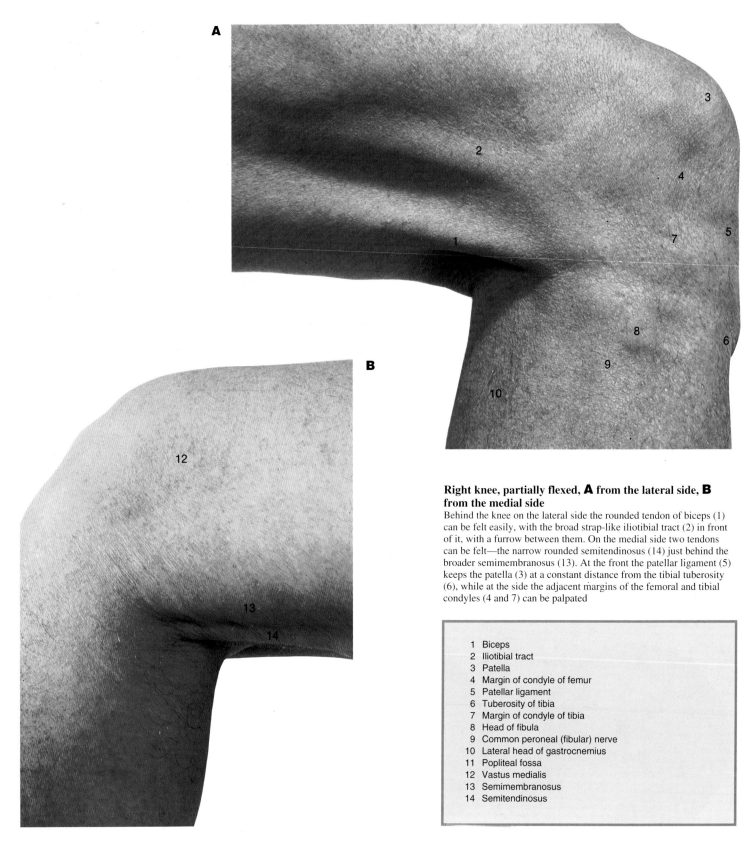

Right knee, partially flexed, A from the lateral side, B from the medial side

Behind the knee on the lateral side the rounded tendon of biceps (1) can be felt easily, with the broad strap-like iliotibial tract (2) in front of it, with a furrow between them. On the medial side two tendons can be felt—the narrow rounded semitendinosus (14) just behind the broader semimembranosus (13). At the front the patellar ligament (5) keeps the patella (3) at a constant distance from the tibial tuberosity (6), while at the side the adjacent margins of the femoral and tibial condyles (4 and 7) can be palpated

1 Biceps
2 Iliotibial tract
3 Patella
4 Margin of condyle of femur
5 Patellar ligament
6 Tuberosity of tibia
7 Margin of condyle of tibia
8 Head of fibula
9 Common peroneal (fibular) nerve
10 Lateral head of gastrocnemius
11 Popliteal fossa
12 Vastus medialis
13 Semimembranosus
14 Semitendinosus

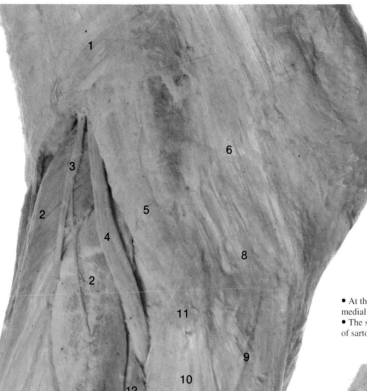

C Right knee, superficial dissection, from the lateral side

D Right knee, superficial dissection, from the medial side

The great saphenous vein (5) runs upwards about a hand's breadth behind the medial border of the patella (1). The saphenous nerve (6) becomes superficial between the tendons of sartorius (4) and gracilis (7), and its infrapatellar branch (10) curls forwards a little below the upper margin of the tibial condyle

1	Patella
2	Vastus medialis
3	Branches of medial femoral cutaneous nerve
4	Sartorius
5	Great saphenous vein
6	Saphenous nerve
7	Gracilis
8	Semitendinosus
9	Medial head of gastrocnemius
10	Infrapatellar branch of saphenous nerve
11	Level of margin of medial condyle of tibia

● At the level of the knee joint the great saphenous vein (5) lies about a hand's breadth behind the medial border of the patella (1); this is the guide for the surface marking of the vessel.
● The saphenous nerve (6) becomes superficial by piercing the deep fascia between the lower ends of sartorius (4) and gracilis (7).

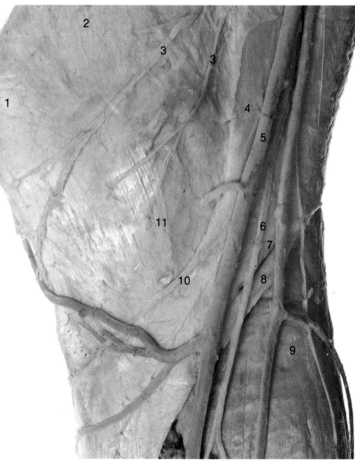

C Right knee, superficial dissection, from the lateral side

The fascia behind biceps (5) has been removed to show the common peroneal (fibular) nerve (4) passing downwards immediately behind the tendon, and then running between the adjacent borders of soleus (12) and peroneus longus (10), under cover of which it lies against the neck of the fibula. Minor superficial vessels and nerves have been removed

1	Fascia lata
2	Lateral head of gastrocnemius
3	Lateral cutaneous nerve of calf
4	Common peroneal (fibular) nerve
5	Biceps
6	Iliotibial tract
7	Patella
8	Attachment of iliotibial tract to tibia
9	Deep fascia overlying extensor muscles
10	Deep fascia overlying peroneus longus
11	Head of fibula
12	Soleus

● The iliotibial tract (6) is the thickened lateral part of the fascia lata (1). At its upper part the tensor fasciae latae and most of gluteus maximus are inserted into it; its lower end is attached to the lateral condyle of the tibia (8).
● Its subcutaneous position and contact with the neck of the fibula make the common peroneal (fibular) nerve (4) the most commonly injured nerve in the lower limb.

A

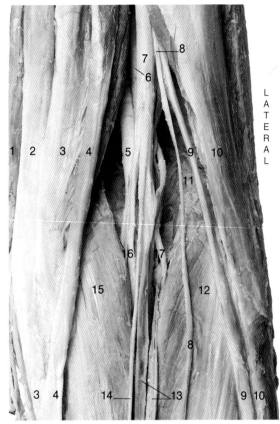

B

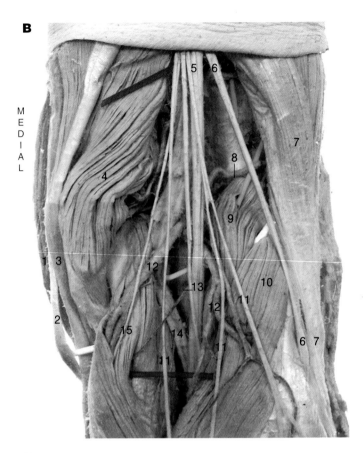

A Right popliteal fossa

The fascia that forms the roof of the diamond-shaped fossa and the fat within it have been removed but the small saphenous vein which pierces the fascia is preserved (13, double in this specimen). The main structures in the fossa are the tibial nerve (7), popliteal vein (6) and popliteal artery (5), which lie in that order from superficial to deep. The common peroneal (fibular) nerve (9) passes laterally behind the posterior border of biceps. Semimembranosus (3) and semitendinosus (4) are on the medial side of the fossa, with the two heads of gastrocnemius (12 and 15) forming the lower boundaries

B Right popliteal fossa. Vessels and nerves

Here the margins of the fossa have been displaced and markers hold various structures apart. The upper red marker passes between the tibial nerve (5) and the underlying popliteal vein (seen lower down, 14). The uppermost blue marker is behind an unlabelled muscular branch of the popliteal artery (seen lower down, 13). The middle blue marker is behind the superior lateral genicular artery (8), and the lateral head of gastrocnemius (10). The lowest blue marker displaces the popliteal vein (14) medially to show the underlying popliteal artery (13). The lower red marker holds the two heads of gastrocnemius apart (10 and 15). The lower white marker (outside the fossa) is between the tendons of gracilis (2) and semitendinosus (3)

1	Sartorius	10	Biceps
2	Gracilis	11	Plantaris
3	Semimembranosus	12	Lateral head of gastrocnemius
4	Semitendinosus	13	Small saphenous vein (double)
5	Popliteal artery	14	Sural nerve
6	Popliteal vein	15	Medial head of gastrocnemius
7	Tibial nerve	16	Nerve to medial head ⎫ of gastroc-
8	Lateral cutaneous nerve of calf	17	Nerve to lateral head ⎭ nemius
9	Common peroneal (fibular) nerve		

1	Sartorius	9	Plantaris
2	Gracilis	10	Lateral head of gastrocnemius
3	Semitendinosus	11	Branches of sural nerve
4	Semimembranosus	12	Sural arteries
5	Tibial nerve	13	Popliteal artery
6	Common peroneal (fibular) nerve	14	Popliteal vein
7	Biceps	15	Medial head of gastrocnemius and nerve
8	Superior lateral genicular artery		

• The sural nerve (B11) has divided at an unusually high level into several branches. The sural communicating branch of the common peroneal (fibular) nerve is not present.
• The principal structures in the middle of the fossa—the tibial nerve (A7 and B5), popliteal vein (A6 and B14) and popliteal artery (A5 and B13)—lie in that order from superficial to deep. The deep position of the artery makes palpation of its pulsation difficult.

• The most lateral branch of the sural nerve (B11) may here take the place of the lateral cutaneous nerve of the calf which normally arises from the common peroneal (fibular) nerve

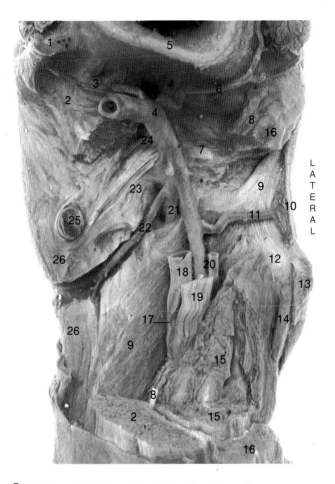

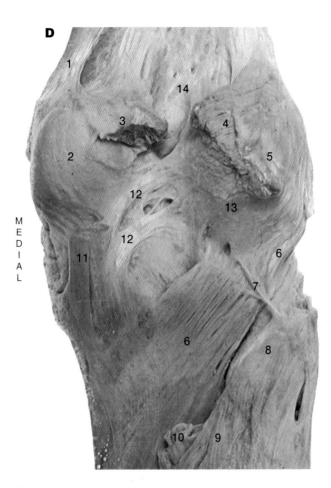

C Right popliteal fossa. Deep dissection of vessels

Most of the superficial muscles have been removed to show the branches of the popliteal artery (4). The knee is flexed so that the artery and the cut end of the femur (5) are seen 'end on'. The artery divides into anterior tibial (21) and posterior tibial (20) branches; usually the anterior tibial passes superficial to popliteus (9) but here the popliteal artery has divided at a high level and the anterior tibial has passed deep to the muscle. The upper pair of superior genicular arteries (3 and 6) run above the heads of gastrocnemius (2 and 16); the inferior pair (22 and 11) pass deep to the tibial and fibular collateral ligaments (26 and 10)

D Right popliteal fossa. Joint capsule and popliteal ligaments

The back of the capsule of the knee joint is shown (13 and 2), reinforced centrally by the oblique popliteal ligament (12) and forming the lower part of the floor of the fossa, with the popliteal surface of the femur (14) in the upper part of the floor

1 Adductor magnus	14 Common peroneal nerve
2 Medial head of gastrocnemius	15 Soleus
3 Superior medial genicular artery	16 Lateral head of gastrocnemius
4 Popliteal artery	17 Nerve to popliteus
5 Popliteal surface of femur in section	18 Popliteal vein
6 Superior lateral genicular artery	19 Tibial nerve
7 Capsule of knee joint	20 Posterior tibial artery and vein
8 Plantaris	21 Anterior tibial artery
9 Popliteus	22 Inferior medial genicular artery
10 Fibular collateral ligament	23 Oblique popliteal ligament
11 Inferior lateral genicular artery	24 Middle genicular artery
12 Head of fibula	25 Semimembranosus
13 Biceps	26 Tibial collateral ligament

1 Adductor magnus	7 Arcuate popliteal ligament
2 Capsule overlying medial condyle of femur	8 Head of fibula
3 Medial head of gastrocnemius	9 Soleus
4 Plantaris	10 Popliteal vessels and tibial nerve
5 Lateral head of gastrocnemius	11 Semimembranosus
6 Popliteus	12 Oblique popliteal ligament
	13 Capsule of knee joint
	14 Popliteal surface of femur

● The oblique popliteal ligament (12) is derived from the semimembranosus tendon (11) and reinforces the central posterior part of the joint capsule (13); it is pierced by the middle genicular artery which passes through the capsule to supply the cruciate ligaments.
● The arcuate popliteal ligament (7) arches over popliteus (6) as it emerges from the capsule.

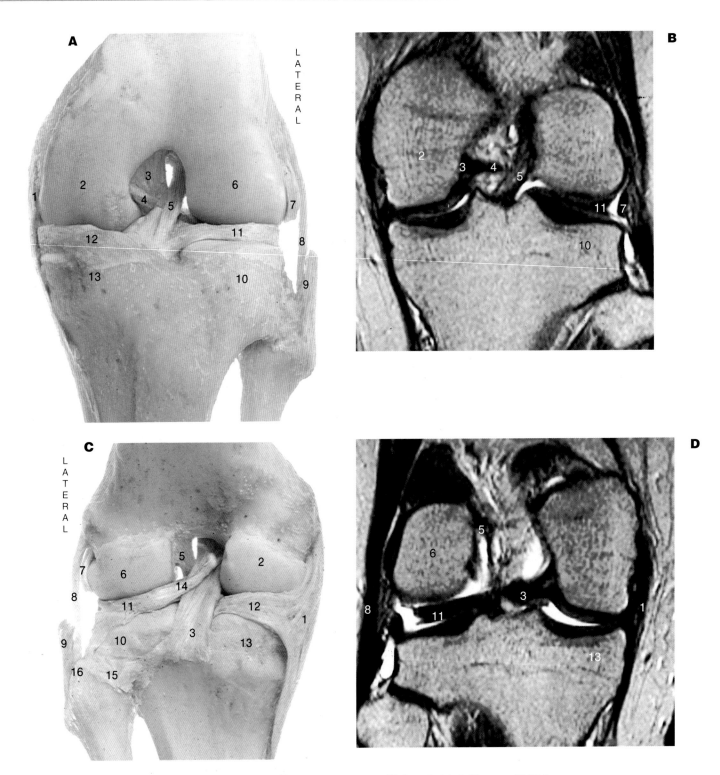

Left knee joint. Ligaments, A from the front, B coronal MR image, C from behind, D coronal MR image
The capsule of the knee joint and all surrounding tissues have been removed, leaving only the ligaments of the joint, which is partially flexed

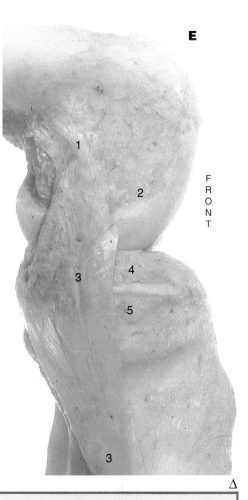

E

FRONT

1 Tibial collateral ligament
2 Medial condyle of femur
3 Posterior cruciate ligament
4 Anterior meniscofemoral ligament
5 Anterior cruciate ligament
6 Lateral condyle of femur
7 Popliteus
8 Fibular collateral ligament
9 Biceps tendon
10 Lateral condyle of tibia
11 Lateral meniscus
12 Medial meniscus
13 Medial condyle of tibia
14 Posterior meniscofemoral ligament
15 Capsule of superior tibiofemoral joint
16 Apex of head of fibula

• The fibular collateral (lateral) ligament (A8) is a rounded cord about 5 cm long, passing from the lateral epicondyle of the femur to the head of the fibula just in front of its apex (C16), largely under cover of the tendon of biceps (C9).

• The medial meniscus (E4 and F4) is attached to the deep part of the tibial collateral ligament (E3 and F21). This helps to anchor the meniscus but makes it liable to become trapped and torn by rotatory movements between the tibia and femur.

• The lateral meniscus (A11) is not attached to the fibular collateral ligament (A8), but is attached posteriorly to the popliteus muscle (F11, and C5 on page 306).

• The anterior and posterior meniscofemoral ligaments (A4 and C14, F9 and F8) are both derived from the lateral meniscus (C11, F13), and are named from their relationships to the posterior cruciate ligament which they embrace (F7).

• The tibial collateral (medial) ligament (E3) is a broad flat band about 12 cm long, passing from the medial epicondyle of the femur (E1) to the medial condyle of the tibia (E5) and an extensive area of the medial surface of the tibia below the condyle (as in the lower part of E).

• The cruciate ligaments are named from their attachments to the tibia.

• The anterior cruciate ligament (A5 and F19) passes upwards, backwards and laterally to be attached to the medial side of the lateral condyle of the femur (C6).

• The posterior cruciate ligament (C3 and F7) passes upwards, forwards and medially to be attached to the lateral surface of the medial condyle of the femur (A2).

• The anterior cruciate ligament (F19) is attached to the intercondylar area of the tibia some distance behind the anterior margin of the bone.

• The attachment of the posterior cruciate ligament overlaps the posterior margin of the bone to extend on to the posterior surface (C3).

• The transverse ligament (small in F18; absent in A) connects the medial and lateral menisci anteriorly.

Left knee joint. Ligaments, E from the medial side, F from above

The same specimen as in A and C is seen from the medial side in E, to show the broad tibial collateral ligament (3). F is the view looking down on the upper surface of the tibia after removing the femur by cutting through the capsule, the collateral ligaments, and the cruciate ligaments. The medial and lateral menisci (4 and 13) remain at the periphery of the articular surfaces of the tibial condyles. The horns of the menisci (20 and 6; 17 and 10) and the cruciate ligaments (19 and 7) are attached to the non-articular intercondylar area of the tibia. Compare with C on page 278

1 Medial epicondyle of femur
2 Medial condyle of femur
3 Tibial collateral ligament
4 Medial meniscus
5 Medial condyle of tibia
6 Posterior horn of medial meniscus
7 Posterior cruciate ligament
8 Posterior ⎱ meniscofemoral
9 Anterior ⎰ ligament
10 Posterior horn of lateral meniscus
11 Attachment of lateral meniscus to popliteus (with underlying marker)
12 Lateral condyle of tibia
13 Lateral meniscus
14 Tendon of popliteus
15 Fibular collateral ligament
16 Tendon of biceps
17 Anterior horn of lateral meniscus
18 Transverse ligament
19 Anterior cruciate ligament
20 Anterior horn of medial meniscus
21 Tibial collateral ligament attached to medial meniscus

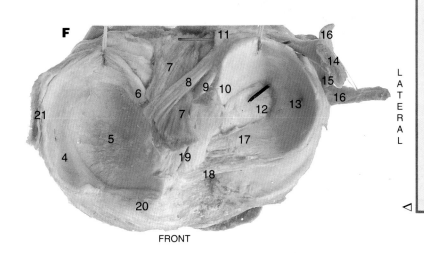

F

LATERAL

FRONT

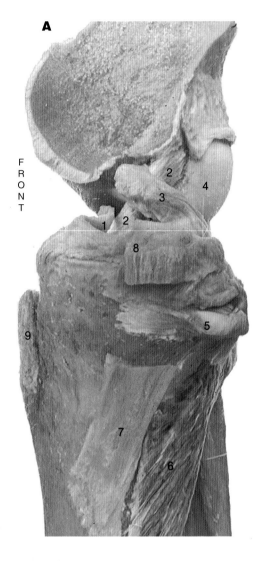

A

FRONT

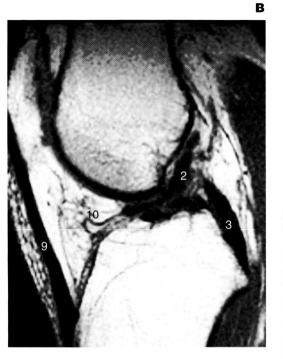

B

Right knee joint. A from the medial side with the medial femoral condyle removed, B sagittal MR image
Removal of the medial half of the lower end of the femur enables the X-shaped crossover of the cruciate ligaments to be seen: the anterior cruciate (2) is passing backwards and laterally, while the posterior cruciate (3) passes forwards and medially. The MR image in B shows the backward projection of the infrapatellar fat pad (10)

1	Transverse ligament (displaced backwards)
2	Anterior cruciate ligament
3	Posterior cruciate ligament
4	Lateral condyle of femur
5	Semimembranosus
6	Popliteus
7	Tibial collateral ligament
8	Medial meniscus and attachment of tibial collateral ligament
9	Patellar ligament
10	Infrapatellar fat pad

C Left knee joint, from behind with the femur removed
This view demonstrates the attachment of the lateral meniscus (5) to popliteus (4). There are markers underneath the attachment and behind the popliteus tendon

1	Head of fibula
2	Biceps
3	Fibular collateral ligament
4	Popliteus tendon
5	Attachment of lateral meniscus to popliteus
6	Anterior cruciate ligament
7	Posterior cruciate ligament
8	Posterior meniscofemoral ligament
9	Medial meniscus attached to tibial collateral ligament
10	Semimembranosus
11	Popliteus
12	Soleus
13	Interosseous membrane

C

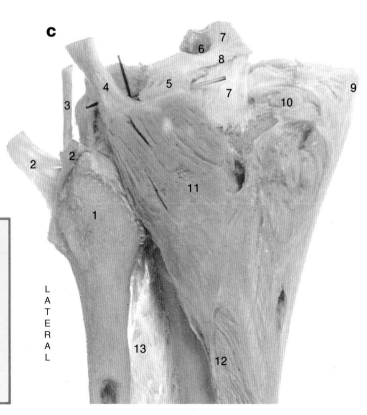

LATERAL

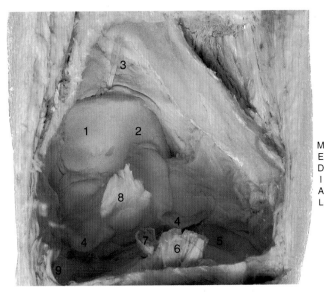

MEDIAL

D Left knee joint, opened from behind with the femur removed
By looking into the joint from behind after removal of the femur, the articular surfaces of the patella (1 and 2) are seen, while below them are the alar and infrapatellar folds (4 and 8)

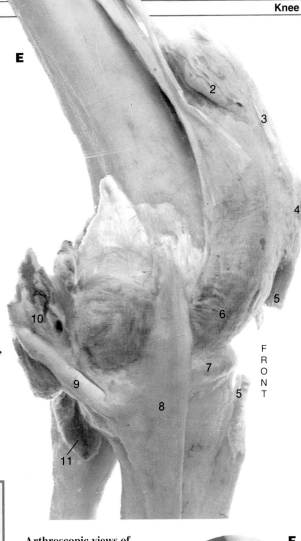

FRONT

E Left knee joint, from the medial side, with synovial and bursal cavities injected
The resin injection has distended the synovial cavity of the joint (6) and extends into the suprapatellar bursa (2), the bursa round the popliteus tendon (11) and the semimembranosus bursa (10)

---

1 Lateral ⎱ articular surface
2 Medial ⎰ of patella
3 Suprapatellar bursa (supported by glass rod)
4 Alar fold
5 Medial meniscus
6 Posterior ⎱ cruciate ligament
7 Anterior ⎰
8 Infrapatellar fold (ligamentum mucosum)
9 Lateral meniscus

---

1 Articularis genu
2 Suprapatellar bursa
3 Quadriceps tendon
4 Patella
5 Patellar ligament
6 Capsule
7 Medial meniscus
8 Tibial collateral ligament
9 Semimembranosus
10 Semimembranosus bursa
11 Bursa of popliteus tendon

• Below the patella (D1 and 2) the synovial membrane is projected backwards by the infrapatellar fat pad, so forming the two alar folds (D4) which have posterior free borders and a central infrapatellar fold (D8). The latter is attached to the front of the intercondylar area of the femur. The folds with their contained fat occupy what would otherwise be the 'dead space' below the curved front parts of the femoral condyles (see B10 on page opposite).

• The normal knee joint (the largest of all synovial joints) contains less than 1 ml of synovial fluid; the joint illustrated in E contains about 80 ml of injected resin which has distended the synovial cavity.
• The suprapatellar bursa (E2) always communicates with the joint cavity. The bursa around the popliteus tendon (E11) usually does so. The semimembranosus bursa (E10) may do so.
• Muscles producing movements at the knee joint:

Flexion: semimembranosus, semitendinosus, biceps, gracilis, sartorius, gastrocnemius and popliteus.
Extension: vastus medialis, intermedius and lateralis, rectus femoris, and tensor fasciae latae and gluteus maximus acting via the iliotibial tract.
Medial rotation of leg: popliteus (when the knee is extended), semimembranosus, semitendinosus, gracilis and sartorius (when the knee is flexed).
Lateral rotation of leg: biceps (when flexed).

Arthroscopic views of the left knee, F antero-lateral approach, G postero-medial approach
Reproduced with kind permission of David J. Dandy from *Current Problems in Orthopaedics: Arthroscopic Management of the Knee,* 2nd Edition, Churchill Livingstone

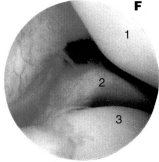

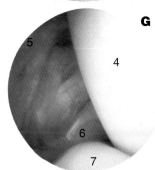

---

1 Lateral condyle of femur
2 Lateral meniscus
3 Lateral condyle of tibia
4 Medial condyle of femur
5 Posterior part of capsule
6 Posterior cruciate ligament
7 Medial meniscus

A

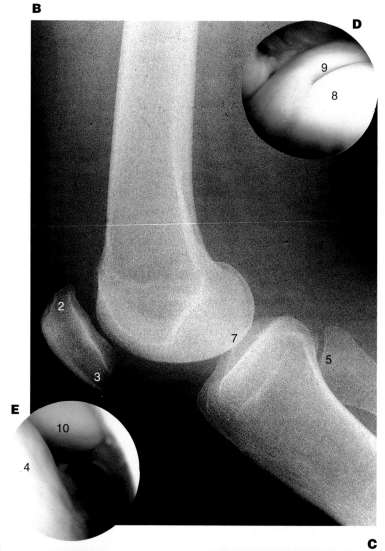

B

D

E

C

Radiographs and arthroscopic views of the knee, A from the front, B from the lateral side in partial flexion, C skyline view projection, D anterolateral approach, E lateral view of patella

 In A the shadow of the patella (2 and 3) is superimposed on that of the femur. The regular space between the condyles of the femur and tibia (1 and 8, 4 and 6) is due to the thickness of the hyaline cartilage on the articulating surface, with the menisci at the periphery. In C with the knee flexed, the view should be compared with the bones seen on page 274, E, and the lateral edge of the patella (11) is seen in the arthroscopic view in E. (D and E reproduced with kind permission of David J. Dandy from *Current Problems in Orthopaedics: Arthroscopic Management of the Knee*, 2nd Edition, Churchill Livingstone.)

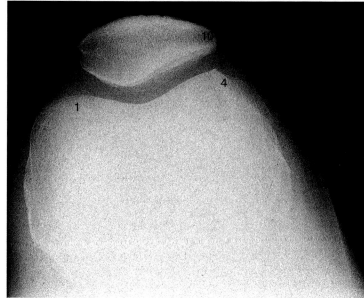

1	Medial condyle of femur	7	Tubercles of intercondylar eminence
2	Base ⎫ of patella	8	Medial condyle of tibia
3	Apex ⎭	9	Medial meniscus
4	Lateral condyle of femur	10	Lateral edge of patella
5	Head of fibula		
6	Lateral condyle of tibia		

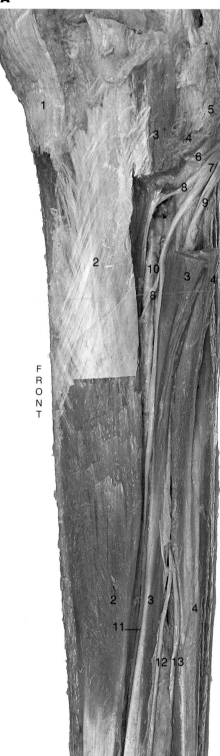

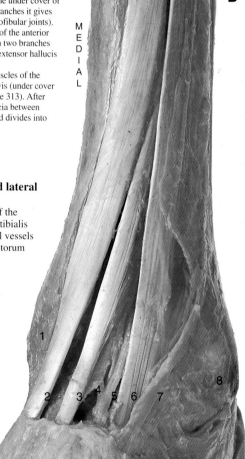

A Left leg, from the front and lateral side
Most of the deep fascia has been removed, and segments of extensor digitorum longus (3) and peroneus longus (4) have been cut out to display the deep (7) and superficial (9) branches of the common peroneal (fibular) nerve just below the head of the fibula (5). The gap between tibialis anterior (2) and extensor digitorum longus (3) has been opened up to show the anterior tibial artery (10)

1 Tuberosity of tibia and patellar ligament
2 Tibialis anterior and overlying fascia
3 Extensor digitorum longus
4 Peroneus longus
5 Head of fibula
6 Recurrent branch of common peroneal (fibular) nerve
7 Deep peroneal (fibular) nerve
8 Branch to tibialis anterior
9 Superficial peroneal (fibular) nerve
10 Anterior tibial artery overlying interosseous membrane
11 Extensor hallucis longus
12 Medial } branch of superficial
13 Lateral } peroneal (fibular) nerve

• The common peroneal (fibular) nerve (page 310, B10) divides into its superficial and deep branches (A9 and A7) below the lateral side of the head of the fibula (A5), where it lies in contact with the neck of the bone under cover of peroneus longus (A4). Just before dividing into its two main branches it gives off a small recurrent branch (A6) (to the knee and superior tibiofibular joints).
• The deep peroneal (fibular) nerve (A7) supplies the muscles of the anterior compartment of the leg—tibialis anterior (A2 and B2, to which two branches are shown here, A8), extensor digitorum longus (A3 and B6), extensor hallucis longus (A11 and B3) and peroneus tertius (page 319, C7).
• The superficial peroneal (fibular) nerve (A9) supplies the muscles of the lateral compartment—peroneus longus (A4) and peroneus brevis (under cover of peroneus longus in A, but its lower end is seen at D7 on page 313). After supplying the peroneal muscles, the nerve pierces the deep fascia between extensor digitorum longus and peroneus longus (A3 and 4), and divides into medial and lateral (cutaneous) branches (A12 and 13).

B Left lower leg and ankle, from the front and lateral side
The deep fascia has been removed to show the order of the structures in front of the ankle: from medial to lateral, tibialis anterior (2), extensor hallucis longus (3), anterior tibial vessels (4), deep peroneal (fibular) nerve (5) and extensor digitorum longus (6)

1 Medial malleolus
2 Tibialis anterior
3 Extensor hallucis longus
4 Anterior tibial vessels
5 Deep peroneal (fibular) nerve
6 Extensor digitorum longus
7 Medial branch of superficial peroneal (fibular) nerve
8 Lateral malleolus

• On the front of the ankle the *extensor hallucis* longus tendon (B3) is immediately adjacent to the *tibialis anterior* tendon (B2). Behind the medial malleolus (D13 on page 313) it is the *flexor digitorum* longus tendon (D1) that lies immediately adjacent to the *tibialis posterior* tendon (D12).

A

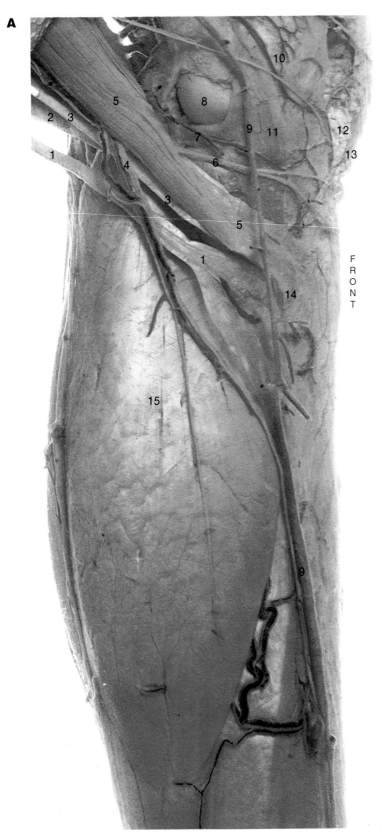
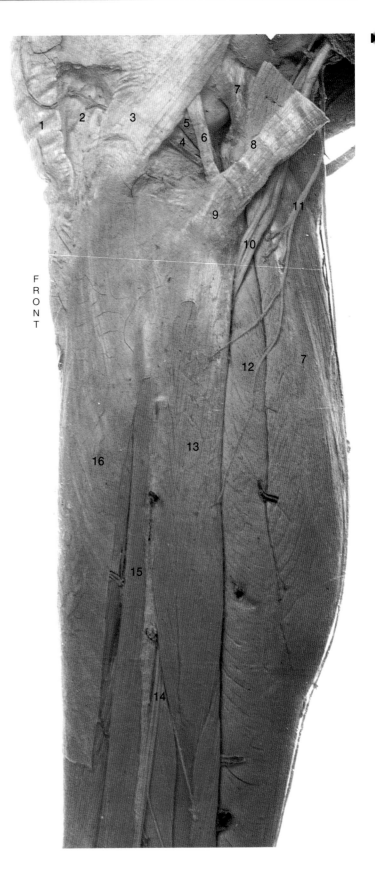

◁ **A** Left knee and leg, from the medial side and behind

A small window has been cut in the capsule of the knee joint to show part of the medial condyle of the femur (8) and the medial meniscus (7). The tendons of sartorius (5), gracilis (3) and semitendinosus (1) gain attachment to the medial surface of the tibia (14). The saphenous nerve (4) becomes superficial between sartorius (5) and gracilis (3) and its infrapatellar branch (6) has pierced sartorius to run forwards immediately below the knee joint and the medial meniscus (7). The great saphenous vein (9) in the region of the knee is unusually small

1	Semitendinosus
2	Semimembranosus
3	Gracilis
4	Saphenous nerve and artery
5	Sartorius
6	Infrapatellar branch of saphenous nerve
7	Branch of saphenous artery overlying medial meniscus
8	Medial condyle of femur (part of capsule removed)
9	Great saphenous vein
10	Branches of superior medial genicular artery
11	Tibial collateral ligament
12	Infrapatellar fat pad
13	Patellar ligament
14	Medial surface of tibia
15	Medial head of gastrocnemius

◁ **B** Left knee and leg, from the lateral side

A small window has been cut in the capsule of the knee joint to show the tendon of popliteus (5) passing deep to the fibular collateral ligament (6). The common peroneal (fibular) nerve (10) runs down behind biceps (8) to pass through the gap between peroneus longus (13) and soleus (12). The superficial peroneal (fibular) nerve becomes superficial between peroneus longus (13) and extensor digitorum longus (15)

1	Patellar ligament
2	Infrapatellar fat pad
3	Iliotibial tract
4	Lateral meniscus
5	Popliteus
6	Fibular collateral ligament
7	Lateral head of gastrocnemius
8	Biceps
9	Head of fibula
10	Common peroneal (fibular) nerve
11	Lateral cutaneous nerve of calf
12	Soleus
13	Peroneus longus
14	Superficial peroneal (fibular)nerve
15	Extensor digitorum longus
16	Fascia overlying tibialis anterior

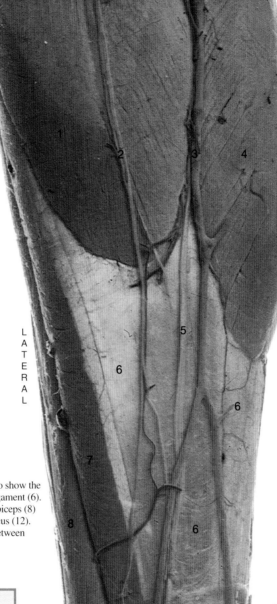

C Left calf, superficial dissection

Most of the deep fascia has been removed, but a small part has been preserved (9) to indicate that the superficial veins and nerves such as the small saphenous vein (3) and sural nerve (5) lie superficial to it

1	Lateral head of gastrocnemius
2	Lateral cutaneous nerve of calf
3	Small saphenous vein
4	Medial head of gastrocnemius
5	Sural nerve
6	Aponeurosis of gastrocnemius
7	Soleus
8	Peroneus longus
9	Deep fascia
10	Tendo calcaneus (Achilles' tendon)

• The medial head of gastrocnemius (C4) extends to a lower level than the lateral head (C1).
• Below knee level the great saphenous vein (A9) is accompanied by the saphenous nerve (A4).
• In the calf the small saphenous vein (C3) is accompanied by the sural nerve (C5).
• On the medial side of the upper leg, sartorius (A5), gracilis (A3) and semitendinosus (A1) all converge on to the medial surface of the tibia.
• On the lateral side of the upper leg, biceps (B8) converges on to the head of the fibula (B9), with the common peroneal (fibular) nerve (B10) behind them. The nerve divides under cover of peroneus longus (B13) and in contact with the neck of the fibula into superficial and deep branches (page 309, A9 and 7).
• The two heads of gastrocnemius join a broad aponeurosis (C6) which lower down unites with the tendon of soleus (C7) to form the tendo calcaneus (Achilles' tendon, C10).

A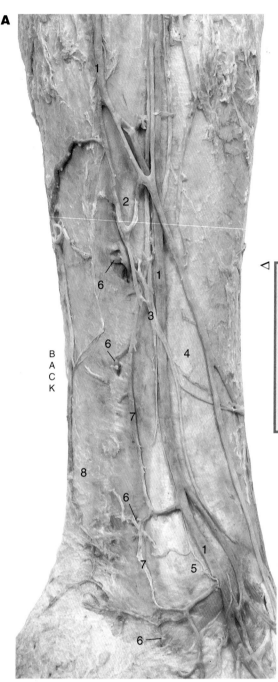

A Left leg and ankle. Superficial veins and nerves, from the medial side

Skin and subcutaneous tissues have been removed, leaving nerves and veins lying on the deep fascia. In A the great saphenous vein (1), with several tributaries at its lower end and elsewhere, runs up in front of the medial malleolus (5). The saphenous nerve (3) accompanies the vein and divides (where labelled) several centimetres above the malleolus into branches which continue down in front of and behind the vein. The rather small (normal) posterior arch vein (7) is joined by several perforating veins (6), typically just below, just above and some distance above, the malleolus (see notes)

◁

1 Great saphenous vein
2 Deep fascia over soleus
3 Saphenous nerve
4 Medial (subcutaneous) surface of tibia
5 Medial malleolus
6 Perforating veins
7 Posterior arch vein
8 Tendo calcaneus (Achilles' tendon)

B Left leg and ankle. Superficial veins and nerves, from behind

In this specimen (different from that in A), the posterior arch vein (4) on the medial side is large and becoming varicose (see notes). The small saphenous vein (3) runs up behind the lateral malleolus (11) and is accompanied on the back of the calf by the sural nerve

▷

1 Deep fascia
2 Sural nerve
3 Small saphenous vein
4 Posterior arch vein
5 A perforating vein
6 Tendo calcaneus (under fascia)
7 Medial malleolus
8 Medial calcanean nerve
9 Posterior surface of calcaneus
10 Fibrofatty tissue of heel
11 Lateral malleolus

B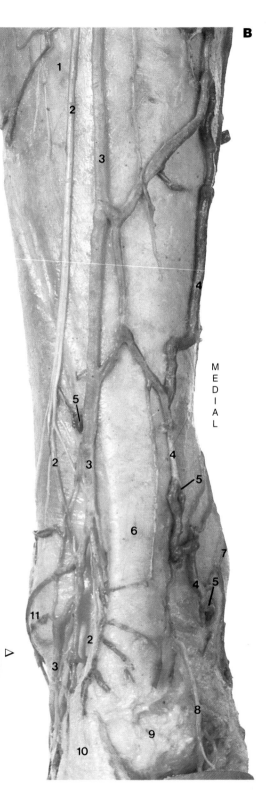

• The perforating veins are communications between the superficial veins (above the deep fascia) and the deep veins (below the fascia). The commonest sites for them are just behind the tibia, behind the fibula and in the adductor canal. These communicating vessels possess valves which direct the blood flow from superficial to deep; venous return from the limb is then brought about by the pumping action of the deep muscles (which are all below the deep fascia). If the valves become incompetent or the deep veins blocked, pressure in the superficial veins increases and they become varicose (dilated and tortuous).
• The posterior arch vein (A7) unites some of the perforating veins and usually drains into the great saphenous (A1).

C

C Right popliteal fossa and upper calf

All vessels and nerves and most parts of the superficial muscles have been removed to show popliteus (7) and the deep muscles of the calf—tibialis posterior (16), flexor digitorum longus (15) and flexor hallucis longus (14)

1	Tibial collateral ligament
2	Medial condyle of femur
3	Medial head of gastrocnemius
4	Capsule of knee joint
5	Plantaris
6	Lateral head of gastrocnemius
7	Popliteus
8	Attachment of popliteus to lateral meniscus
9	Fibular collateral ligament
10	Biceps
11	Soleus
12	Peroneus longus
13	Posterior surface of fibula (soleus removed)
14	Flexor hallucis longus
15	Flexor digitorum longus
16	Tibialis posterior
17	Semitendinosus
18	Gracilis
19	Sartorius
20	Semimembranosus

D Right lower calf and ankle

All vessels and nerves have been removed to show the order of the structures behind the ankle: from medial to lateral behind the medial malleolus (13), tibialis posterior (12), flexor digitorum longus (1), posterior tibial vessels and tibial nerve (11) and flexor hallucis longus (3). Behind the lateral malleolus (5), peroneus brevis (7) lies against the bone with peroneus longus (4) behind it

1	Flexor digitorum longus
2	Fascia overlying tibialis posterior
3	Flexor hallucis longus
4	Peroneus longus
5	Lateral malleolus
6	Superior peroneal retinaculum
7	Peroneus brevis
8	Posterior talofibular ligament
9	Tendo calcaneus (Achilles' tendon)
10	Part of flexor retinaculum
11	Position of posterior tibial vessels and tibial nerve
12	Tibialis posterior
13	Medial malleolus

D

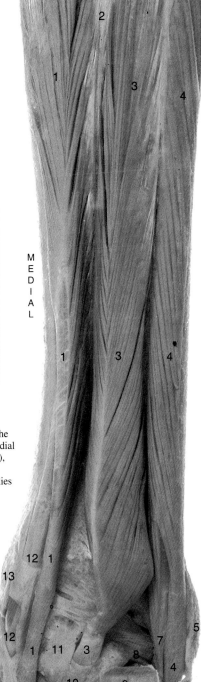

- Tibialis posterior (C16, D12) is the deepest muscle of the calf.
- Flexor hallucis longus (C14, D3), although passing to the great toe on the *medial* side of the foot, arises from the fibula on the *lateral* side of the leg.

313

A

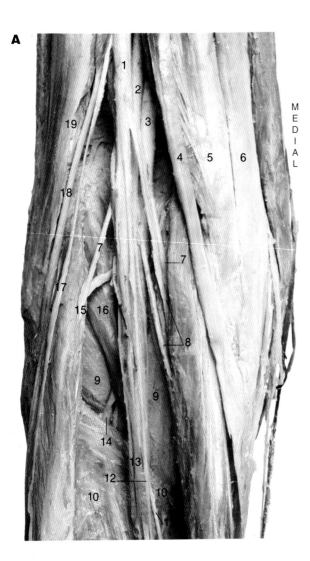

B

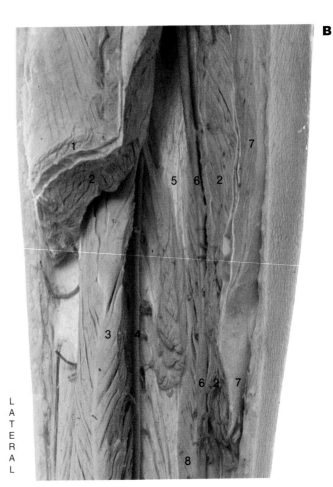

M
E
D
I
A
L

L
A
T
E
R
A
L

A Left popliteal fossa and upper calf

Gastrocnemius has been incised longitudinally and the two heads (8 and 15) split apart to reveal plantaris (16) and its thin tendon (11), popliteus (9) and the upper part of soleus (10). The sural nerve (12) and small saphenous vein (13) remain in the midline and obscure the lower part of the tibial nerve (1)

B Left calf. Deep dissection of muscles and arteries

In the middle of the calf most of gastrocnemius (1 and 7) and soleus (2) have been removed with nerves and veins. The peroneal artery (4) runs down the medial crest of the fibula between flexor hallucis longus (3) and tibialis posterior (5). The posterior tibial artery (6) runs down behind the tibia on tibialis posterior (5) and flexor digitorum longus (8) and under cover of soleus (2). Compare with the cross section in D

1	Tibial nerve	12	Sural nerve
2	Popliteal vein	13	Small saphenous vein (double)
3	Popliteal artery	14	Nerve to soleus
4	Semitendinosus	15	Lateral head of gastrocnemius and nerve
5	Semimembranosus		
6	Gracilis	16	Plantaris
7	Sural artery	17	Lateral cutaneous nerve of calf
8	Medial head of gastrocnemius and nerves		
		18	Common peroneal (fibular) nerve
9	Popliteus		
10	Soleus	19	Biceps
11	Plantaris tendon		

1	Lateral head of gastrocnemius	
2	Soleus	
3	Flexor hallucis longus	
4	Peroneal (fibular) artery	
5	Tibialis posterior	
6	Posterior tibial artery	
7	Medial head of gastrocnemius	
8	Flexor digitorum longus	

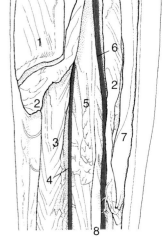

● Flexor hallucis longus, going to the great toe on the medial side of the foot, arises from the fibula on the lateral side of the leg; the tendon crosses to the medial side in the sole (page 318, B6).

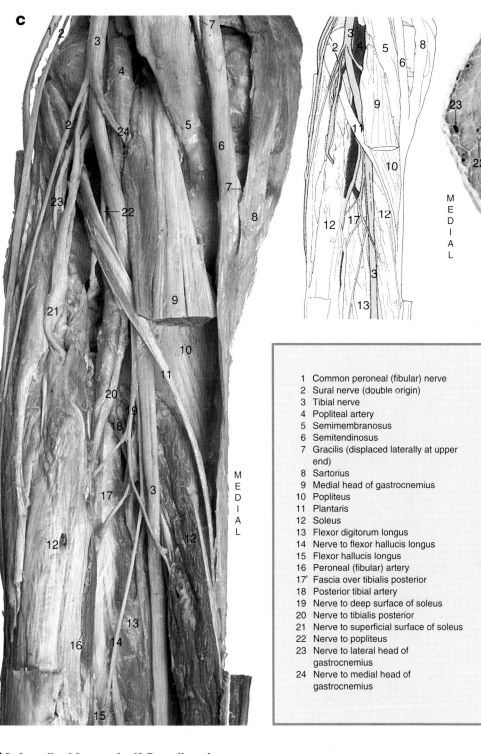

C

D

D Cross section of the left leg, from below

The section is viewed looking from the ankle to the knee. Behind the interosseous membrane (5), tibialis posterior (13) is the deepest of the calf muscles, with the tibial nerve (19) behind it and the posterior tibial vessels (20) more medially, between flexor digitorum longus (21) and soleus (14). The peroneal artery (12) is adjacent to flexor hallucis longus (11) behind the fibula (8). Note the (unlabelled) large veins within and deep to soleus (14; see note). In the anterior compartment, the anterior tibial vessels (3) and deep peroneal nerve (4) are between tibialis anterior (2) and extensor hallucis longus (6)

MEDIAL

1	Common peroneal (fibular) nerve
2	Sural nerve (double origin)
3	Tibial nerve
4	Popliteal artery
5	Semimembranosus
6	Semitendinosus
7	Gracilis (displaced laterally at upper end)
8	Sartorius
9	Medial head of gastrocnemius
10	Popliteus
11	Plantaris
12	Soleus
13	Flexor digitorum longus
14	Nerve to flexor hallucis longus
15	Flexor hallucis longus
16	Peroneal (fibular) artery
17	Fascia over tibialis posterior
18	Posterior tibial artery
19	Nerve to deep surface of soleus
20	Nerve to tibialis posterior
21	Nerve to superficial surface of soleus
22	Nerve to popliteus
23	Nerve to lateral head of gastrocnemius
24	Nerve to medial head of gastrocnemius

1	Tibia
2	Tibialis anterior
3	Anterior tibial vessels
4	Deep peroneal (fibular) nerve
5	Interosseous membrane
6	Extensor hallucis longus
7	Extensor digitorum longus
8	Fibula
9	Superficial peroneal (fibular) nerve
10	Peroneus longus and brevis
11	Flexor hallucis longus
12	Peroneal (fibular) artery
13	Tibialis posterior
14	Soleus
15	Gastrocnemius
16	Plantaris tendon
17	Sural nerve
18	Small saphenous vein
19	Tibial nerve
20	Posterior tibial vessels
21	Flexor digitorum longus
22	Saphenous nerve
23	Great saphenous vein

C Left popliteal fossa and calf. Deep dissection

Soleus (12) has been bisected in the midline and displaced to each side to show the branches of the tibial nerve (3). (The knee joint was injected with orange resin and the capsule removed.)

• The deep veins of the calf, deep to and within soleus, are sites for potentially dangerous venous thrombosis.

A

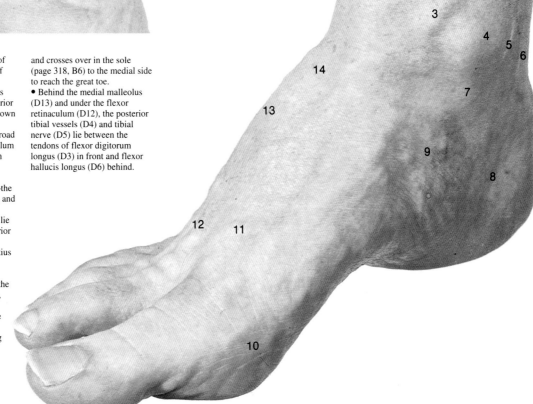

A Right ankle and foot, from the lateral side

The most prominent surface features are the lateral malleolus (3), the tendo calcaneus (1) at the back and the tendon of tibialis anterior (4) at the front

B Right ankle and foot, from the front and medial side

The most prominent surface features are the medial malleolus (4), the tendo calcaneus (6) at the back and the tendons of tibialis anterior (2) and extensor hallucis longus (1) at the front. The dorsalis pedis artery (14) can be palpated where labelled, as may the long tendons

1	Tendo calcaneus (Achilles' tendon)
2	Peroneus longus and brevis
3	Lateral malleolus
4	Tibialis anterior
5	Extensor digitorum brevis
6	Tuberosity of base of fifth metatarsal
7	Small saphenous vein

1	Extensor hallucis longus
2	Tibialis anterior
3	Great saphenous vein
4	Medial malleolus
5	Posterior tibial artery
6	Tendo calcaneus (Achilles' tendon)
7	Tibialis posterior
8	Calcaneus
9	Tuberosity of navicular
10	Head of first metatarsal
11	Dorsal venous arch
12	Extensor digitorum longus
13	Extensor digitorum brevis
14	Dorsalis pedis artery

● The great saphenous vein (B3) runs upwards in front of the medial malleolus (B4).
● The small saphenous vein (A7) runs upwards behind the lateral malleolus (A3).

● Behind the lateral malleolus (C11) the tendon of peroneus brevis (C4) lies in front of the tendon of peroneus longus (C5). As they pass under the superior peroneal retinaculum (C14) both tendons are in a single synovial sheath, but under the inferior peroneal retinaculum (C15) they each have their own synovial sheath.
● The superior extensor retinaculum (C12) is a broad transverse band but the inferior extensor retinaculum is like a capital Y on its side, with the single stem (C13) on the lateral side (continuous with the inferior peroneal retinaculum, C15), and the two limbs passing as bands across to the medial side–the upper band (D18) to the medial malleolus (D13), and the lower (D15) to the fascia of the sole.
● Under the extensor retinacula the long tendons lie in the order (from medial to lateral): tibialis anterior (D16), extensor hallucis longus (D17 and C20), extensor digitorum longus (C3) and peroneus tertius (C17).
● Behind the medial malleolus (D13) under the flexor retinaculum (D12) the long tendons lie in the order (from front to back): tibialis posterior (D2), flexor digitorum longus (D3) and flexor hallucis longus (D6). The hallucis tendon for the great toe thus appears to be 'out of order', but the muscle arises from the fibula on the lateral side of the leg

and crosses over in the sole (page 318, B6) to the medial side to reach the great toe.
● Behind the medial malleolus (D13) and under the flexor retinaculum (D12), the posterior tibial vessels (D4) and tibial nerve (D5) lie between the tendons of flexor digitorum longus (D3) in front and flexor hallucis longus (D6) behind.

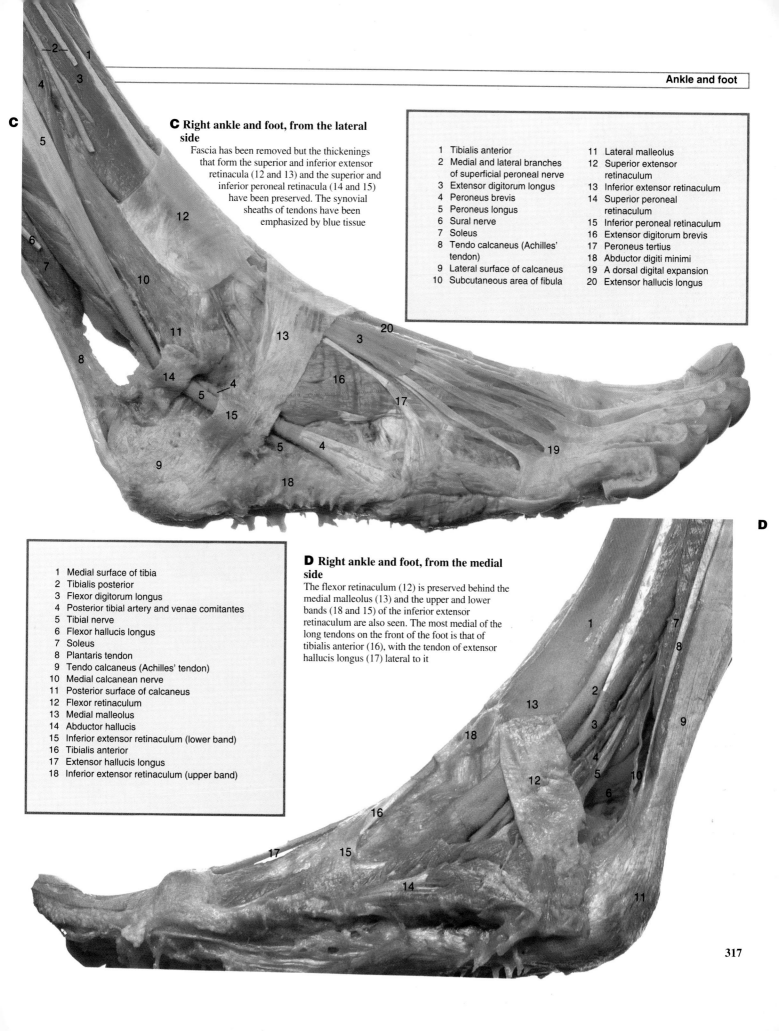

C Right ankle and foot, from the lateral side

Fascia has been removed but the thickenings that form the superior and inferior extensor retinacula (12 and 13) and the superior and inferior peroneal retinacula (14 and 15) have been preserved. The synovial sheaths of tendons have been emphasized by blue tissue

1	Tibialis anterior	11	Lateral malleolus
2	Medial and lateral branches of superficial peroneal nerve	12	Superior extensor retinaculum
3	Extensor digitorum longus	13	Inferior extensor retinaculum
4	Peroneus brevis	14	Superior peroneal retinaculum
5	Peroneus longus	15	Inferior peroneal retinaculum
6	Sural nerve	16	Extensor digitorum brevis
7	Soleus	17	Peroneus tertius
8	Tendo calcaneus (Achilles' tendon)	18	Abductor digiti minimi
9	Lateral surface of calcaneus	19	A dorsal digital expansion
10	Subcutaneous area of fibula	20	Extensor hallucis longus

1 Medial surface of tibia
2 Tibialis posterior
3 Flexor digitorum longus
4 Posterior tibial artery and venae comitantes
5 Tibial nerve
6 Flexor hallucis longus
7 Soleus
8 Plantaris tendon
9 Tendo calcaneus (Achilles' tendon)
10 Medial calcanean nerve
11 Posterior surface of calcaneus
12 Flexor retinaculum
13 Medial malleolus
14 Abductor hallucis
15 Inferior extensor retinaculum (lower band)
16 Tibialis anterior
17 Extensor hallucis longus
18 Inferior extensor retinaculum (upper band)

D Right ankle and foot, from the medial side

The flexor retinaculum (12) is preserved behind the medial malleolus (13) and the upper and lower bands (18 and 15) of the inferior extensor retinaculum are also seen. The most medial of the long tendons on the front of the foot is that of tibialis anterior (16), with the tendon of extensor hallucis longus (17) lateral to it

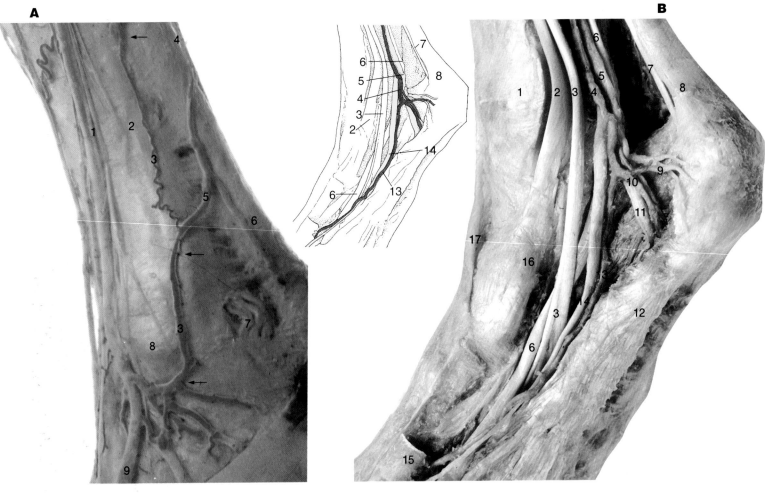

A Right lower leg and ankle, from the medial side and behind

The deep fascia remains intact apart from a small window cut to show the position of the posterior tibial vessels and tibial nerve (7). The great saphenous vein (1) runs upwards in front of the medial malleolus (8) with the posterior arch vein (3) behind it. The arrows indicate common levels for perforating veins (page 312, A6 and B5)

B Right ankle and sole, from the medial side and below

The foot is in plantar flexion, and the flexor retinaculum and most of abductor hallucis (15) have been removed to show how the tendon of flexor hallucis longus (6) passes deep to flexor digitorum longus (3) in the sole to run towards the great toe

1	Great saphenous vein and saphenous nerve	6	Tendo calcaneus (Achilles' tendon)
2	Tibialis posterior and flexor digitorum longus underlying deep fascia	7	Posterior tibial vessels and tibial nerve
3	Posterior arch vein	8	Medial malleolus
4	Small saphenous vein	9	Dorsal venous arch
5	Communication with small saphenous vein		

1	Medial malleolus	10	Lateral plantar artery
2	Tibialis posterior	11	Lateral plantar nerve
3	Flexor digitorum longus	12	Plantar aponeurosis overlying flexor digitorum brevis
4	Posterior tibial artery	13	Medial plantar artery
5	Tibial nerve	14	Medial plantar nerve
6	Flexor hallucis longus	15	Abductor hallucis
7	Plantaris tendon	16	Tuberosity of navicular
8	Tendo calcaneus (Achilles' tendon)	17	Tibialis anterior
9	Calcanean nerves and vessels		

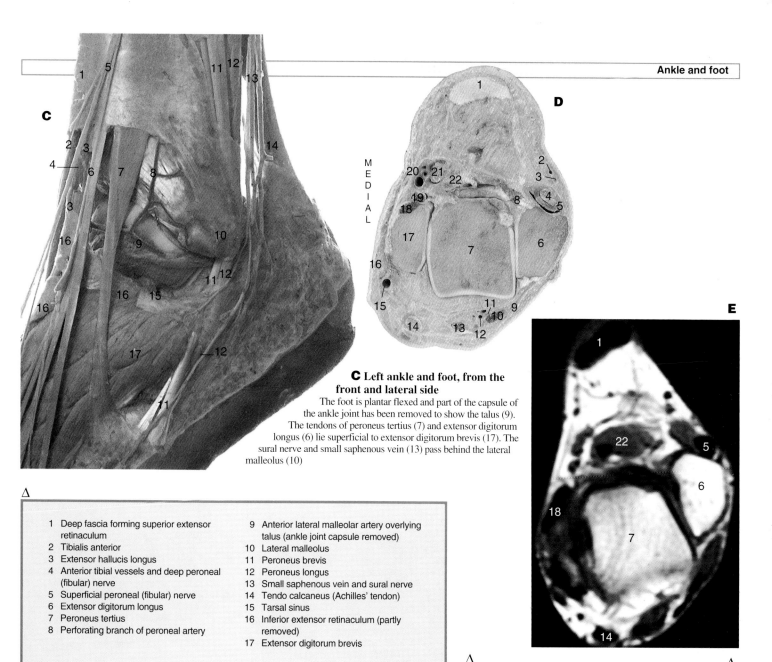

C Left ankle and foot, from the front and lateral side

The foot is plantar flexed and part of the capsule of the ankle joint has been removed to show the talus (9). The tendons of peroneus tertius (7) and extensor digitorum longus (6) lie superficial to extensor digitorum brevis (17). The sural nerve and small saphenous vein (13) pass behind the lateral malleolus (10)

1 Deep fascia forming superior extensor retinaculum	9 Anterior lateral malleolar artery overlying talus (ankle joint capsule removed)
2 Tibialis anterior	10 Lateral malleolus
3 Extensor hallucis longus	11 Peroneus brevis
4 Anterior tibial vessels and deep peroneal (fibular) nerve	12 Peroneus longus
5 Superficial peroneal (fibular) nerve	13 Small saphenous vein and sural nerve
6 Extensor digitorum longus	14 Tendo calcaneus (Achilles' tendon)
7 Peroneus tertius	15 Tarsal sinus
8 Perforating branch of peroneal artery	16 Inferior extensor retinaculum (partly removed)
	17 Extensor digitorum brevis

• Muscles producing movements at the ankle joint:

Dorsiflexion: tibialis anterior, extensor digitorum longus, extensor hallucis longus and peroneus tertius.

Plantar flexion: gastrocnemius, soleus, plantaris, tibialis posterior, flexor digitorum longus, flexor hallucis longus, peroneus longus and peroneus brevis.

Left ankle, D cross section, E axial MR image

This section, looking down from above, emphasizes the positions of tendons, vessels and nerves in the ankle region. The talus (7) is in the centre, with the medial malleolus (17) on the left of the picture and the lateral malleolus (6) on the right. The great saphenous vein (15) and saphenous nerve (16) are in front of the medial malleolus, with the tendon of tibialis posterior (18) immediately behind it. The small saphenous vein (2) and the sural nerve (3) are behind the lateral malleolus, with the tendons of peroneus longus (4) and peroneus brevis (5) intervening. At the front of the ankle the dorsalis pedis vessels (12) and deep peroneal (fibular) nerve (11) are between the tendons of extensor hallucis longus (13) and extensor digitorum longus (10). Behind the medial malleolus (17) and tibialis posterior (18), the posterior tibial vessels (20) and tibial nerve (21) are between the tendons of flexor digitorum longus (19) and flexor hallucis longus (22)

1 Tendo calcaneus (Achilles' tendon)	12 Dorsalis pedis artery and venae comitantes
2 Small saphenous vein	13 Extensor hallucis longus
3 Sural nerve	14 Tibialis anterior
4 Peroneus longus	15 Great saphenous vein
5 Peroneus brevis	16 Saphenous nerve
6 Lateral malleolus of fibula	17 Medial malleolus of tibia
7 Talus	18 Tibialis posterior
8 Posterior talofibular ligament	19 Flexor digitorum longus
9 Peroneus tertius	20 Posterior tibial artery and venae comitantes
10 Extensor digitorum longus	21 Tibial nerve
11 Deep peroneal (fibular) nerve	22 Flexor hallucis longus

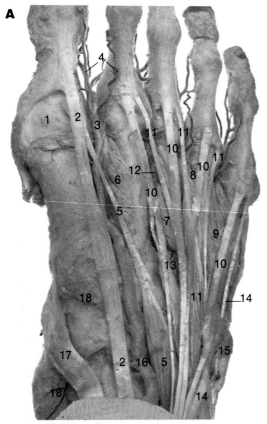

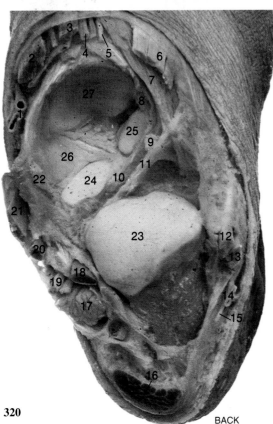

A Dorsum of the right foot
Fascia and superficial nerves have been removed to show tendons and arteries

1 First metatarsophalangeal joint	11 Extensor digitorum brevis
2 Extensor hallucis longus	12 Second dorsal metatarsal artery
3 First dorsal metatarsal artery	13 Arcuate artery
4 Digital arteries	14 Peroneus tertius
5 Extensor hallucis brevis	15 Tuberosity of base of fifth metatarsal and
6 First ⎫	peroneus brevis
7 Second ⎬ dorsal interosseous	16 Dorsalis pedis artery
8 Third ⎪	17 Tibialis anterior
9 Fourth ⎭	18 Tarsal arteries
10 Extensor digitorum longus	

● Extensor digitorum longus (10) sends its tendons to the four lateral toes, while extensor digitorum brevis (11) sends its tendons to the four medial toes; the part of extensor digitorum brevis that goes to the great toe is often known as extensor hallucis brevis (5).

B Right talocalcanean and talocalcaneonavicular joints
The talus has been removed to show the articular surfaces of the calcaneus (23, 24 and 25), navicular (27) and plantar calcaneonavicular (spring) ligament (26)

1 Dorsal venous arch	15 Sural nerve
2 Tibialis anterior	16 Tendo calcaneus (Achilles' tendon)
3 Extensor hallucis longus	17 Abductor hallucis
4 Dorsalis pedis artery and vena comitans	18 Flexor hallucis longus
5 Deep peroneal (fibular) nerve	19 Posterior tibial vessels and medial and
6 Extensor digitorum longus	lateral plantar nerves
7 Extensor digitorum brevis	20 Flexor digitorum longus
8 Calcaneonavicular part of bifurcate	21 Tibialis posterior
ligament	22 Deltoid ligament
9 Cervical ligament	23 Posterior ⎫ articular surface
10 Interosseous talocalcanean ligament	24 Middle ⎬ on calcaneus
11 Inferior extensor retinaculum	25 Anterior ⎭ for talus
12 Peroneus brevis	26 Plantar calcaneonavicular (spring)
13 Peroneus longus	ligament
14 Small saphenous vein	27 Articular surface on navicular for talus

● There are two joints beneath the talus (page 286, A and B). The more posterior is the talocalcanean joint, between the posterior articular surfaces of the calcaneus and talus.; this joint is sometimes known anatomically as the subtalar joint.
● The more anterior joint, the talocalcaneonavicular, is between (a) the middle and anterior articular surfaces of the talus and calcaneus and the upper surface of the plantar calcaneonavicular (spring) ligament, all of which constitute the talocalcanean part of the joint, and (b) the head of the talus and the posterior articular surface of the navicular, which constitute the talonavicular part of the joint. The two parts of the joint share one synovial cavity.
● Do not confuse the talocalcanean joint with the talocalcanean part of the talocalcaneonavicular joint.
● Clinicians sometimes use the term subtalar joint as a combined name for both the talocalcanean joint and the talocalcanean part of the talocalcaneonavicular joint, because it is at both these joints beneath the talus at which most of the movements of inversion and eversion of the foot occur.
● Muscles producing inversion of the foot: tibialis anterior and tibialis posterior.
● Muscles producing eversion of the foot: peroneus longus, peroneus brevis and peroneus tertius.
● The deltoid ligament (C3) is the medial ligament of the ankle joint. On the lateral side of the joint there are three separate ligaments—anterior and posterior talofibular (D12 and E23) and calcaneofibular (D14).

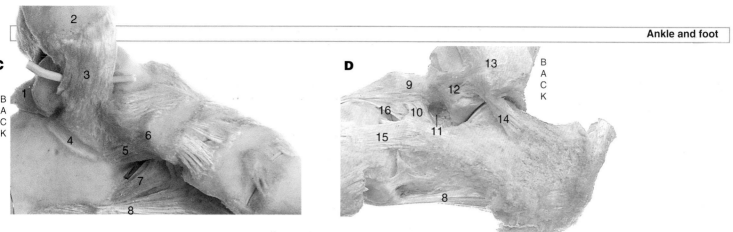

Ligaments of the left ankle and foot. C from the medial side, D from the lateral side, E from behind

In C the marker below the medial malleolus (2) passes between the superficial and deep parts of the deltoid ligament (3). The marker below the tuberosity of the navicular (6) passes between the plantar calcaneonavicular (spring) and calcaneocuboid (short plantar) ligaments (5 and 7)

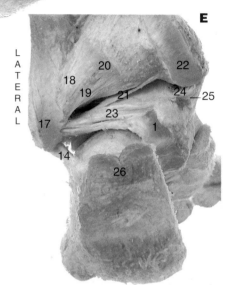

1	Groove on talus for flexor hallucis longus	
2	Medial malleolus	
3	Deltoid ligament	
4	Groove below sustentaculum tali for flexor hallucis longus	
5	Plantar calcaneonavicular (spring) ligament	
6	Tuberosity of navicular	
7	Plantar calcaneocuboid (short plantar) ligament	
8	Long plantar ligament	
9	Neck of talus	
10	Cervical ligament	
11	Tarsal sinus	
12	Anterior talofibular ligament	
13	Lateral malleolus	

14	Calcaneofibular ligament
15	Calcaneocuboid ⎫ parts of
16	Calcaneonavicular ⎭ bifurcate ligament
17	Groove on lateral malleolus for peroneus brevis
18	Posterior tibiofibular ligament
19	Inferior transverse ligament
20	Groove on tibia for flexor hallucis longus
21	Tibial slip of posterior talofibular ligament
22	Groove on medial malleolus for tibialis posterior
23	Posterior talofibular ligament
24	Posterior tibiotalal ⎫ parts of deltoid
25	Tibiocalcanean ⎭ ligament
26	Tendo calcaneus (Achilles' tendon)

F Sagittal section of the left foot, from the right

The section is through the medial side of the foot, passing through the great toe and first metatarsal (17), medial cuneiform (15), navicular (13), talus (3) and calcaneus (6)

1	Tibia	12	Talonavicular part of talocalcaneonavicular joint
2	Tibiotalal part of ankle joint		
3	Talus	13	Navicular
4	Talocalcanean (subtalar) joint	14	Cuneonavicular joint
5	Interosseous talocalcanean ligament	15	Medial cuneiform
6	Calcaneus	16	First tarsometatarsal (cuneometatarsal) joint
7	Tendo calcaneus (Achilles' tendon)	17	First metatarsal
8	Flexor accessorius	18	Sesamoid bone
9	Flexor digitorum brevis	19	Metatarsophalangeal joint of great toe
10	Plantar aponeurosis	20	Proximal phalanx
11	Plantar calcaneonavicular (spring) ligament	21	Interphalangeal joint
		22	Distal phalanx

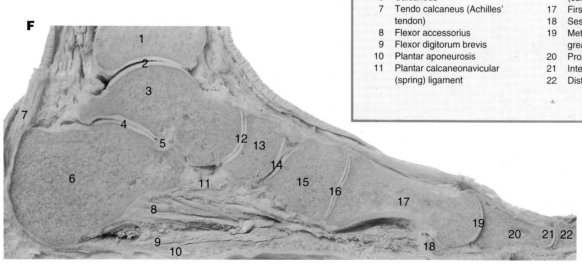

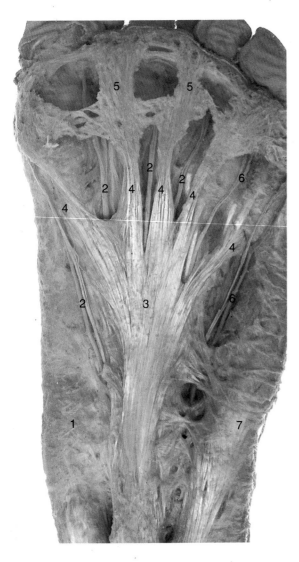

A Sole of the left foot. Plantar aponeurosis

Skin and connective tissue of the sole have been removed to show the tough central part of the plantar aponeurosis (3) which divides into slips (4) for each toe, and thinner medial and lateral parts overlying abductor hallucis (1) and abductor digiti minimi (7) respectively

1 Medial part of aponeurosis overlying abductor hallucis
2 Digital branches of medial plantar nerve and artery
3 Central part of aponeurosis overlying flexor digitorum brevis
4 Digital slip of central part of aponeurosis
5 Superficial stratum of digital slip of aponeurosis
6 Digital branches of lateral plantar nerve and artery
7 Lateral part of aponeurosis overlying abductor digiti minimi

B Sole of the left foot, with the plantar aponeurosis removed

The central muscle is flexor digitorum brevis (19), and passing forwards from beneath its borders are various digital vessels and nerves (such as 24 and 11) which arise from the medial and lateral plantar vessels and nerves still largely under cover of the muscle

1	Plantar digital nerve of great toe	12	Fourth dorsal interosseous
2	Plantar digital nerves of first cleft	13	Third plantar interosseous
3	Superficial transverse metatarsal ligament	14	Plantar digital nerve of fifth toe
4	Fibrous flexor sheath	15	Flexor digiti minimi brevis
5	First lumbrical	16	Abductor digiti minimi
6	Second lumbrical	17	Deep branch of lateral plantar nerve
7	Third lumbrical	18	Lateral plantar artery
8	Fourth lumbrical	19	Flexor digitorum brevis
9	Third plantar metatarsal artery	20	Plantar aponeurosis
10	A superficial digital branch of medial plantar artery	21	Abductor hallucis
		22	Flexor hallucis brevis
11	Fourth common plantar digital nerve	23	Flexor hallucis longus
		24	First common plantar digital nerve

C Sole of the left foot, with flexor digitorum brevis removed

Flexor accessorius (11) joins the lateral side of flexor digitorum longus whose tendon to the little toe (1) is the most clearly seen. One of the cut tendons of flexor digitorum brevis is labelled at 4. The medial and lateral plantar nerves (10 and 12) are now displayed; their accompanying arteries have been removed. The deep branch of the lateral plantar nerve (15) reaches the deeper part of the sole by curling round the lateral border of flexor accessorius (11)

1	Fourth tendon of flexor digitorum longus (fourth lumbrical absent)	9	Abductor hallucis
		10	Medial plantar nerve
2	Common plantar digital branch of lateral plantar nerve	11	Flexor accessorius
		12	Lateral plantar nerve
3	Transverse head of adductor hallucis	13	Long plantar ligament
4	Third tendon of flexor digitorum brevis (cut)	14	Abductor digiti minimi
		15	Deep branch of lateral plantar nerve
5	Second lumbrical and common plantar digital branch of medial plantar nerve	16	Second plantar interosseous
		17	Fourth dorsal interosseous
6	Oblique head of adductor hallucis	18	Third plantar interosseous
7	Flexor hallucis brevis	19	Flexor digiti minimi brevis
8	Flexor hallucis longus		

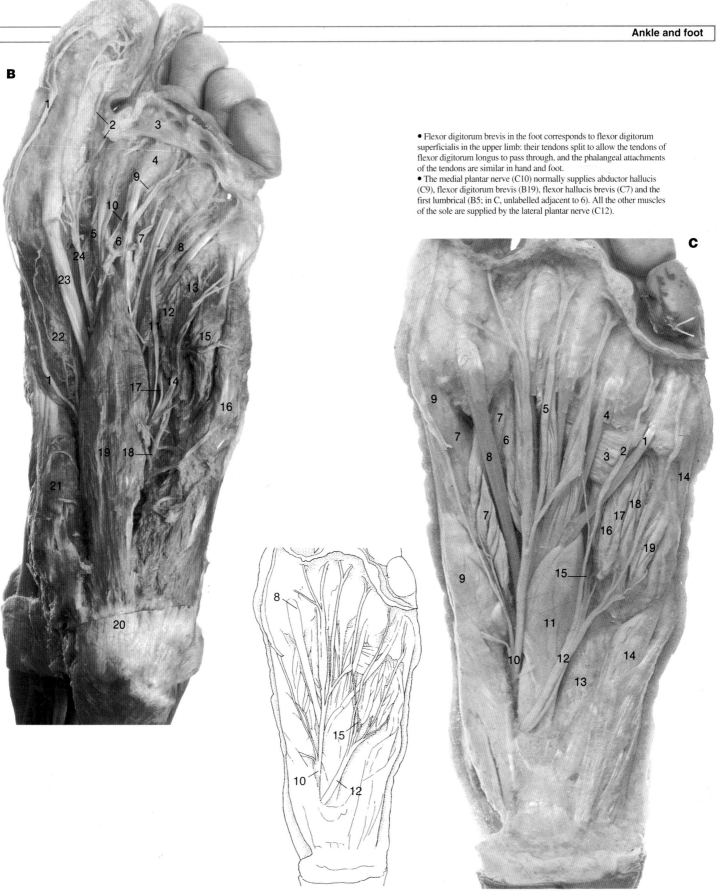

• Flexor digitorum brevis in the foot corresponds to flexor digitorum superficialis in the upper limb: their tendons split to allow the tendons of flexor digitorum longus to pass through, and the phalangeal attachments of the tendons are similar in hand and foot.

• The medial plantar nerve (C10) normally supplies abductor hallucis (C9), flexor digitorum brevis (B19), flexor hallucis brevis (C7) and the first lumbrical (B5; in C, unlabelled adjacent to 6). All the other muscles of the sole are supplied by the lateral plantar nerve (C12).

A

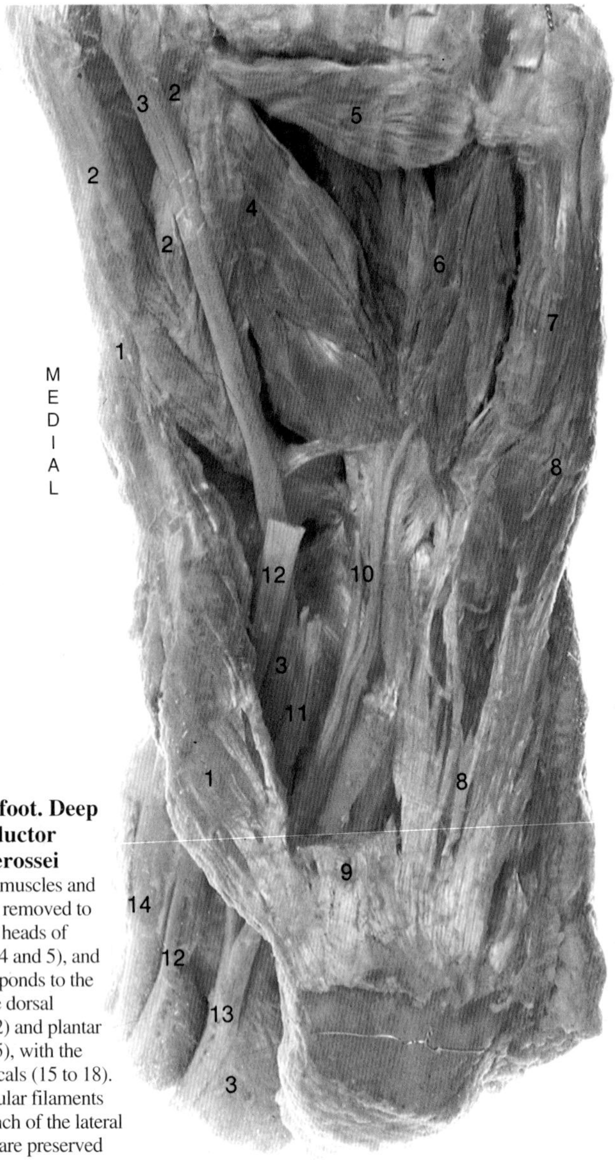

B

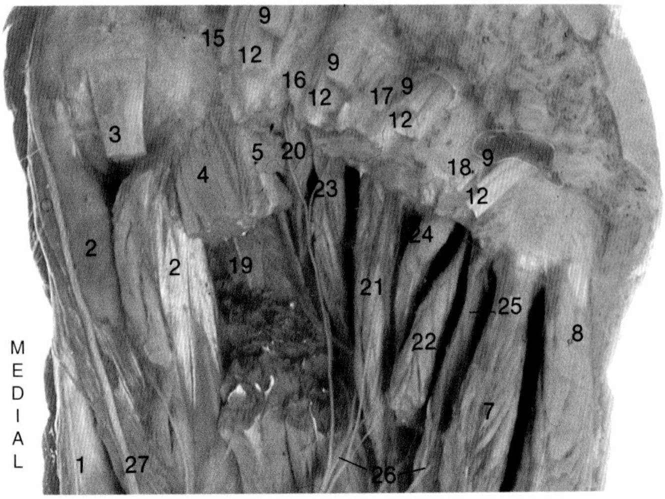

C

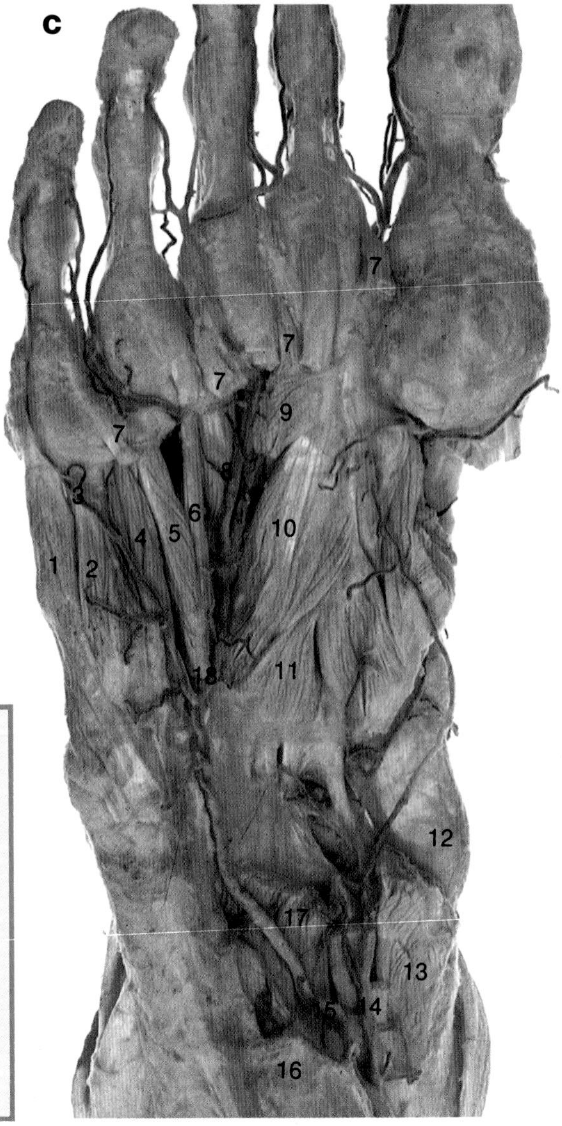

Sole of the left foot. Deep muscles, A adductor hallucis, B interossei

Most of the flexor muscles and tendons have been removed to show in A the two heads of adductor hallucis (4 and 5), and in B (which corresponds to the front part of A) the dorsal interossei (19 to 22) and plantar interossei (23 to 25), with the ends of the lumbricals (15 to 18). Many of the muscular filaments from the deep branch of the lateral plantar nerve (26) are preserved

- 1 Abductor hallucis
- 2 Flexor hallucis brevis
- 3 Flexor hallucis longus
- 4 Oblique } head of adductor hallucis
- 5 Transverse } head of adductor hallucis
- 6 Interossei
- 7 Flexor digiti minimi brevis
- 8 Abductor digiti minimi
- 9 Flexor digitorum brevis
- 10 Deep branch of lateral plantar nerve
- 11 Medial plantar nerve
- 12 Flexor digitorum longus
- 13 Tibial nerve
- 14 Tibialis posterior
- 15 First } lumbrical
- 16 Second } lumbrical
- 17 Third } lumbrical
- 18 Fourth } lumbrical
- 19 First } dorsal interosseous
- 20 Second } dorsal interosseous
- 21 Third } dorsal interosseous
- 22 Fourth } dorsal interosseous
- 23 First } plantar interosseous
- 24 Second } plantar interosseous
- 25 Third } plantar interosseous
- 26 Branches of deep branch of lateral plantar nerve
- 27 Plantar digital nerve of great toe

D

D Sole of the left foot. Ligaments and tendons

The anterior end of the long plantar ligament (8) forms with the groove of the cuboid (E7) a tunnel for the peroneus longus tendon (7) which runs to the medial cuneiform (3) and the base of the first metatarsal (5). Peroneus brevis passes to the tuberosity of the base of the fifth metatarsal (10). The main attachment of tibialis posterior (1) is to the tuberosity of the navicular (2), while tibialis anterior is attached to the medial cuneiform (3) and the base of the first metatarsal (5)

M
E
D
I
A
L

◁

1	Tibialis posterior
2	Tuberosity of navicular
3	Medial cuneiform
4	Tibialis anterior
5	Base of first metatarsal
6	Flexor hallucis longus
7	Peroneus longus
8	Long plantar ligament
9	Plantar calcaneocuboid (short plantar) ligament
10	Tuberosity of base of fifth metatarsal
11	Peroneus brevis

E

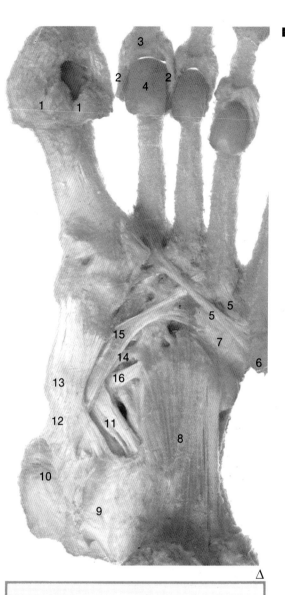

C Sole of the right foot. Plantar arch

Most of the flexor muscles and tendons have been removed to show the lateral plantar artery (15) crossing flexor accessorius (17) to become the plantar arch (18) which would lie deep to the flexor tendons

◁

1	Abductor digiti minimi
2	Flexor digiti minimi brevis
3	Plantar digital artery
4	Third plantar interosseous
5	Fourth dorsal interosseous
6	Second plantar interosseous
7	Lumbrical
8	Plantar metatarsal artery
9	Transverse } head of adductor hallucis
10	Oblique }
11	Flexor hallucis brevis
12	Tuberosity of navicular
13	Abductor hallucis
14	Medial plantar artery and nerve
15	Lateral plantar artery
16	Flexor digitorum brevis
17	Flexor accessorius
18	Plantar arch

• Tibialis anterior (D4) is attached to the medial sides of the medial cuneiform and base of the first metatarsal (D3 and 5); peroneus longus (D7) is attached to the lateral sides of the same bones.
• The plantar calcaneonavicular ligament (E11), commonly called the spring ligament, is one of the most important in the foot. It stretches between the sustentaculum tali (E9) and the tuberosity of the navicular (E13), blending on its medial side with the deltoid ligament of the ankle joint and supporting on its upper surface (page 320, B26) part of the head of the talus.
• The plantar calcaneocuboid ligament (D9), commonly called the short plantar ligament, is largely covered by the long plantar ligament (D8).

E Sole of the left foot. Ligaments

The anterior end of the long plantar ligament (8) has been removed to show the groove for peroneus longus on the cuboid (7). The tibialis posterior tendon (12) is attached to the tuberosity of the navicular (13). The deltoid ligament of the ankle joint is labelled (10) where it passes from the lower margin of the medial malleolus to the sustentaculum tali (9) of the calcaneus

Δ

1	Sesamoid bone
2	Collateral ligament of metatarsophalangeal joint
3	Base of proximal phalanx
4	Head of second metatarsal
5	Plantar metatarsal ligament
6	Tuberosity of base of fifth metatarsal
7	Groove on cuboid for peroneus longus
8	Deep fibres of long plantar ligament
9	Groove on sustentaculum tali for flexor hallucis longus
10	Deltoid ligament
11	Plantar calcaneonavicular (spring) ligament
12	Tibialis posterior
13	Tuberosity of navicular
14	Plantar cuneonavicular ligament
15	Fibrous slip from tibialis posterior
16	Plantar cuboideonavicular ligament

B

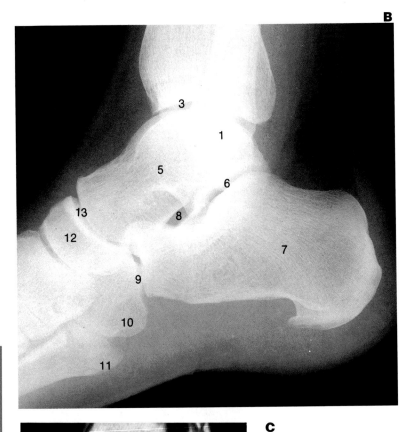

A

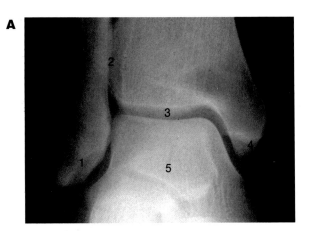

Ankle and foot, A anteroposterior radiograph, B lateral radiograph, C axial MR image
The side view in B shows a small calcanean spur (about 2 cm below the label 7)

1	Lateral malleolus	12	Navicular
2	Inferior tibiofibular syndesmosis	13	Talonavicular part of talocalcaneonavicular joint
3	Ankle joint	14	Medial
4	Medial malleolus	15	Intermediate } cuneiform
5	Talus	16	Lateral
6	Talocalcanean (subtalar) joint	17	First metatarsal
		18	Shaft of metatarsal
7	Calcaneus	19	Proximal phalanx of great toe
8	Tarsal sinus		
9	Calcaneocuboid joint	20	Abductor digiti minimi
10	Cuboid	21	Tibialis anterior
11	Tuberosity of base of fifth metatarsal	22	Peroneus brevis

C

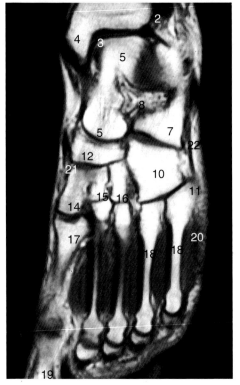

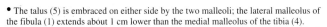

- The talus (5) is embraced on either side by the two malleoli; the lateral malleolus of the fibula (1) extends about 1 cm lower than the medial malleolus of the tibia (4).
- The calcaneocuboid joint (B9) and the talonavicular part of the talocalcaneonavicular joint (B13) together form the midtarsal joint.
- For notes on the joints beneath the talus see page 320.

Appendix

A

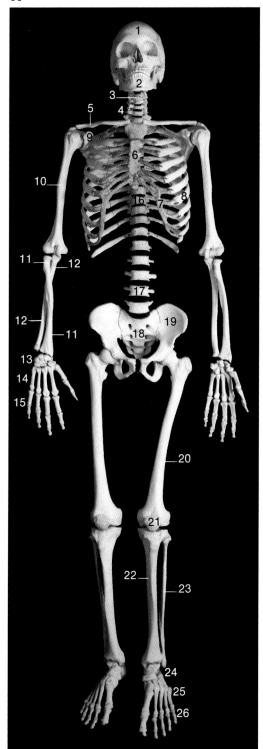

Skeleton

A from the front, **B** from behind.
The left forearm is in the position of
supination, the right in pronation

1 Skull
2 Mandible
3 Hyoid bone
4 Cervical vertebrae
5 Clavicle
6 Sternum
7 Costal cartilages
8 Ribs
9 Scapula
10 Humerus
11 Radius
12 Ulna
13 Carpal bones
14 Metacarpal bones
15 Phalanges of thumb and fingers
16 Thoracic vertebrae
17 Lumbar vertebrae
18 Sacrum
19 Hip bone
20 Femur
21 Patella
22 Tibia
23 Fibula
24 Tarsal bones
25 Metatarsal bones
26 Phalanges of toes
27 Coccyx

B

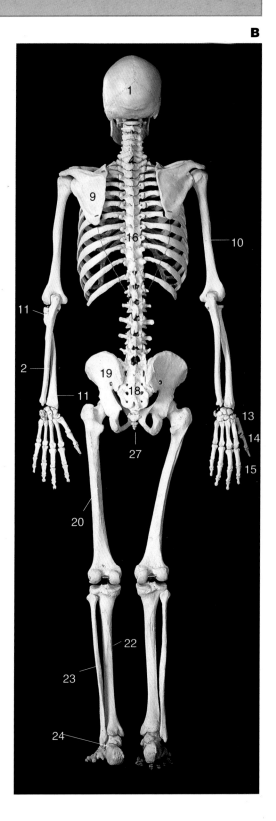

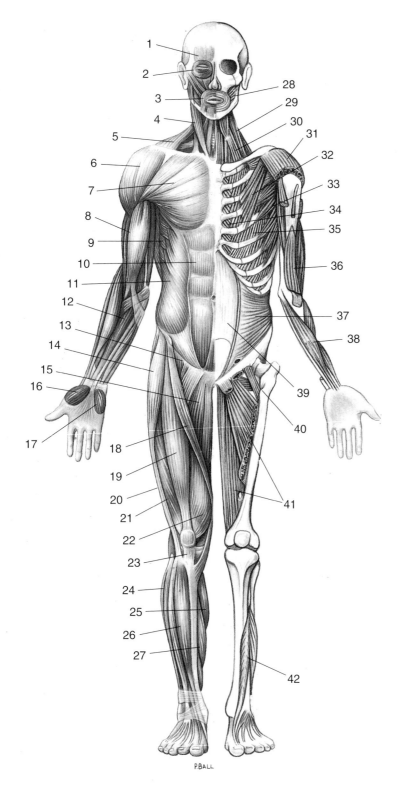

P.BALL

Muscles

From the front. Superficial muscles on the right side of the body, deep muscles on the left side

1 Frontalis
2 Orbicularis oculi
3 Orbicularis oris
4 Sternocleidomastoid
5 Trapezius
6 Deltoid
7 Pectoralis major
8 Biceps brachii
9 Serratus anterior
10 Rectus abdominis
11 External oblique
12 Superficial flexor muscles of forearm
13 Inguinal ligament
14 Tensor fasciae latae
15 Adductor muscles
16 Thenar muscles
17 Hypothenar muscles
18 Sartorius
19 Rectus femoris
20 Iliotibial tract
21 Vastus lateralis
22 Vastus medialis
23 Patellar ligament
24 Peroneal muscles
25 Gastrocnemius
26 Extensor muscles of leg
27 Soleus
28 Buccinator
29 Levator scapulae
30 Scalenus anterior
31 Deltoid
32 Pectoralis minor
33 Serratus anterior
34 Internal intercostal
35 External intercostal
36 Brachialis
37 Internal oblique
38 Deep flexor muscles of forearm
39 Rectus sheath
40 Psoas major and iliacus
41 Adductor magnus
42 Extensor hallucis longus

Muscles

From the back. Superficial muscles on the left side of the body, deep muscles on the right side

1 Sternocleidomastoid
2 Trapezius
3 Spine of scapula
4 Deltoid
5 Infraspinatus
6 Latissimus dorsi
7 Triceps
8 External oblique
9 Iliac crest
10 Gluteus medius
11 Superficial extensor muscles of forearm
12 Gluteus maximus
13 Ilotibial tract
14 Biceps femoris
15 Semimembranosus
16 Semitendinosus
17 Gastrocnemius
18 Soleus
19 Tendo calcaneus (Achilles' tendon)
20 Semispinalis capitis
21 Splenius
22 Levator scapulae
23 Supraspinatus
24 Rhomboid minor
25 Infraspinatus
26 Teres minor
27 Rhomboid major
28 Teres major
29 Erector spinae
30 Triceps
31 Deep extensor muscles of forearm
32 Gluteus medius
33 Piriformis
34 Obturator internus
35 Quadratus femoris
36 Adductor magnus
37 Semimembranosus
38 Biceps femoris
39 Popliteus
40 Soleus
41 Deep flexor muscles of leg
42 Flexor hallucis longus

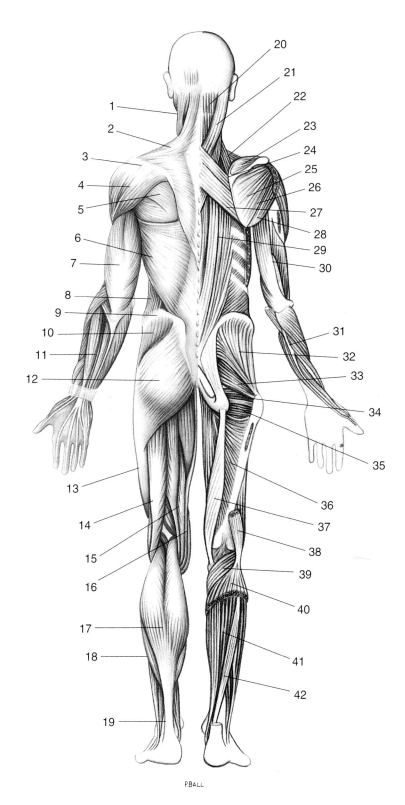

P.BALL

Arteries

Veins

Arteries

Some major arteries, from the front

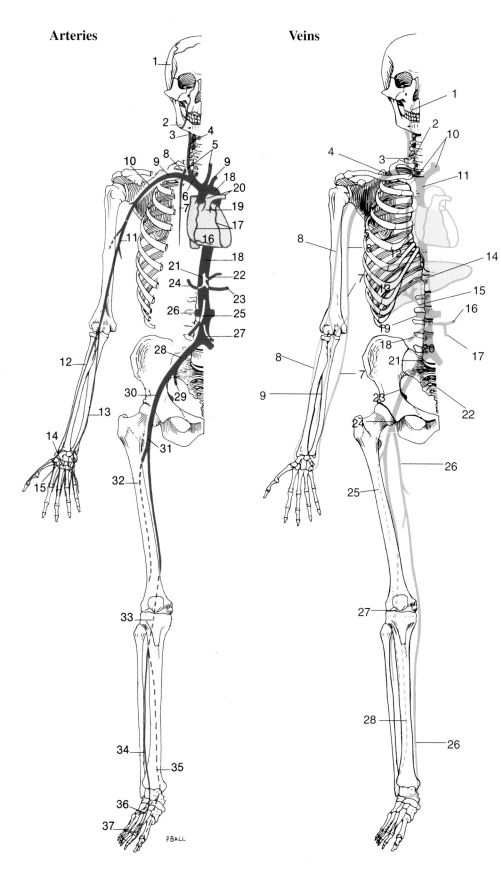

1	Superficial temporal a.	18	Aorta
2	Facial a.	19	Pulmonary trunk
3	Internal carotid a.	20	Pulmonary a.
4	External carotid a.	21	Coeliac trunk
5	Common carotid a.	22	Left gastric a.
		23	Splenic a.
6	Brachiocephalic trunk	24	Common hepatic a.
7	Internal thoracic a.	25	Superior mesenteric a.
8	Vertebral a.	26	Renal a.
9	Subclavian a.	27	Inferior mesenteric a.
10	Axillary a.	28	Common iliac a.
11	Brachial a.	29	Internal iliac a.
12	Radial a.	30	External iliac a.
13	Ulnar a.	31	Femoral a.
14	Deep palmar arch	32	Profunda femoris a.
15	Superficial palmar arch	33	Popliteal a.
		34	Anterior tibial a.
16	Heart	35	Posterior tibial a.
17	Coronary a.	36	Dorsalis pedis a.
		37	Plantar arch

Veins

Some major veins, from the front
(The pulmonary veins enter the left atrium at the back of the heart and are not shown)

1	Facial v.	16	Splenic v.
2	Internal jugular v.	17	Inferior mesenteric v.
3	External jugular v.	18	Superior mesenteric v.
4	Subclavian v.	19	Renal v.
5	Axillary v.	20	Inferior vena cava
6	Brachial v.	21	Common iliac v.
7	Basilic v.	22	Internal iliac v.
8	Cephalic v.	23	External iliac v.
9	Median forearm v.	24	Femoral v.
10	Brachiocephalic v.	25	Profunda femoris v.
11	Superior vena cava	26	Great saphenous v.
12	Azygos v.	27	Popliteal v.
13	Liver	28	Small saphenous v.
14	Hepatic v.		
15	Portal v.		

P.BALL

Nerves

The facial nerve and some major branches of the brachial, lumbar and sacral plexuses, A from the front, B from the back

1 Facial n.
2 Brachial plexus
3 Musculocutaneous n.
4 Median n.
5 Ulnar n.
6 Lumbar plexus
7 Obturator n.
8 Femoral n.
9 Saphenous n.
10 Common peroneal (fibular) n.
11 Superficial peroneal (fibular) n.
12 Deep peroneal (fibular) n.
13 Axillary n.
14 Radial n.
15 Sacral plexus
16 Superior gluteal n.
17 Inferior gluteal n.
18 Pudendal n.
19 Posterior femoral cutaneous n.
20 Sciatic n.
21 Tibial n.
22 Sural n.

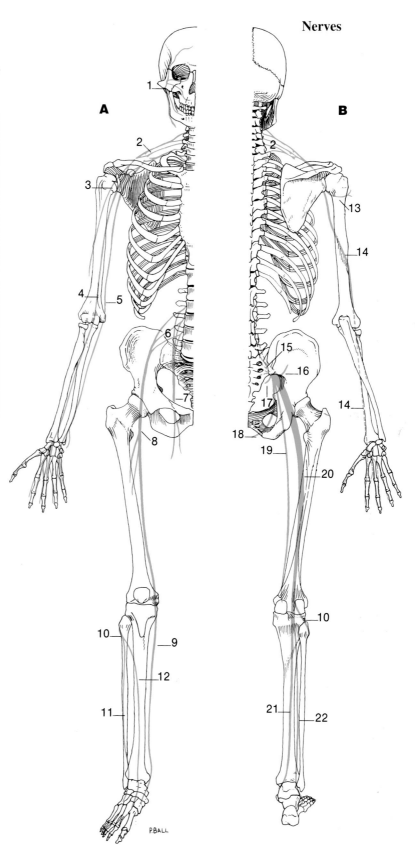

Nerves

A

B

P.BALL

The reference lists of vessels and nerves have been arranged for quick identification of parent trunks and branches. Thus, the left common carotid artery is one of the three branches of the arch of the aorta, while the right common carotid is one of the branches of the brachiocephalic trunk.

The arrows indicate a continuity (instead of branching) with a change of name.

The generally accepted standard pattern has been given. For common variations, which are particularly frequent among veins, reference should be made to standard texts. (The articular and vascular branches of nerves have been omitted.)

The inclusion of items in these lists does not necessarily imply that they are illustrated in the atlas; many of the smaller and less important items are not shown but have been included in the lists for reference purposes.

For skull foramina, two lists are given: one of the principal foramina and their contents, which most students would be expected to know, and another giving more specialized details for those who require them.

Arteries

AORTA AND BRANCHES

Ascending aorta → arch of aorta → thoracic aorta → abdominal aorta

Ascending aorta
Right coronary
    Conus
    Sinuatrial nodal (55%)
    Atrial
    Right marginal
    Posterior interventricular
        Septal
    Atrioventricular nodal (90%)
Left coronary
    Anterior interventricular
        Conus
        Diagonal
        Septal
    Circumflex
        Sinuatrial nodal (45%)
        Atrioventricular nodal (10%)
        Atrial
        Left marginal

Arch of aorta
Brachiocephalic trunk
    Right common carotid
        Right internal carotid
        Right external carotid
    Right subclavian → axillary → brachial
    Thyroidea ima (occasional)
Left common carotid
    Left internal carotid
    Left external carotid
Left subclavian → axillary → brachial

Thoracic aorta
Pericardial
Left bronchial
Oesophageal
Mediastinal
Phrenic
Posterior intercostal (3 to 11)
    Right bronchial (from third)
Subcostal

Abdominal aorta
Coeliac trunk
Superior mesenteric
Inferior mesenteric
Middle suprarenal
Renal
    Inferior suprarenal
Testicular (ovarian)
Inferior phrenic
    Superior suprarenal
Lumbar
Median sacral
Common iliac
    Internal iliac
    External iliac → femoral

CAROTID ARTERIES AND BRANCHES

Internal carotid
Caroticotympanic
Pterygoid
Cavernous
Hypophysial
Meningeal
Ophthalmic
    Central of retina
    Lacrimal
        Lateral palpebral
        Zygomatic
        Recurrent meningeal
    Muscular
        Anterior ciliary
    Long posterior ciliary
    Short posterior ciliary
    Supra-orbital
    Posterior ethmoidal
    Anterior ethmoidal
    Anterior meningeal
    Medial palpebral
    Supratrochlear
    Dorsal nasal
Anterior cerebral
    Striate (and others)
Middle cerebral
    Striate (and others)
Posterior communicating
Anterior choroidal

External carotid
Ascending pharyngeal
Superior thyroid
    Infrahyoid
    Sternocleidomastoid
    Superior laryngeal
    Cricothyroid
Lingual
Facial
    Ascending palatine
    Tonsillar
    Glandular
    Submental
    Inferior labial
    Superior labial
        Septal
    Lateral nasal
Occipital
Posterior auricular
Superficial temporal
    Transverse facial
Maxillary → sphenopalatine
    Deep auricular
    Anterior tympanic
    Middle meningeal
    Accessory meningeal
    Inferior alveolar
        Dental
        Mylohyoid
        Mental
    Deep temporal
    Pterygoid
    Masseteric
    Buccal
    Infra-orbital
        Anterior superior alveolar
        Dental
    Posterior superior alveolar
        Dental
    Greater palatine
        Lesser palatine
    Pharyngeal
    Artery of pterygoid canal

SUBCLAVIAN ARTERY AND BRANCHES

Subclavian → axillary → brachial
Vertebral
    Spinal
    Meningeal
    Anterior spinal
    Posterior spinal
    Posterior inferior cerebellar
Internal thoracic
    Pericardiacophrenic
    Mediastinal
    Thymic
    Sternal
    Perforating
        Mammary
    Anterior intercostal
    Musculophrenic
    Superior epigastric
Thyrocervical trunk
    Inferior thyroid
        Ascending cervical
        Inferior laryngeal
        Glandular
        Pharyngeal
        Oesophageal
        Tracheal
    Suprascapular
    Superficial cervical
Costocervical trunk
    Superior intercostal
    Deep cervical
Dorsal scapular (sometimes from superficial cervical)

Basilar (union of vertebrals)
Pontine
Labyrinthine
Anterior inferior cerebellar
Superior cerebellar
Posterior cerebral

AXILLARY ARTERY AND BRANCHES

Axillary → brachial
Superior thoracic
Thoraco-acromial
    Acromial
    Clavicular
    Deltoid
    Pectoral
Lateral thoracic
    Lateral mammary
Subscapular
    Circumflex scapular
    Thoracodorsal
Anterior circumflex humeral
Posterior circumflex humeral

Brachial
Profunda brachii
    Posterior descending
    Radial collateral
Nutrient
Superior ulnar collateral
Inferior ulnar collateral
Radial
    Radial recurrent
    Palmar carpal
    Superficial palmar
    Dorsal carpal
    Dorsal metacarpal
        Dorsal digital
    First dorsal metacarpal
    Princeps pollicis
    Radialis indicis
    Deep palmar arch
        Palmar metacarpal
        Perforating
Ulnar
    Anterior ulnar recurrent
    Posterior ulnar recurrent
    Common interosseous
        Anterior interosseous
            Median
        Posterior interosseous
            Interosseous recurrent
    Palmar carpal
    Dorsal carpal
    Deep carpal
    Superficial palmar arch
        Common palmar digital
        Palmar digital

SOME BRANCHES OF THE ABDOMINAL AORTA

Coeliac trunk
Left gastric
    Oesophageal
Common hepatic
    Hepatic
        Right hepatic
            Cystic
        Left hepatic
    Gastroduodenal
        Right gastro-epiploic
        Superior pancreaticoduodenal
        Supraduodenal
    Right gastric
Splenic
    Pancreatic
    Short gastric
    Left gastro-epiploic

Superior mesenteric
Inferior pancreaticoduodenal
Jejunal and ileal
Ileocolic
    Ascending
    Anterior caecal
    Posterior caecal
        Appendicular
    Ileal
Right colic
Middle colic

Inferior mesenteric
Left colic
Sigmoid
Superior rectal

Internal iliac
Anterior trunk
    Superior vesical → obliterated umbilical
    Artery to ductus deferens (sometimes from
    inferior vesical)
Inferior vesical
    Middle rectal
    Uterine
    Vaginal
    Obturator
    Internal pudendal
        Inferior rectal
        Perineal
        Artery of the bulb
        Urethral
        Deep artery of the penis (clitoris)
        Dorsal artery of the penis (clitoris)
    Inferior gluteal
Posterior trunk
    Iliolumbar
    Lateral sacral
    Superior gluteal

External iliac → femoral
Inferior epigastric
    Cremasteric
    Pubic (accessory obturator)
Deep circumflex iliac

FEMORAL ARTERY AND BRANCHES

Femoral → popliteal
Superficial epigastric
Superficial circumflex iliac
Superficial external pudendal
Deep external pudendal
Profunda femoris
    Lateral circumflex femoral
    Medial circumflex femoral
    Perforating
Descending genicular

Popliteal
Sural
Superior genicular
Middle genicular
Inferior genicular
Anterior tibial → dorsalis pedis
    Posterior tibial recurrent
    Anterior tibial recurrent
    Anterior medial malleolar
    Anterior lateral malleolar
    Dorsalis pedis → plantar arch
        Tarsal
        First dorsal metatarsal
            Dorsal digital
        Arcuate
            Dorsal metatarsal (2–4)
                Dorsal digital
Posterior tibial
    Circumflex fibular
    Peroneal
        · Nutrient
        Perforating
        Communicating
        Lateral malleolar
        Calcanean
    Nutrient
    Communicating
    Medial malleolar
    Calcanean
    Medial plantar
        Superficial digital
    Lateral plantar → plantar arch
        Superficial digital
        Plantar metatarsal
            Common plantar digital
                Plantar digital
        Perforating

Veins

TRIBUTARIES OF MAJOR VEINS

SUPERIOR VENA CAVA

Superior vena cava
Left brachiocephalic
    Left internal jugular
    Left subclavian
    Left vertebral
    Left supreme (first posterior) intercostal
    Left superior intercostal (2–4)
    Inferior thyroid
    Thymic
    Pericardial
Right brachiocephalic
    Right internal jugular
    Right subclavian
    Right vertebral
    Right supreme (first posterior) intercostal
Azygos
    Right superior intercostal (2–4)
    Right posterior intercostal (5–11)
    Right subcostal
    Right ascending lumbar and/or lumbar azygos
    Right bronchial
    Oesophageal
    Pericardial
    Mediastinal
    Vertebral venous plexuses
    Hemi-azygos
        Left ascending lumbar and/or lumbar azygos
        Left subcostal
        Left posterior intercostal (9–11)
        Oesophageal
        Pericardial
        Mediastinal
        Vertebral venous plexuses
    Accessory hemi-azygos
        Left posterior intercostal (5–8)
        Left bronchial
        Oesophageal
        Pericardial
        Mediastinal
        Vertebral venous plexuses

INFERIOR VENA CAVA

Inferior vena cava
Common iliac (right and left)
Fourth lumbar (right and left)
Third lumbar (right and left)
Testicular (ovarian) (right)
Renal (right and left)
Suprarenal (right)
Inferior phrenic (right and left)
Hepatic (right, middle and left)
(Upper lumbar veins join ascending lumbar. Left
    testicular or ovarian and suprarenal veins join left
    renal)

INTERNAL JUGULAR VEIN

Internal jugular
Inferior petrosal sinus
Pharyngeal
Lingual
Facial
Superior thyroid
Middle thyroid

EXTERNAL JUGULAR VEIN

External jugular
Posterior auricular
Posterior branch of retromandibular
Occipital
Posterior external jugular
Suprascapular
Superficial cervical
Anterior jugular

RETROMANDIBULAR VEIN

Retromandibular
Superficial temporal
Maxillary
Transverse facial
Pterygoid plexus
    Middle meningeal
    Greater palatine
    Sphenopalatine
    Buccal
    Dental
    Deep facial
    Inferior ophthalmic
Anterior branch to join facial
Posterior branch to external jugular

FACIAL VEIN

Facial
Supratrochlear
Supra-orbital
Superior ophthalmic
Palpebral
External nasal
Labial
Deep facial
Submental
Submandibular
Tonsillar
External palatine (paratonsillar)

GREAT SAPHENOUS VEIN

Great saphenous
Dorsal venous arch
Posterior arch
    Perforating
Perforating
Accessory saphenous
Anterior femoral cutaneous
Superficial epigastric
Superficial circumflex iliac
Superficial external pudendal
Deep external pudendal
(Small saphenous vein communicates with great
saphenous but usually drains to popliteal vein)

CARDIAC VEINS

Coronary sinus
Great cardiac
Middle cardiac
Small cardiac
Posterior of left ventricle
Oblique of left atrium

Anterior cardiac

Venae cordis minimae

DURAL VENOUS SINUSES

Posterosuperior group
Superior sagittal
Inferior sagittal
Straight
Transverse
Sigmoid
Petrosquamous
Occipital

Antero-inferior group
Cavernous
Intercavernous
Inferior petrosal
Superior petrosal
Sphenoparietal
Basilar
Middle meningeal veins

HEPATIC PORTAL SYSTEM

Portal vein
Superior mesenteric
    Jejunal and ileal
    Right gastro-epiploic
    Pancreatic
    Pancreaticoduodenal
    Ileocolic
        Caecal
        Appendicular
    Right colic
    Middle colic
Splenic
    Pancreatic
    Short gastric
    Left gastro-epiploic
    Inferior mesenteric
        Left colic
        Sigmoid
        Superior rectal
Left gastric
Right gastric
    Prepyloric
Para-umbilical (to left branch)
Cystic (to right branch)

PORTAL-SYSTEMIC ANASTOMOSES

Oesophageal branches of the left gastric vein with the
    hemi-azygos vein
Superior rectal branch of the inferior mesenteric vein with
    the middle and inferior rectal veins (internal iliac)
Para-umbilical veins of the falciform ligament with
    anterior abdominal wall veins
Retroperitoneal colonic veins with posterior abdominal
    wall veins
Bare area of the liver with diaphragmatic veins

Lymphatic system

THORACIC DUCT AND CISTERNA CHYLI TRIBUTARIES

Thoracic duct
Left jugular trunk
Left subclavian trunk
Left bronchomediastinal trunk

Right lymphatic duct
Right jugular trunk
Right subclavian trunk
Right bronchomediastinal trunk

Cisterna chyli
Left lumbar trunk
Right lumbar trunk
Intestinal trunks

LYMPH NODES OF THE HEAD AND NECK

Deep cervical
Superior (including jugulodigastric)
Inferior (including jugulo-omohyoid)

Draining superficial tissues in the head
Occipital
Retro-auricular (mastoid)
Parotid
Buccal (facial)

Draining superficial tissues in the neck
Submandibular
Submental
Anterior cervical
Superficial cervical

Draining deep tissues in the neck
Retropharyngeal
Paratracheal
Lingual
Infrahyoid
Prelaryngeal
Pretracheal

LYMPH NODES OF THE UPPER LIMB AND MAMMARY GLAND

Draining the upper limb
Axillary
    Apical
    Central
    Lateral
    Pectoral (anterior)
    Subscapular (posterior)
Infraclavicular
Supratrochlear
Cubital

Draining the mammary gland
Pectoral
Subscapular
Apical
Parasternal
Intercostal

LYMPH NODES OF THE THORAX

Draining thoracic walls
Superficial
    Pectoral
    Subscapular
    Parasternal
    Inferior deep cervical
Deep
    Parasternal
    Intercostal
    Phrenic
    Diaphragmatic

Draining thoracic contents
Brachiocephalic
Posterior mediastinal
Tracheobronchial
    Paratracheal
    Superior tracheobronchial
    Inferior tracheobronchial
    Bronchopulmonary
    Pulmonary

LYMPH NODES OF THE ABDOMEN AND PELVIS

Lumbar
    Pre-aortic
        Coeliac
            Gastric
                Left gastric
                Right gastro-epiploic
                Pyloric
            Hepatic
            Pancreaticosplenic
        Superior mesenteric
        Inferior mesenteric
    Lateral aortic
        Common iliac
        External iliac
        Internal iliac
        Inferior epigastric
        Circumflex iliac
        Sacral
    Retro-aortic

LYMPH NODES OF THE LOWER LIMB

Superficial inguinal
    Upper
    Lower
Deep inguinal
Popliteal

Nerves

CRANIAL NERVES AND BRANCHES

I Olfactory (from olfactory mucous membrane)

II Optic (from retina)

III Oculomotor
Superior ramus (to superior rectus and levator palpebrae superioris)
Inferior ramus (to medial rectus, inferior rectus, inferior oblique and ciliary ganglion)

IV Trochlear (to superior oblique)

V Trigeminal
Ophthalmic
    Lacrimal
    Frontal
        Supratrochlear
        Supra-orbital
    Nasociliary → anterior ethmoidal → external
        nasal
        Internal nasal (from anterior ethmoidal)
        Ciliary ganglion
        Long ciliary
        Infratrochlear
        Posterior ethmoidal
Maxillary → infra-orbital
    Meningeal
    Pterygopalatine
        Orbital
        Palatine
        Nasal
        Pharyngeal
    Zygomatic
        Zygomaticotemporal
        Zygomaticofacial
    Posterior superior alveolar
    Middle superior alveolar
    Anterior superior alveolar
    Palpebral ⎫
    Nasal   ⎬ (from infra-orbital)
    Superior labial ⎭
Mandibular
    Meningeal
    Nerve to medial pterygoid (and tensor veli palatini and tensor tympani)
    Anterior trunk
        Buccal
        Masseteric
        Deep temporal
        Nerve to lateral pterygoid
    Posterior trunk
        Auriculotemporal
        Lingual
        Inferior alveolar
            Nerve to mylohyoid
            Mental

VI Abducent (to lateral rectus)

VII Facial
Greater petrosal
Nerve to stapedius
Chorda tympani
Posterior auricular (to occipitalis and auricular muscles)
Nerve to posterior belly of digastric
Nerve to stylohyoid
Temporal
Zygomatic   ⎫
Buccal   ⎬ to frontalis and muscles of facial expression
Marginal mandibular
Cervical   ⎭

VIII Vestibulocochlear
Cochlear (from coils of cochlea)
Vestibular (from utricle, saccule and ampullae of semicircular ducts)

IX Glossopharyngeal
Tympanic
    Lesser petrosal
Carotid sinus
Pharyngeal
Muscular (to stylopharyngeus)
Tonsillar
Lingual

X Vagus
Meningeal
Auricular
Pharyngeal (to muscles of pharynx and soft palate except stylopharyngeus and tensor veli palatini)
Carotid body
Superior laryngeal
    Internal laryngeal
    External laryngeal (to cricothyroid)
Right recurrent laryngeal (to muscles of larynx except cricothyroid)
Cardiac (cervical)
Cardiac (thoracic)
Left recurrent laryngeal (to muscles of larynx except cricothyroid)
Pulmonary
Oesophageal
Anterior trunk
    Gastric
    Hepatic
Posterior trunk
    Coeliac
    Gastric

XI Accessory
Cranial root (to muscles of palate and possibly larynx via vagus)
Spinal root (to sternocleidomastoid and trapezius)

XII Hypoglossal
Meningeal
Descending (upper root of ansa cervicalis, from C1 to superior belly of omohyoid, then forming ansa cervicalis – see cervical plexus)
Nerve to thyrohyoid (from C1)
Muscular (to geniohyoid from C1 and to muscles of tongue except palatoglossus)

SOME HEAD AND NECK NERVE SUPPLIES

All the muscles of	Supplied by	Except	Supplied by
Pharynx	Pharyngeal plexus	Stylopharyngeus	Glosso-pharyngeal nerve
Palate	Pharyngeal plexus	Tensor veli palatini	Nerve to medial pterygoid
Larynx	Recurrent laryngeal nerve	Cricothyroid	External laryngeal nerve
Tongue	Hypoglossal nerve	Palatoglossus	Pharyngeal plexus
Facial expression (including buccinator)	Facial nerve		
Mastication	Mandibular nerve		

CERVICAL PLEXUS AND BRANCHES

Lesser occipital C2
Great auricular C2, 3
Transverse cervical C2, 3
Supraclavicular C3, 4
Phrenic (to diaphragm) C3, 4, 5
Communicating (with vagus and hypoglossal nerves and superior cervical sympathetic ganglion)
Muscular (to rectus capitis lateralis, rectus capitis anterior, longus capitis and longus colli, and by lower root of ansa cervicalis and ansa itself to sternohyoid, sternothyroid and inferior belly of omohyoid) C2, 3

TYPICAL THORACIC NERVE BRANCHES

Thoracic spinal nerve
Dorsal ramus
    Medial
    Lateral
Ventral ramus → anterior cutaneous
    Recurrent
    Collateral
    Lateral cutaneous
        Posterior
        Anterior

BRACHIAL PLEXUS AND BRANCHES

Supraclavicular branches
From the roots
    To scalenes and longus colli C5, 6, 7, 8
    To join phrenic nerve C5
    Dorsal scapular (to rhomboids) C5
    Long thoracic (to serratus anterior) C5, 6, 7

From the upper trunk
    Nerve to subclavius C5, 6
    Suprascapular (to supraspinatus and infra-
      spinatus) C5, 6

Infraclavicular branches
From the lateral cord
    Lateral pectoral (to pectoralis major and minor)
      C5, 6, 7
    Musculocutaneous C5, 6, 7
    Lateral root of the median C(5), 6, 7

From the medial cord
    Medial pectoral (to pectoralis major and minor)
      C8, T1
    Medial root of the median C8, T1
    Medial cutaneous of arm C8, T1
    Medial cutaneous of forearm C8, T1
    Ulnar C(7), 8, T1

From the posterior cord
    Upper subscapular (to subscapularis) C5, 6
    Thoracodorsal (to latissimus dorsi) C6, 7, 8
    Lower subscapular (to subscapularis and teres
      major) C5, 6
    Axillary C5, 6
    Radial C5, 6, 7, 8, T1

Musculocutaneous C5, 6, 7
Muscular (to coracobrachialis, biceps and brachialis)
Lateral cutaneous of forearm

Median C(5), 6, 7, 8, T1
In the arm
    To pronator teres (occasional)
In the forearm
    Muscular (to pronator teres, flexor carpi radialis,
      palmaris longus and flexor digitorum
      superficialis)
    Anterior interosseous (to flexor pollicis longus,
      flexor digitorum profundus and pronator
      quadratus)
    Palmar cutaneous
    Communicating (with ulnar nerve)
In the hand
    Muscular (to abductor pollicis brevis, flexor
      pollicis brevis, opponens pollicis and the two
      lateral lumbricals)
    Common palmar digital
      Palmar digital

Ulnar C7, 8, T1
Muscular (to flexor carpi ulnaris and flexor digitorum
    profundus)
Palmar cutaneous
Dorsal
    Dorsal digital
Superficial terminal
    Nerve to palmaris brevis
    Common palmar digital
      Palmar digital
Deep terminal (to abductor digiti minimi, opponens
    digiti minimi, flexor digiti minimi brevis, adductor
    pollicis, all the interossei and the two medial
    lumbricals)

Axillary C5, 6
Muscular (to deltoid and teres minor)
Upper lateral cutaneous of arm

Radial C5, 6, 7, 8, T1
Muscular (to triceps, anconeus, brachioradialis,
    extensor carpi radialis longus and brachialis)
Posterior cutaneous of arm
Lower lateral cutaneous of arm
Posterior cutaneous of forearm
Superficial terminal
    Dorsal digital
Deep terminal (posterior interosseous) (to extensor
    carpi radialis brevis, supinator, extensor digitorum,
    extensor digiti minimi, extensor carpi ulnaris,
    extensor pollicis longus, extensor indicis, abductor
    pollicis longus and extensor pollicis brevis)

LUMBAR PLEXUS AND BRANCHES

Muscular (to psoas major and minor, quadratus
    lumborum and iliacus) T12, L1, 2, 3, 4
Iliohypogastric (to part of internal oblique and
    transversus abdominis) L1
Ilio-inguinal (to part of internal oblique and
    transversus abdominis) L1
Genitofemoral L1, 2
    Genital branch (to cremaster)
    Femoral branch
Lateral cutaneous of thigh L2, 3
Femoral L2, 3, 4
    Nerve to pectineus
    Anterior division
      Intermediate femoral cutaneous
      Medial femoral cutaneous
      Nerve to sartorius
    Posterior division
      Saphenous
      Nerves to quadriceps femoris
Obturator L2, 3, 4
    Anterior branch
      Muscular (to adductor longus, adductor
      brevis and gracilis)
    Posterior branch
      Muscular (to obturator externus and adductor
      magnus)
Accessory obturator (occasional) (to pectineus) L3, 4

SACRAL PLEXUS AND BRANCHES

Nerve to quadratus femoris and inferior gemellus L4,
    5, S1
Nerve to obturator internus and superior gemellus L5,
    S1, 2
Nerve to piriformis S(1), 2
Superior gluteal (to gluteus medius and minimus and
    tensor fasciae latae) L4, 5, S1
Inferior gluteal (to gluteus maximus) L5, S1, 2
Posterior femoral cutaneous S2, 3
Sciatic L4, 5, S1, 2, 3
Muscular (to biceps, semitendinosus,
    semimembranosus and adductor magnus)
Tibial L4, 5, S1, 2, 3
    Muscular (to gastrocnemius, plantaris, soleus,
      popliteus, tibialis posterior, flexor digitorum
      longus and flexor hallucis longus)
    Sural
    Medial calcanean
    Medial plantar
      Common plantar digital
        Plantar digital
      Muscular (to abductor hallucis, flexor
        digitorum brevis, flexor hallucis brevis
        and first lumbrical)
Lateral plantar
    Muscular (to flexor accessorius and abductor
      digiti minimi)
    Superficial
      Muscular (to flexor digiti minimi brevis, and
        fourth dorsal and third plantar interossei)
      Common plantar digital
        Plantar digital
    Deep (to adductor hallucis, first to third dorsal
      and first and second plantar interossei, and
      second to fourth lumbricals)
Common peroneal (fibular) L4, 5, S1, 2
    Recurrent
    Lateral cutaneous of calf
    Sural communicating
    Superficial peroneal (fibular)
      Muscular (to peroneus longus and peroneus
        brevis)
      Medial dorsal cutaneous
      Intermediate dorsal cutaneous
        Dorsal digital
    Deep peroneal (fibular)
      Muscular (to tibialis anterior, extensor
        hallucis longus, extensor digitorum
        longus, peroneus tertius and extensor
        digitorum brevis)
      Dorsal digital
Perforating cutaneous S2, 3
Pudendal S2, 3, 4
    Inferior rectal (to external anal sphincter)
    Perineal
      Posterior scrotal (labial)
      Muscular (to perineal muscles)
      Dorsal nerve of penis (clitoris)
Nerves to levator ani and coccygeus S3 and 4
Pelvic splanchnics (nervi erigentes) S2, 3, (4)

Muscles

MUSCLES OF THE HEAD

Muscles of the scalp
Epicranius
    Occipitofrontalis
    Temporoparietalis

Muscles of the nose
Procerus
Nasalis (compressor and dilator naris)
Depressor septi

Muscles of the eyelids
Orbicularis oculi
Corrugator supercilii
Levator palpebrae superioris (see Muscles of the Orbit)

Muscles of mastication
Masseter
Temporalis
Lateral pterygoid
Medial pterygoid

Muscles of the mouth
Levator labii superioris alaeque nasi
Levator labii superioris
Zygomaticus minor
Zygomaticus major
Levator anguli oris
Mentalis
Depressor labii inferioris
Depressor anguli oris
Buccinator
Orbicularis oris
Risorius

MUSCLES OF THE NECK

Superficial and lateral muscles
Platysma
Sternocleidomastoid
Trapezius (see upper limb)

Anterior vertebral muscles
Longus colli
Longus capitis
Rectus capitis anterior
Rectus capitis lateralis

Lateral vertebral muscles
Scalenus anterior
Scalenus medius
Scalenus posterior

Suprahyoid muscles
Digastric
Stylohyoid
Mylohyoid
Geniohyoid

Infrahyoid muscles
Sternohyoid
Sternothyroid
Thyrohyoid
Omohyoid

MUSCLE GROUPS IN HEAD AND NECK

Muscles of the pharynx
Superior constrictor
Middle constrictor
Inferior constrictor
Stylopharyngeus
Palatopharyngeus
Salpingopharyngeus

Muscles of the palate
Palatoglossus
Palatopharyngeus
Tensor veli palatini
Levator veli palatini
Musculus uvulae

Muscles of the larynx
Cricothyroid
Posterior crico-arytenoid
Lateral crico-arytenoid
Transverse arytenoid
Oblique arytenoid
Aryepiglottic
Thyro-arytenoid and vocalis
Thyro-epiglottic

Muscles of the tongue
Extrinsic
    Genioglossus
    Hyoglossus and chondroglossus
    Styloglossus
    Palatoglossus
Intrinsic
    Superior longitudinal
    Inferior longitudinal
    Transverse
    Vertical

Muscles of the orbit
Levator palpebrae superioris
Orbitalis
Muscles of the eyeball
    Superior rectus
    Inferior rectus
    Medial rectus
    Lateral rectus
    Superior oblique
    Inferior oblique

MUSCLES OF THE TRUNK

Suboccipital muscles
Rectus capitis posterior major
Rectus capitis posterior minor
Obliquus capitis inferior
Obliquus capitis superior

Deep muscles of the back
Splenius capitis
Splenius cervicis
Erector spinae
    Iliocostalis
    Longissimus
    Spinalis
Transversospinalis
    Semispinalis
    Multifidus
    Rotator
Interspinal
Intertransverse

Muscles of the thorax
External intercostal
Internal intercostal
Innermost intercostal
Subcostal
Transversus thoracis
Levatores costarum
Serratus posterior superior
Serratus posterior inferior
Diaphragm

Muscles of the abdomen
Anterolateral muscles
    External oblique
    Internal oblique
    Cremaster
    Transversus abdominis
    Rectus abdominis
    Pyramidalis
Posterior muscles
    Psoas major
    Psoas minor
    Iliacus
    Quadratus lumborum

Muscles of the pelvis
Piriformis
Obturator internus
Levator ani
Coccygeus

Muscles of the perineum
Anal muscle
    External anal sphincter
Urogenital muscles
    Superficial transverse perinei
    Bulbospongiosus
    Ischiocavernosus
    Deep transverse perinei
    Sphincter urethrae

MUSCLES OF THE UPPER LIMB

Connecting limb and vertebral column
Trapezius
Latissimus dorsi
Levator scapulae
Rhomboid major
Rhomboid minor

Connecting limb and thoracic wall
Pectoralis major
Pectoralis minor
Subclavius
Serratus anterior

Scapular muscles
Deltoid
Subscapularis
Supraspinatus
Infraspinatus
Teres minor
Teres major

Muscles of the upper arm
Biceps brachii
Coracobrachialis
Brachialis
Triceps

Muscles of the forearm
Anterior forearm muscles
    Superficial flexor group
        Pronator teres
        Flexor carpi radialis
        Palmaris longus
        Flexor carpi ulnaris
        Flexor digitorum superficialis
    Deep flexor group
        Flexor digitorum profundus
        Flexor pollicis longus
        Pronator quadratus
Posterior forearm muscles
    Superficial extensor group
        Brachioradialis
        Extensor carpi radialis longus
        Extensor carpi radialis brevis
        Extensor digitorum
        Extensor digiti minimi
        Extensor carpi ulnaris
        Anconeus
    Deep extensor group
        Supinator
        Abductor pollicis longus
        Extensor pollicis brevis
        Extensor pollicis longus
        Extensor indicis

Muscles of the hand
Thenar group
    Abductor pollicis brevis
    Flexor pollicis brevis
    Opponens pollicis
Adductor pollicis
Lumbricals (four)
Dorsal interossei (four)
Palmar interossei (four)
Hypothenar group
    Palmaris brevis
    Abductor digiti minimi
    Flexor digiti minimi brevis
    Opponens digiti minimi

MUSCLES OF THE LOWER LIMB

Muscles of the iliac region
Psoas major
Psoas minor
Iliacus

Muscles of the gluteal region
Gluteus maximus
Gluteus medius
Gluteus minimus
Piriformis
Obturator internus
Superior gemellus
Inferior gemellus
Quadratus femoris
Obturator externus

Muscles of the thigh
Anterior femoral group
    Tensor fasciae latae
    Sartorius
    Quadriceps femoris
        Rectus femoris
        Vastus lateralis
        Vastus medialis
        Vastus intermedius
    Articularis genu
Medial femoral group
    Gracilis
    Pectineus
    Adductor longus
    Adductor brevis
    Adductor magnus
Posterior femoral group
    Biceps femoris
    Semitendinosus
    Semimembranosus

Muscles of the leg
Anterior muscles
    Tibialis anterior
    Extensor hallucis longus
    Extensor digitorum longus
    Peroneus tertius
Lateral muscles
    Peroneus longus
    Peroneus brevis
Posterior muscles
    Superficial group
        Gastrocnemius
        Soleus
        Plantaris
    Deep group
        Popliteus
        Flexor hallucis longus
        Flexor digitorum longus
        Tibialis posterior

Muscles of the foot
Dorsal muscle— extensor digitorum brevis
Plantar muscles
    First layer
        Abductor hallucis
        Flexor digitorum brevis
        Abductor digiti minimi
    Second layer
        Flexor accessorius
        Lumbricals (four)
    Third layer
        Flexor hallucis brevis
        Adductor hallucis
        Flexor digiti minimi brevis
    Fourth layer
        Dorsal interossei (four)
        Plantar interossei (three)

Skull foramina

PRINCIPAL FORAMINA AND CONTENTS
(For a more detailed list, see pages 340 to 341)

Supra-orbital foramen
Supra-orbital nerve and vessels

Infra-orbital foramen
Infra-orbital nerve and vessels

Mental foramen
Mental nerve and vessels

Mandibular foramen
Inferior alveolar nerve and vessels

Optic canal
Optic nerve
Ophthalmic artery

Superior orbital fissure
Ophthalmic nerve and veins
Oculomotor, trochlear and abducent nerves

Inferior orbital fissure
Maxillary nerve

Sphenopalatine foramen
Sphenopalatine artery
Nasal branches of pterygopalatine ganglion

Foramen rotundum
Maxillary nerve

Foramen ovale
Mandibular and lesser petrosal nerves

Foramen spinosum
Middle meningeal vessels

Foramen lacerum
Internal carotid artery (entering from behind and
    emerging above)
Greater petrosal nerve (entering from behind and
    leaving anteriorly as the nerve of the pterygoid
    canal)

Carotid canal
Internal carotid artery and sympathetic plexus

Jugular foramen
Inferior petrosal sinus
Glossopharyngeal, vagus and accessory nerves
Internal jugular vein (emerging below)

Internal acoustic meatus
Facial and vestibulocochlear nerves
Labyrinthine artery

Hypoglossal canal
Hypoglossal nerve

Stylomastoid foramen
Facial nerve

Foramen magnum
Medulla oblongata and meninges
Vertebral and anterior and posterior spinal arteries
Accessory nerves (spinal parts)

Skull foramina (detailed list)

INSIDE THE SKULL

MIDDLE CRANIAL FOSSA

Optic canal: in the sphenoid between the body and the two roots of the lesser wing
Optic nerve
Ophthalmic artery

Superior orbital fissure: in the sphenoid between the body and greater and lesser wings, with a fragment of the frontal bone at the lateral extremity
Oculomotor, trochlear and abducent nerves
Lacrimal, frontal and nasociliary nerves
Filaments from the internal carotid (sympathetic) plexus
Orbital branch of the middle meningeal artery
Recurrent branch of the lacrimal artery
Superior ophthalmic vein

Foramen rotundum: in the greater wing of the sphenoid
Maxillary nerve

Foramen ovale: in the greater wing of the sphenoid
Mandibular nerve
Lesser petrosal nerve (usually)
Accessory meningeal artery
Emissary veins (from cavernous sinus to pterygoid plexus)

Foramen spinosum: in the greater wing of the sphenoid
Middle meningeal vessels
Meningeal branch of the mandibular nerve

Venous (emissary sphenoidal) foramen: in 40% of skulls, in the greater wing of the sphenoid medial to the foramen ovale
Emissary vein (from the cavernous sinus to the pterygoid plexus)

Petrosal (innominate) foramen: occasional, in the greater wing of the sphenoid, medial to the foramen spinosum
Lesser petrosal nerve (if not through foramen ovale)

Foramen lacerum: between the sphenoid, apex of the petrous temporal and the basilar part of the occipital
Internal carotid artery (entering from behind and emerging above)
Greater petrosal nerve (entering from above and behind, and leaving anteriorly as nerve of pterygoid canal)
Nerve of pterygoid canal (leaving through anterior wall)
A meningeal branch of the ascending pharyngeal artery
Emissary veins (from the cavernous sinus to the pterygoid plexus)

Hiatus for the greater petrosal nerve: in the tegmen tympani of the petrous temporal, in front of the arcuate eminence
Greater petrosal nerve
Petrosal branch of the middle meningeal artery

Hiatus for the lesser petrosal nerve: in the tegmen tympani of the petrous temporal, about 3 mm in front of the hiatus for the greater petrosal nerve
Lesser petrosal nerve

ANTERIOR CRANIAL FOSSA

Foramina in the cribriform plate of the ethmoid
Olfactory nerve filaments
Anterior ethmoidal nerve and vessels

Foramen caecum: between the frontal crest of the frontal bone and the ethmoid in front of the crista galli
Emissary vein (between nose and superior sagittal sinus)

POSTERIOR CRANIAL FOSSA

Internal acoustic meatus: in the posterior surface of the petrous temporal
Facial nerve
Vestibulocochlear nerve
Labyrinthine artery

Aqueduct of the vestibule: in the petrous temporal about 1 cm behind the internal acoustic meatus
Endolymphatic duct and sac
A branch from the meningeal branch of the occipital artery
A vein (from the labyrinth and vestibule to the sigmoid sinus)

Jugular foramen: between the jugular fossa of the petrous temporal and the occipital bone
Glossopharyngeal, vagus and accessory nerves
Meningeal branches of the vagus nerve
Inferior petrosal sinus
Internal jugular vein
A meningeal branch of the occipital artery

Hypoglossal canal: in the occipital bone above the anterior part of the condyle
Hypoglossal nerve and its (recurrent) meningeal branch
A meningeal branch of the ascending pharyngeal artery
Emissary vein (from the basilar plexus to the internal jugular vein)

Condylar canal: occasional, from the lower part of the sigmoid groove in the lateral part of the occipital bone to the condylar fossa on the external surface of the occipital bone behind the condyle
Emissary vein (from the sigmoid sinus to occipital veins)
A meningeal branch of the occipital artery

Mastoid foramen: in the petrous temporal near the posterior margin of the lower part of the sigmoid groove, passing backwards to open behind the mastoid process
Emissary vein (from the sigmoid sinus to occipital veins)
A meningeal branch of the occipital artery

Foramen magnum: in the occipital bone
Apical ligament of the dens of the axis
Tectorial membrane
Medulla oblongata and meninges (including first digitations of denticulate ligaments)
Spinal parts of the accessory nerves
Meningeal branches of the upper cervical nerves
Vertebral arteries
Anterior spinal artery
Posterior spinal arteries

IN THE BASE OF THE SKULL EXTERNALLY

Foramen lacerum
Foramen ovale
Foramen spinosum
Jugular foramen — see INSIDE THE SKULL
Hypoglossal canal
Condylar canal
Mastoid foramen
Foramen magnum

Inferior orbital fissure—see IN THE ORBIT

Lateral incisive foramen: opens into the incisive fossa, in the midline at the front of the hard palate
Nasopalatine nerve
Greater palatine vessels

Greater palatine foramen: between the maxilla and the palatine bone at the lateral border of the hard palate behind the palatomaxillary fissure
Greater palatine nerve and vessels

Lesser palatine foramina: two or three, in the inferior and medial aspects of the pyramidal process of the palatine bone
Lesser palatine nerves and vessels

Palatovaginal canal: between lower surface of the vaginal process of the root of the medial pterygoid plate and the upper surface of the sphenoidal process of the palatine bone
Pharyngeal branch of the pterygopalatine ganglion
Pharyngeal branch of the maxillary artery

Vomerovaginal canal: occasional, medial to the palatovaginal canal, between the upper surface of the vaginal process of the root of the medial pterygoid plate and the lower surface of the ala of the vomer
Pharyngeal branch of the sphenopalatine artery

Petrosquamous fissure: between the squamous temporal and the tegmen tympani
Petrosquamous vein

Petrotympanic fissure: between the tympanic part of the temporal bone and the tegmen tympani
Chorda tympani
Anterior ligament of the malleus
Anterior tympanic branch of the maxillary artery

Cochlear canaliculus: in the petrous temporal, at the apex of a notch in front of the medial part of the jugular fossa
Perilymphatic duct
Emissary vein (from the cochlea to the internal jugular vein or inferior petrosal sinus)

Carotid canal: in the inferior surface of the petrous temporal
Internal carotid artery
Internal carotid (sympathetic) plexus
Internal carotid venous plexus (from the cavernous sinus to the internal jugular vein)

Tympanic canaliculus: in the inferior surface of the petrous temporal, on the ridge of bone between the carotid canal and the jugular fossa
Tympanic branch of the glossopharyngeal nerve
Inferior tympanic branch of the ascending pharyngeal artery

Mastoid canaliculus: in the inferior surface of the petrous temporal, on the lateral wall of the jugular fossa
Auricular branch of the vagus nerve

Stylomastoid foramen: between the styloid and mastoid processes of the temporal bone
Facial nerve
Stylomastoid branch of the posterior auricular artery

IN THE ORBIT

Superior orbital fissure — see INSIDE THE SKULL
Optic canal

Frontal notch or foramen: in the supra-orbital margin of the frontal bone one finger's breadth from the midline
Supratrochlear nerve and vessels

Supra-orbital notch or foramen: in the supra-orbital margin of the frontal bone two fingers' breadths from the midline
Supra-orbital nerve and vessels

Anterior ethmoidal foramen: in the medial wall of the orbit between the orbital part of the frontal bone and the ethmoid labyrinth
Anterior ethmoidal nerve and vessels

Posterior ethmoidal foramen: occasional, 1 to 2 cm behind the anterior ethmoidal foramen
Posterior ethmoidal nerve and vessels

Zygomatico-orbital foramen: in the orbital surface of the zygomatic bone
Zygomatic branch of the maxillary nerve

Nasolacrimal canal: at the front, lower, medial corner of the orbit formed by the lacrimal bone and maxilla
Nasolacrimal duct

Inferior orbital fissure: towards the back of the orbit, between the maxilla and the greater wing of the sphenoid
Maxillary nerve
Zygomatic nerve
Orbital branches of the pterygopalatine ganglion
Infra-orbital vessels
Inferior ophthalmic veins

Infra-orbital canal: in the orbital surface of the maxilla
Infra-orbital nerve and vessels

MISCELLANEOUS

Infra-orbital foramen: the anterior opening of the infra-orbital canal, in the maxilla below the infra-orbital margin
Infra-orbital nerve and vessels

Mental foramen: on the outer surface of the body of the mandible below the second premolar tooth or slightly more anteriorly
Mental nerve and vessels

Mandibular foramen: on the inner surface of the ramus of the mandible, overlapped anteriorly and medially by the lingula
Inferior alveolar nerve and vessels

Foramina in the infratemporal (posterior) surface of the maxilla
Posterior superior alveolar nerves and vessels

Pterygomaxillary fissure: between the lateral pterygoid plate and the infratemporal (posterior) surface of the maxilla, and continuous above with the posterior end of the inferior orbital fissure
Maxillary artery (entering pterygopalatine fossa)
Maxillary nerve (entering inferior orbital fissure)
Sphenopalatine veins

Sphenopalatine foramen: at the upper end of the perpendicular plate of the palatine between its orbital and sphenoidal processes and (above) the body of the sphenoid; in the medial wall of the pterygopalatine fossa (viewed laterally through the pterygomaxillary fissure) and lateral wall of the nasal cavity (viewed medially)
Nasopalatine and posterior superior nasal nerves
Sphenopalatine vessels

Foramina in the perpendicular plate of the palatine
Posterior inferior nasal nerves

Pterygoid canal: at the root of the pterygoid process of the sphenoid in line with the medial pterygoid plate, leading from the anterior wall of the foramen lacerum to the posterior wall of the pterygopalatine fossa (and only clearly seen in a disarticulated sphenoid)
Nerve of the pterygoid canal
Artery of the pterygoid canal

Musculotubular canal: at the lateral side of the apex of the petrous temporal, at the junction of the petrous and squamous parts, and divided by a bony septum into upper and lower semicanals
Tensor tympani (upper semicanal)
Auditory tube (lower semicanal)

Parietal foramen: in the parietal bone near the posterosuperior (occipital) angle
Emissary vein (from the superior sagittal sinus to the scalp)

Index